Nutrition and Human Reproduction

Nutrition and Human Reproduction

Edited by
W. Henry Mosley

The Johns Hopkins University
School of Hygiene and Public Health
Baltimore, Maryland

Plenum Press · New York and London

Library of Congress Cataloging in Publication Data

Conference on Nutrition and Human Reproduction, National Institutes of
Health, 1977.
    Nutrition and human reproduction.

    Papers presented at the Conference on Nutrition and Human Reproduc-
tion held at the National Institute of Health, Bethesda, Md. Feb. 1977,
organized by the National Institute of Child Health and Human Development and the Subcommittee on Nutrition and Fertility of the Committee
on International Nutrition Programs of the National Research Council.
    Includes index.
    1. Human reproduction — Nutritional aspects — Congresses. 2. Fertility,
Human — Nutritional aspects — Congresses. 3. Breast feeding — Congresses.
I. Mosley, Wiley H., 1933-   II. United States. National Institute of
Child Health and Human Development. III. National Research Council.
Subcommittee on Nutrition and Fertility. IV. Title.
QP251.C675 1977   612.6   77-28738
ISBN-13: 978-1-4684-0792-1   e-ISBN-13: 978-1-4684-0790-7
DOI: 10.1007/978-1-4684-0790-7

Proceedings of a Conference on Nutrition and Human Reproduction,
supported and organized by the National Institutes of Child Health
and Human Development, held at the National Institutes of
Health, Bethesda, Maryland, February 14—16, 1977

© 1978 Plenum Press, New York
Softcover reprint of the hardcover 1st edition 1978
A Division of Plenum Publishing Corporation
227 West 17th Street, New York, N.Y. 10011

PREFACE

This book is the product of the Conference on Nutrition and
Human Reproduction, supported and organized by the National Insti-
tutes of Child Health and Human Development, and held at the
National Institutes of Health, Bethesda, Maryland, in February
1977. The genesis of this Conference came from the work of the
Subcommittee on Nutrition and Fertility of the Committee on
International Nutrition Programs of the National Research Council.

The purpose of the Conference was to assemble scientists and
program planners from a broad range of fields including nutrition,
epidemiology, demography, endocrinology, sociology, economics,
anthropology, biostatistics and public health. Each individual
brought his or her analytical skills and perspective to the meeting,
with the goal of developing a more coherent picture of the many
facets of nutrition and reproduction. The approach was to get a
more comprehensive view by:

1. Clarifying terminology and definitions.

2. Reviewing recent and current work on the biological
   basis for nutrition-fertility interactions.

3. Reviewing biomedical and socioeconomic factors related
   to breast-feeding to assess how this practice relates to
   maternal and infant nutrition and fertility.

4. Assessing some current analytical models for defining
   nutrition-fertility interrelationships.

5. Reviewing recent field studies from Africa, Asia and
   Latin America which are examining the interrelationships
   of nutrition and reproduction.

The papers in this volume were specially prepared for the
Conference by the authors. The range of topics represents the
effort by the Subcommittee on Nutrition and Fertility to bring

together scientists from a variety of disciplines who are actively
working on questions relating to how nutrition affects reproduction
in human populations. Such topics as the nutritional requirements
of pregnancy and lactation, or the effect of high fertility on
nutritional status were selectively excluded since these topics are
covered elsewhere. Special effort was made to include reports from
ongoing field investigations. Since this is a relatively new
topic of research, some of the reports give only preliminary
results, but they provide important documentation of field research
methodologies.

Special acknowledgement for the success of this Conference
must go to several persons. The work of the Subcommittee on
Nutrition and Fertility would not have begun without the initiative
of Dr. Nevin Scrimshaw, Chairman of the parent Committee on International Nutrition Programs, NRC. Dr. Philip Corfman, Director of
the Center for Population Research, National Institute for Child
Health and Human Development, took an active role with the Subcommittee in organizing the Conference. The Subcommittee is
indebted to Mrs. Joan MacDonald, Administrator in the Center for
Population Research, for her outstanding work in managing and
organizing the travel and other arrangements for the Conference.

I am especially indebted to Mrs. Marta Pramschufer for almost
all the secretarial work leading up to the production of this
volume, ranging from the management of correspondence, files, and
communications to the ultimate preparation of the typescript in
this book. Her reliability and the quality of her work has made
my own task much easier.

W. Henry Mosley

CONTENTS

INTRODUCTION

ISSUES, DEFINITIONS, AND AN ANALYTIC FRAMEWORK

W. Henry Mosley

The Johns Hopkins University

Baltimore, Maryland

INTRODUCTION

Rapid population growth and limited world food supplies are universally recognized as two of the major global problems confronting mankind in this generation. The interdependence of population growth and food has been recognized since Malthus; however, the focus of interest has largely centered on nutrition and mortality. Only recently has it been recognized that nutrition can play a major role as a determinant of birth rates as well.

Many questions relating to the interactions of nutrition and fertility have major programmatic and policy implications, particularly for developing countries. For example, it is not clear what effects improvement in nutrition will have on reproductive performance in chronically malnourished populations. Currently, birth spacing typically extends beyond three years in many developing countries particularly where breast-feeding is universal and prolonged. How much of this suppression of fertility is due to malnutrition, and what change in birth rates might be anticipated with nutrition programs are important questions that often spark heated debates.

Another issue relates to the interactions of fertility control programs with nutrition. Two dimensions are important here, one relates to how the modern contraceptive technologies may affect the marginal nutritional status of women in poorer countries. A second and increasingly important question is what will be the impact on nutrition (particularly infant nutrition) of the changing social roles for women that are facilitated by fertility control programs.

1

Policy makers and program planners also need to know what the potentials are for reinforcing the naturally beneficial interactions between nutrition and fertility control. Our interest here is the important role of breast-feeding, both in infant nutrition and in birth spacing. The physiological mechanisms of both lactation and lactational amenorrhea are poorly understood, particularly as they relate to maternal nutritional status. The possibility of promoting both infant nutrition and birth spacing through the program of improving maternal nutrition and encouraging breast-feeding, possibly coupled with an oral hormone designed to help maintain lactation and amenorrhea, is an avenue that has been almost totally ignored by contraceptive research efforts in the developed world; yet, such an approach could be appropriate for a large majority of reproducing women in the world today.

There is little information on many of these complex questions, in part because disciplinary barriers result in limited communication between the biomedical scientists who concentrate on nutrition research and the social scientists who are studying human reproduction. In 1964 an interdisciplinary meeting somewhat similar to this Conference was held, bringing together demographers and social scientists with biologists, physicians, statisticians and public health workers to discuss research issues in public health and population change (1). It was noted at that time that one of the formidable barriers to communication among scholars from different fields is semantics. Put simply, "One man's precision is another man's jargon." The appeal of that symposium for an international interdisciplinary body to work towards removing the terminological confusion was at least heard, and the International Union for the Scientific Study of Population has undertaken the task of attempting to standardize demographic terminology relating to the field of human reproduction (2). Unfortunately, the results of their effort have not yet permeated into the teaching and research literature of the various disciplinary fields concerned with the study of human reproduction, so that interdisciplinary communication remains difficult.

Another problem is the lack of general and universally accepted conceptual models which encompass all of the specific concerns that various disciplines seek to address as they examine the problems of human reproduction from their own perspectives. In the absence of a concensus on an analytical framework, it is often difficult for one disciplinary group to fully appreciate the relevance and significance of contributions that are made by scientists in another field.

This paper will seek to clarify some of the major areas of confusion in terminology. Further, since there have been efforts at developing general conceptual models in the demographic field that encompass both the biological and social determinants of fertility, this will be briefly described to provide a general frame of reference for the reports that follow.

TERMINOLOGY

Workers in fields relating to human reproduction from all disciplines are urged to refer to the IUSSP publications as a point of reference for standard usage of demographic terminology (2). Efforts have been made to see that most of the terminology in this book is consistent with demographic usage as given by the IUSSP definitions; however, in some of the review articles referring to older work, there will be a lack of consistency. Unfortunately, at times it may be impossible to determine what writers in the past meant to say. As an example, the term completed family size in the demographic literature typically refers to the total number of live births a woman has had throughout her reproductive years, irrespective of whether they are surviving or dead at the time the information is obtained. In some references in the older literature, one may find such expressions as "poorly nourished women have smaller families than well nourished women." Without further clarification, such a statement may be impossible to interpret, since the writer may be referring to fewer surviving children rather than fewer live births.

The word fertility requires special mention. Fertility is used consistently in the demographic literature to refer to the production of live births. Thus, to the demographer, an infertile woman is a woman who has never had a live birth, irrespective of the number of pregnancies she may have had resulting in fetal wastages or stillbirths. A fertility rate relates only to the number of live births per woman (or per 1000 women).

In the biomedical literature, the term fertility generally relates to the physiological capacity of a person (or animal) to reproduce. Thus, an infertile woman is one who cannot conceive. The demographers use the term fecundity to refer to the physiological capacity or potential of a person to produce live born children. A woman is said to be fecundable when she is capable of conceiving, i.e., of reproductive age and neither pregnant nor in a state of postpartum sterility. Sterility is the antonym to fecundity in the strict demographic sense.

There is also confusion with the term parity. To the demographer parity refers to the number of live births that a woman has had while to the physician parity or para number refers to the number of pregnancies a woman has had which reach the point of viability (generally 28 weeks or more) irrespective of whether the

outcome is a live birth or a still birth. The reason for this
distinction is that the physician is concerned with the effect of
a succession of pregnancies on the woman's physiological status
while the demographer is concerned with the effect of a series of
live births on population change.

NATURAL FERTILITY

Natural fertility is a fundamental demographic concept introduced by Louis Henry (3) which provides the foundation for any
population-based research effort that seeks to relate variation in
nutritional levels to reproductive performance. Natural fertility
is defined as the fertility of persons or populations in which
deliberate control of child bearing is not practiced. It is
important to note that under this definition deliberate birth control relates only to modification of behaviour that is influenced
by the number of children already born and the number desired.

Although natural fertility is "uncontrolled" fertility, it is
not synonymus with the maximum fertility biologically possible.
This is because natural fertility can be affected by many social
as well as biological factors unrelated to behaviour explicitly
directed at fertility control. Among these are a delay in marriage,
postpartum abstinence or abstinence for religious reasons, temporary
separations for work, divorce, seasonal variations in coital frequency, breast-feeding practices, diseases, and other factors.

Natural fertility will vary widely between different populations
as well as between social and cultural groups within populations.
Generally, the frame of reference for the level of natural fertility
that approaches the highest biological limits for a population is
the Hutterites (4). This is a religious sect in North America in
which the women average more than ten live births over a reproductive
life beginning at age 20. Essentially every other non-contracepting
population, both historically and in modern times, has had lower
fertility levels (3).

A logical approach to understanding natural fertility has been
an analysis of birth intervals since the cumulative number of live
births a woman can have over her reproductive life is function of
the spacing between births. In the original report by Henry, he
suggested that the major source of variation in fertility levels
between different non-contracepting populations was due to variations in the length of lactational amenorrhea, presumably related
to variations in breast-feeding practices (3). Several studies
have confirmed this basic observation (5,6,7).

An important question that is being addressed by this Conference is to what degree is the prolongation of lactation amenorrhea

and of birth spacing that is typically found in the non-contracepting populations in many developing countries related to the chronic malnutrition. Information on this question has obvious policy and programmatic relevance for health and nutrition programs in the developing countries.

A GENERAL ANALYTIC FRAMEWORK

Because of the multiplicity of factors that can affect human reproductive performance, and their complex interactions, it is useful to have a general conceptual framework to organize these factors for a more coherent discussion. Davis and Blake provided an excellent and simple systematic classification by identifying three basic biological mechanisms through which all social and biological factors that affect live birth rates must operate (8). These requirements are:

1) Exposure to intercourse,
2) Exposure to conception, and
3) Successful gestation.

Within this framework they identified those social and biological factors regulating the production of a live birth. To encompass fully the factors affecting the cumulative production of surviving offspring (net reproduction), this framework can be expanded to include the duration of the reproductive lifespan and the survival probability of the births to reproductive age (9).

Figure 1 is a diagramatic representation of this analytic framework. The central line identifies the successive biological steps required for a woman to produce surviving offspring. She must reach sexual maturation and enter into a sexual union. Both of these factors are required and these determine the duration of effective reproductive life (R). With menstruation, she will presumably be susceptible to pregnancy at monthly intervals; the duration of the susceptible period, or menstruating interval (M), is determined by the number of months until a recognized conception. The period of gestation (G), if successful, terminates in a live birth. This can result in a survivor to the next generation. With each pregnancy termination there follows a period of postpartum sterility and/or lactational amenorrhea (A). The woman then re-enters the susceptible state and the reproductive cycle is maintained until the sexual union is broken or sterility intervenes. The left side of the figure identifies the biological or health factors that can affect reproductive performance; the right side of the figure identifies the social factors, i.e., those factors that are subject to behavioral control.

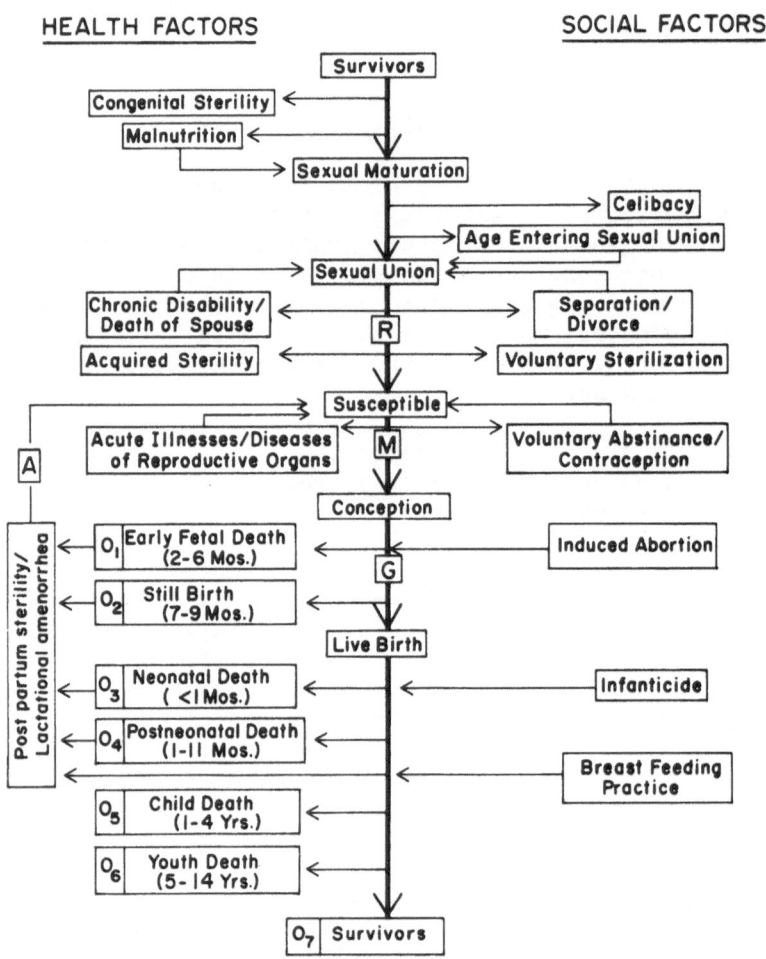

Figure 1. A Model of Human Reproduction. The relevant biological variables are: R - duration of effective reproductive life; M - duration of the menstruating interval; G - duration of gestation; A - duration of postpartum and lactational amenorrhea; O - proportion of pregnancies with a given outcome. The health factors affecting reproduction are shown on the left side, the social/behavioural factors on the right.

This framework is useful in a discussion of the effects of nutrition on reproduction since it permits one to specifically identify where and how in the reproductive cycle various states of malnutrition actually affect the reproductive process in a given population. More significantly, by identifying how health and social factors actually operate on the reproductive process through the same basic biological mechanisms, it highlights some of the problems that are encountered in population-based studies which attempt to determine whether variations in fertility levels are actually due to biological factors, such as malnutrition, or behavioral changes which can also operate through many of the same mechanisms.

References

1. Sheps, M. C. and Ridley, J. C., eds. Public Health and Population Change. University of Pittsburgh Press, Pittsburgh, Pa., 1965.

2. Grebenik, E. and Hill, A. International Demographic Terminology: Fertility, Family Planning and Nuptiality. International Union for the Scientific Study of Population, Liege, Belgium, 1974.

3. Henry, Louis. Some Data on Natural Fertility. Eugenics Quarterly 8: 81-91, 1961.

4. Sheps, M. An Analysis of Reproductive Patterns in an American Isolate. Population Studies 19: 65-80, 1965.

5. Potter, R. C., Wyon, J. B., Parker, M. and Gordon, J. E. A Case Study of Birth Interval Dynamics. Population Studies 19: 81-96, 1965.

6. Chen, L. C., Ahmed, S., Gesche, M. and Mosley, W. H. A Prospective Study of Birth Interval Dynamics in Rural Bangladesh. Population Studies 28, 277-297, 1974.

7. Van Ginneken, J. K. Prolonged Breast Feeding as a Birth Spacing Method. Studies in Family Planning 5, 201, 1974.

8. Davis, K. and Blake, J. Social Structure and Fertility: An Analytic Framework. Econ. Dev. and Cultural Change 4, 211-235, 1956.

9. Mosley, W. H. and Chen, L. C. Health and Human Reproduction in Developing Countries. In preparation, Cholera Research Laboratory, Dacca, Bangladesh, 1976.

NUTRITION AND ENDOCRINE FUNCTION

INTRODUCTORY STATEMENT

John Stanbury

Massachusetts Institute of Technology

Cambridge, Massachusetts

This symposium on nutrition and fertility begins appropriately with an examination of available and recent information on the influences of the nutritional state on the endocrine system. Nutritional factors may influence endocrine function at many levels. They may have effects on synthesis and secretion of the hypothalamic releasing hormones, on synthesis, storage and release of the hormones of the pituitary, on the responses of peripheral endocrine glands such as the thyroid, adrenal cortex and gonads to the respective tropic hormones, or finally on the responsiveness of peripheral cells to effector hormones. Nutritional factors may also have important indirect effects. For example, infant nutrition by influencing the vigor of breastfeeding may affect ovulation.

The postpartum period of infertility accompanying lactation is nature's provision of a respite from pregnancy after delivery. It has not been clear whether protein or calorie malnutrition of the nursing mother prolongs this period of infertility, or whether by improving nutrition one enhances nursing performance and gives more effective inhibition of gonadotropin secretion. In the first contribution to this section of the symposium Tyson and Perez examine the neuroendocrine control of lactation and gonadotropin secretion. They show that the pattern of nursing is important in inhibiting the secretion of gonadotropin-releasing factor. On the other hand, if milk is ample in volume and composition, nursing time and duration may be short, and ovulatory breakthrough may occur earlier than otherwise. Thus, the frequency and duration of nursing as well as the volume and composition of the milk control the resumption of ovulatory activity. Prolactin, stimulated by nursing, may also interfere with gonadotropin at the level of the ovary, perhaps by competitive binding, and may also inhibit secretion of

9

gonadotropin releasing hormone. Tyson and Perez are hopeful that more knowledge of the neuroendocrinology of the reproductive system and lactation may lead to new safe and effective non-steroidal contraception.

Many of the components of the endocrine system are sensitive to the nutritional state. Dr. Brasel has presented a systematic analysis of existing information and summarized the lacunae which need to be filled. Surprisingly, our knowledge of the relationships between nutrition and gonadal function is most deficient. Curiously, in protein malnutrition, when protein synthesis is generally reduced, growth hormone, and possibly ACTH and the gonadotropins, are synthesized and secreted in increased amounts. The endocrinology of anorexia nervosa cannot be equated with imposed protein or calorie malnutrition.

The final paper in this section focuses on the interactions between the oral contraceptives and a variety of micronutrients as observed in an American urban community. In general, the differences between a privileged and less privileged resulting from use of oral contraceptives were few, but this may have been related to the fact that the groups chosen for the study may not have been very different nutritionally. Possibly the effects of the contraceptive steroids would be more significant when used by subjects with limiting amounts of the micronutrients. Thus, for example, the steroids might have important effects when B-6 intake is marginal or insufficient, but no effect when it is only lower than optimal.

These three papers provide the endocrine base for further consideration of the present state of knowledge of the interactions of nutrition and fertility.

THE MAINTENANCE OF INFECUNDITY IN POSTPARTUM WOMEN

John E. Tyson and A. Perez

The Johns Hopkins University, Baltimore, Maryland

The Catholic University of Chile, Santiago, Chile

INTRODUCTION

The duration of postpartum infertility in nursing women relies heavily upon the effectiveness of the nursing stimulus (1), which in turn provokes the secretion of the pituitary hormone prolactin (PRL). This secretion is induced by a neural reflex arc and a change in hypothalamic dopamine turnover (2-4). While the influence of this change is poorly understood, there is evidence to suggest that the peripheral plasma concentration of PRL modulates both hypothalamic and ovarian function (5), including the attenuation of cyclic luteinizing hormone releasing hormone secretion via a positive short loop feedback (6) and a tonic inhibition of ovarian steroidogenesis (7). Furthermore, PRL may block FSH activity at the ovary (8,9). The priority of these several mechanisms remains elusive. The duration of postpartum infertility apparently varies both with the type of nursing and the PRL response to such nursing (10). Thus, lactation has been considered a poor method of contraception. The following studies extend our observations on the hormonal mechanisms relating nursing to postpartum infertility.

MATERIALS AND METHODS

The studies were performed in both Santiago, Chile and Baltimore, Maryland. Each group engaged women of middle socioeconomic class where nutrition was presumed adequate. All women were advised of the nature of the studies and the possible hazards. Informed consent was obtained in each instance. Only healthy

nursing and non-nursing mothers who had completed an uncomplicated
gestation followed by vaginal delivery were selected for these
studies. All nursing was on demand except where otherwise noted
in the text. Any augmentation of daily nourishment consisted of
fruit juices and water.

Blood was drawn at periodic intervals throughout the various
studies and was centrifuged immediately at 4°C. Plasma was then
separated and stored at -20°C until assayed for plasma hormones.

PRL was measured by a modification of the radioimmunoassay
method of Hwang et al. (11), using the iodination technique of
Greenwood et al. (12). Plasma LH and FSH were measured by a modification of the double antibody radioimmunoassay method of Midgely
(13) and the LH standard utilized was LER 907 in addition to the
Second International Reference Preparation for Human Menopausal
Gonadotropin (2nd IRP-HMG). The final antibody dilution for these
antisera was 1:12,000. FSH was iodinated and applied in a similar
manner.

There were four study groups. In the first group, thirty
Chilean women in full nursing were instructed in the use of the
basal temperature thermometer and asked to record their oral
temperature daily before rising. They were asked to continue
their breastfeeding in the usual manner but were seen at weekly
intervals for 15 weeks in the Obstetric Clinic where their basal
temperature chart was evaluated and blood samples were taken before
and after 30 minutes of nursing. The technique used was reported
previously from this laboratory (10).

A second study was designed to evaluate the periodicity and
duration of each nursing and its impact on PRL and gonadotropin
secretion. Seven full nursing North American women volunteered
for periodic blood sampling throughout an 8-10 hour daytime period
during which time infants nursed ad libitum. The women were housed
in attractive surroundings and served regular meals. Blood was
obtained at 15-20 minute intervals and every 5 minutes during nursing. A #19 gauge needle was secured in a forearm vein and attached
to a 3-way stopcock. Blood obtained from a side port on the stopcock was placed in heparinized tubes. The system was then flushed
with 2 ml of physiologic saline containing 1:100,000 sodium
heparin.

These two studies began between 8 a.m. and 9 a.m., at least
two hours after the last nursing event. Infants were nursed until
satisfied. Four were weighed before and after each feeding.

In the third study, five nursing mothers received an intravenous injection of LHRH (100 ug) between the 34th and 87th

postpartum day. The mean gonadotropin response was compared to
that obtained from a group of four bottle-feeding women.

The fourth study involved a more heterogeneous population
where breastfeeding was reportedly impaired. Their PRL and lactational response to the ingestion of oral thyroptropin releasing
hormone (TRH) was measured.

RESULTS

Basal Prolactin Levels

In the study of 30 Chilean women, none of the women in full
breastfeeding displayed a biphasic temperature chart and uterine
bleeding was absent. The cumulative mean weekly basal PRL concentration over 15 weeks was 33.0 ± 2.1 ng/ml as compared to $21.3 \pm$
3.4 ng/ml for 15 bottle-feeding mothers sampled over the same time
frame ($p<.01$). When the nursing was reduced or considered insufficient, supplemental foods were added. These additions were
accompanied by a smaller number of nursing events and a fall in
mean basal PRL to 20 ng/ml. These results substantiated previous
data which found fully breastfeeding women have higher basal PRL
concentrations than those who breastfeed on a more casual schedule
(2,3).

Hormonal Response to Periodic Nursing

In the second study, seven women were evaluated between the
32nd-58th postpartum days, a time when the PRL response to nipple
stimulation is greatest (14). Breastfeeding intervals were evaluated. Each feeding varied from 8-38 minutes with a mean of $19 \pm$
2 minutes. The duration of each feeding was unrelated to the time
of day.

Figures 1,2,3 present three profiles of gonadotropin and PRL
secretion obtained during this study. In Figure 1, five feedings
of variable length were associated with PRL increments, three of
which peaked after the period of sucking. PRL levels in Figure 2
reflect accurately the lack of vigorous sucking by this infant
even though its weight following each feeding indicated an intake
of at least 40 ml. This suggests that an infant may extract
adequate nutrition from the breast in some cases in spite of less
intense suckling. The PRL response most typical of the remaining
five women is demonstrated in Figure 3. Increasing increments
in PRL associated with broader areas under the curve were seen
throughout the day. The initial mean basal PRL concentration in
this group was 84.6 ± 31.3 ng/ml while the mean of the lowest daily

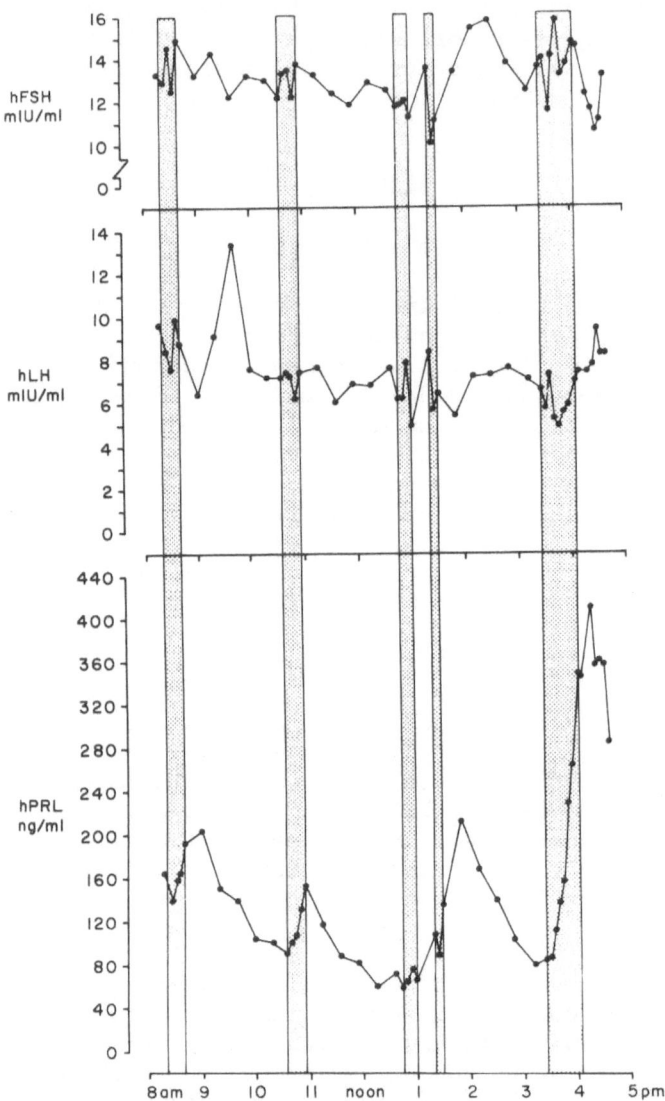

Figure 1. Plasma gonadotropin and prolactin profiles in one woman during demand breastfeeding. The postpartum duration is 32 days. The shaded areas represent the duration of each nursing event during which blood samples were obtained at five minute intervals. All remaining blood samples were drawn at least 15 minutes apart.

PRL level was 19.1 ± 7.6 ng/ml.

Since the number of feedings varied from woman to woman, we calculated the PRL response to the first and last feeding of the day. The mean maximal PRL increment during the first feeding was 36.4 ± 13.6 ng/ml compared to 179.0 ± 37.3 ng/ml for the last (p < .01). The number and duration of daily feedings failed to influence the PRL response at the end of the day. Overall, a substantial mean PRL increment of 89.5 ± 19.5 ng/ml was calculated for

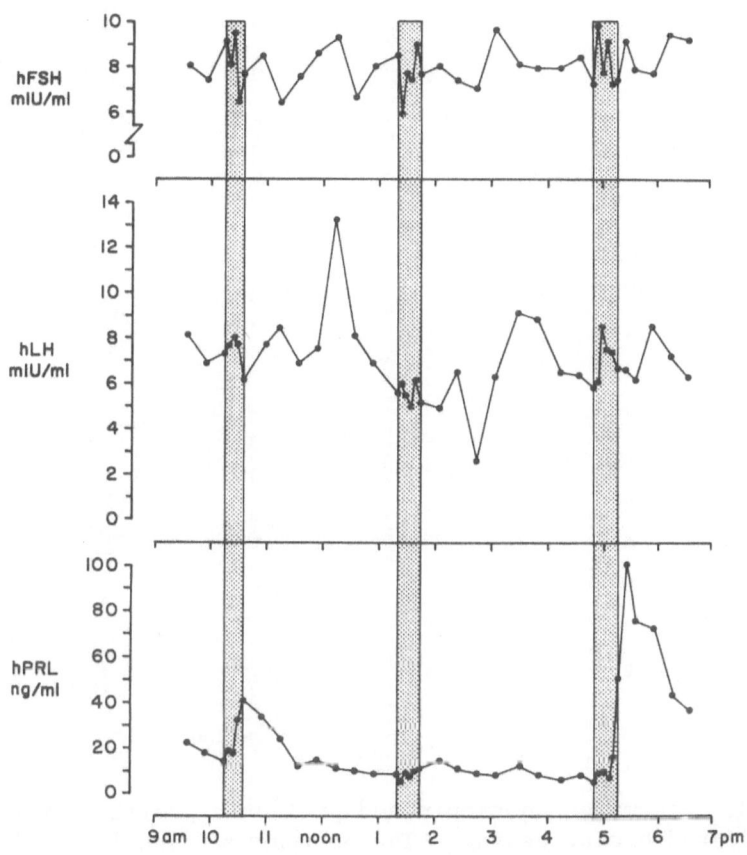

Figure 2. Plasma gonadotropin and prolactin profiles in one woman during demand breastfeeding. The postpartum duration is 36 days. The shaded areas represent the duration of each nursing event during which blood samples were obtained at five minute intervals. All remaining blood samples were drawn at least 15 minutes apart.

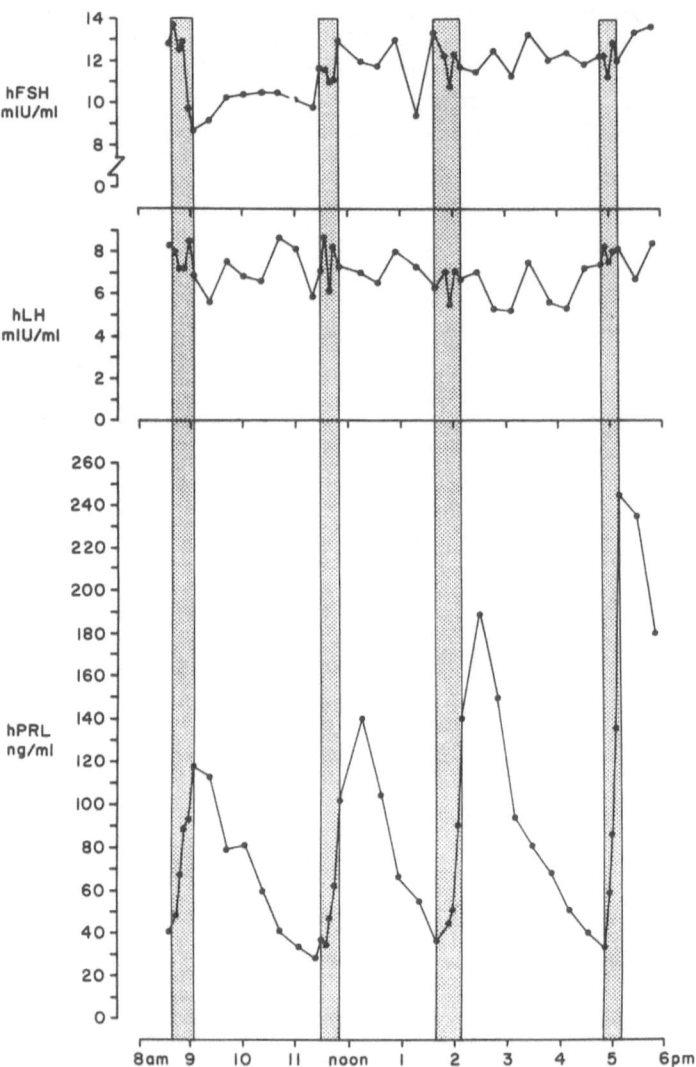

Figure 3. Plasma gonadotropin and prolactin profiles in one woman
during demand breastfeeding. The postpartum duration is 39 days.
The shaded areas represent the duration of each nursing event during which blood samples were obtained at five minute intervals.
All remaining blood samples were drawn at least 15 minutes apart.

all feedings of the group.

Plasma LH and FSH failed to display any consistent secretory pattern. The amplitude of episodic peaks was much lower than those of normally menstruating women (15). Plasma LH fluctuated widely with inconsistent variations in amplitude relative to PRL secretion; specifically, mean basal LH for the seven women prior to nursing was 10.8 ± 1.3 mIU/ml with a fall in the first 40 minutes following nursing to 8.8 ± 0.9 mIU/ml.

Gonadotropin Response to LHRH

The results of study 3, examining the gonadotropin responses to 100 ug LHRH in nursing and non-nursing mothers are shown in Figure 4. Basal pretest levels of LH and FSH were the same in both groups. The increment in LH and FSH were largest in nursing women. The response in nursers suggests adequate stores of gonadotropin were present. Thus, it would appear that some alteration in the cyclic release mechanism is involved, resulting in a pattern of episodic gonadotropin secretion in these studies that is different from those observed in normally menstruating women.

Return of Gonadotropin Secretion

We have studied women who continue to breastfeed beyond 200 postpartum days (1). In these women, the episodic secretion of gonadotropins appears to be inversely related to the secretion of PRL and further the periodicity of secretion appears to be incongruent with increased ovarian function. In one case, a healthy mother who had been breastfeeding her child for 210 postpartum days began oral contraception in anticipation of weaning. She voluntarily discontinued the pills 28 days later and withdrawal bleeding occurred in 48 hours. She continued to breastfeed her child for 14 additional days when she was studied for PRL secretion.

Figure 5 displays her hormonal profile on postpartum day 271. Basal gonadotropins were markedly elevated and the amplitude and frequency of each gonadotropin peak was greater than that observed previously in this case. In contrast, post-nursing PRL responses were modest. A second study was performed seven days later (Figure 6). This time nursing had ceased five days earlier. Basal gonadotropins were considerably lower while basal PRL had now fallen to within the range for menstruating women (0-25 ng/ml). Followup uterine bleeding occurred seven days after the second study. This was her first spontaneous menstrual period, lasting four days.

Study one was apparently coincidentally performed during the first postpartum midcycle gonadotropin peak (day 271). These

results suggest that cyclic gonadotropin secretion leading to menstrual cycles may occur if nursing frequency is reduced. Further,
cessation of nursing leads to a rapid fall in basal PRL concentrations to normal levels.

TRH Stimulation of PRL Release

TRH stimulates the release of PRL in postpartum women (10,16,

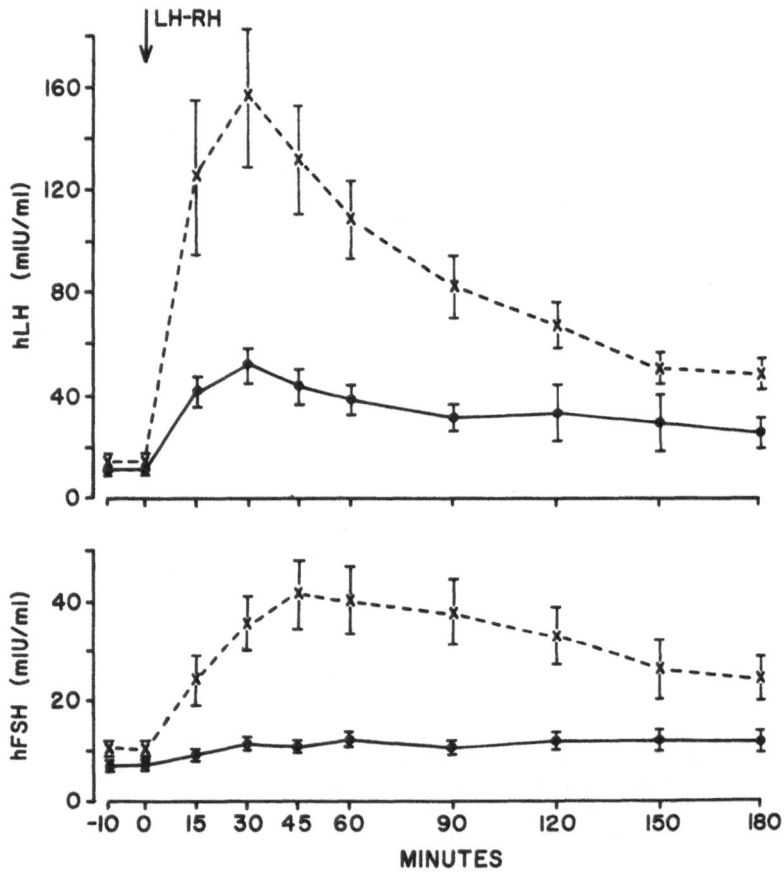

Figure 4. Mean ± SE plasma gonadotropin responses to the intravenous injection of 100 ug LH-RH in women beyond 5 weeks postpartum.
The x - - x represents nursing mothers (n=5) and the o———o
represents non-nursing women (n=4). The peak LH response is
significantly different between the two groups (p < .02) and likewise, the FSH response is significantly different (p < .02).
(Reprinted from J. Clin. Endocrinol. Metab. 42: 1114, 1976).

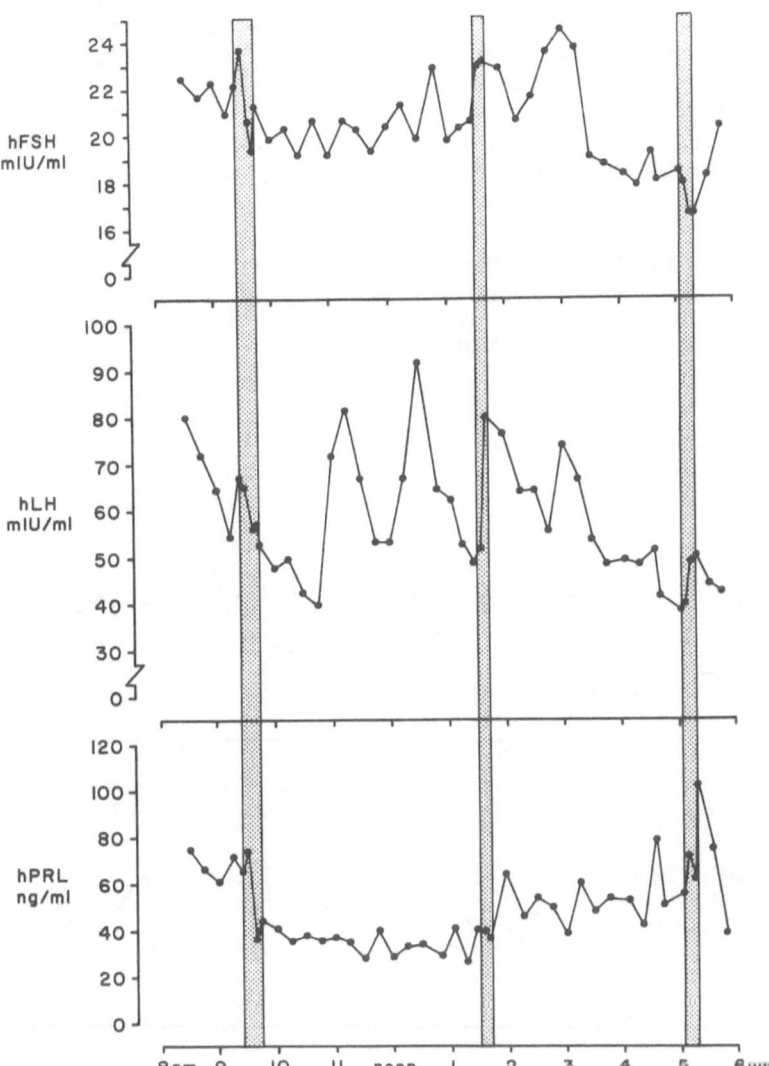

Figure 5. Prolactin and gonadotropin responses to nursing in a woman at 271 days postpartum. Oral contraception had been used for one month but was withdrawn 14 days before this study. The profile of gonadotropin secretion and the concentrations of gonadotropin suggests that this patient was sampled during her midcycle gonadotropin peak.

18). It is not surprising that several investigators have
attempted to augment the human lactational response by administer-
ing oral TRH to nursing mothers (10,16). Table 1 summarizes the
PRL response to oral TRH in 9 postpartum women with poor milk
production. When used postpartum, as little as 20 mg of oral TRH
increased mean basal PRL concentrations 2-3 fold. There was an
immediate increase in milk volume. Milk composition did not change
but full nursing was reestablished. On the other hand, the administration of TRH to women in full nursing with an adequate PRL
response had no effect (10).

We have previously reported that lactation may be induced in
normally menstruating women who are appropriately prepared with
estrogens and TRH. It is also well known that nipple stimulation
alone will provoke lactation.

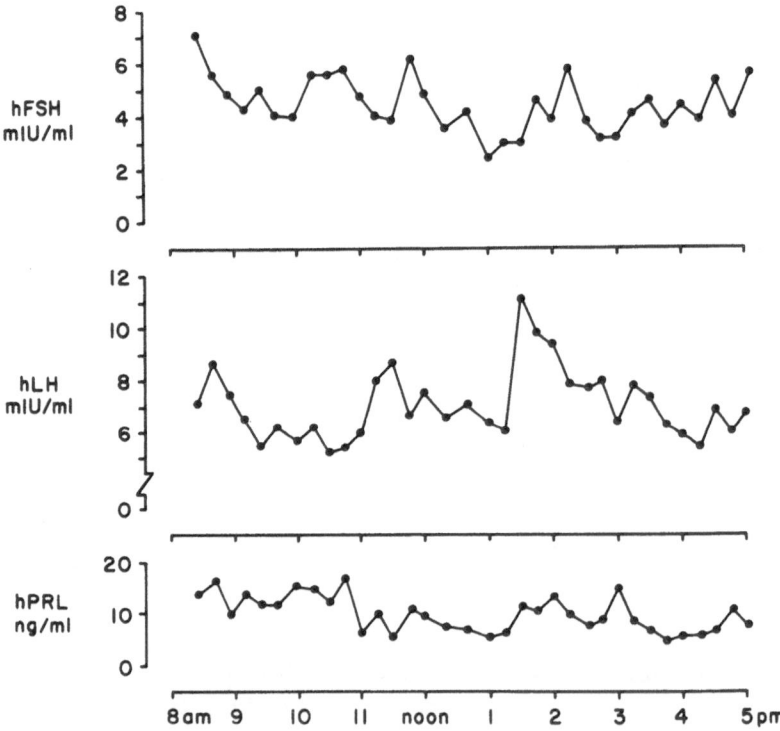

Figure 6. Prolactin and gonadotropin concentrations in the same
woman as outlined in Figure 3 when sampled seven days later and
five days after nursing had ceased. Basal PRL concentrations
are in the range of normal as are LH and FSH values.

Table 1

Mean basal plasma prolactin concentrations in nine healthy postpartum women who had a demonstrable impairment of milk supply.
Oral TRH (5 mg twice daily) was administered beginning on day 1
after the first basal blood sample was drawn. Milk yield in each
instance was increased within the first 24 hours and was associated with an increased frequency and duration of nursing by the
respective infants.

			Days				
Lactation	Days post-partum	Milk Yield	1	2	3	4	5
			PRL ng/ml				
Partial	13	↑	43.0	70.5	114.0	26.5	56.5
Partial	16	↑	22.8	64.0	62.0	25.5	19.2
Partial	17	↑	57.5	81.0	49.0	41.5	28.0
Partial	30	↑	32.5	69.0	33.5	37.8	80.0
Partial	35	↑	7.8	23.5	27.2	18.5	18.5
Partial	38	↑	29.5	65.8	113.2	43.0	122.2
Full	41	↑	15.5	48.5	39.0	60.0	22.0
Partial	70	↑	11.2	43.5	60.0	56.5	-
Partial	71	↑	30.0	23.5	88.0	88.2	92.0
	mean		27.8	53.1	73.3	44.1	54.8
	± s.e.m.		±5.3	±8.7	±12.4	±7.0	±13.9
	p value			(<.0005)	(<.005)	(NS)	(NS)

A 35-year-old diabetic who had suffered from previous stillbirths and abortions adopted a child approximately two years after
she had undergone tubal ligation. In an attempt to nurse the
adopted newborn, she placed the child at the breast frequently for
approximately two weeks. Soon after, breast secretion began. She
was followed regularly and was in excellent diabetic control.
While she had experienced regular menstrual periods prior to nipple
stimulation, three cycles which followed the onset of breast milk
production were shorter and lighter.

Figure 7 illustrates the gonadotropin and PRL profile during
a nursing interval. Basal PRL was elevated at 39.2 ng/ml. A
modest PRL response was observed during nursing and at no time did
the PRL concentration fall to within the normal nonpregnant range.
She received 10 mg or oral TRH on two occasions 12 hours apart
beginning at 8:00 p.m. the evening of the first test. On the
second day, the test was repeated. While there was a slight
elevation in the PRL concentration, there was a dramatic increase

in milk production. The time limitations of the study prevent any
determination of the overall PRL secretory profile during the 12
hour period the patient ingested oral TRH. However, in other
studies we have shown that the basal PRL concentration gradually
rises over three hours when oral TRH is ingested (Figure 8).

DISCUSSION

We have sought to identify factors responsible for the pro-

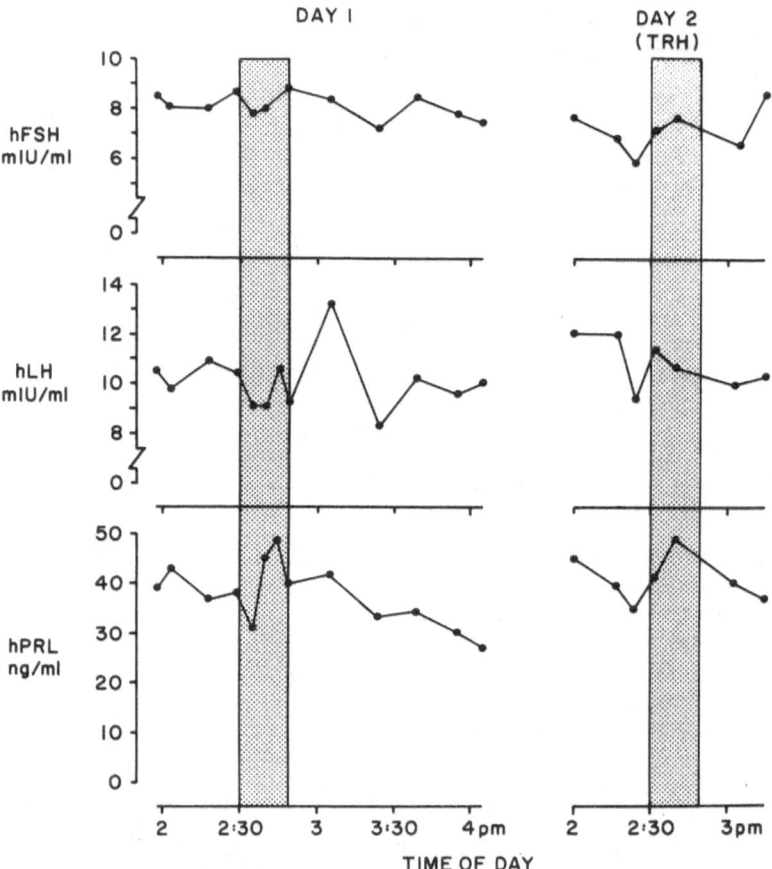

Figure 7. Plasma gonadotropin and PRL responses during one nursing event in a woman experiencing induced lactation. Sampling on
day one was performed before the ingestion of TRH. Sampling on
day two was performed after the ingestion of 10 mg oral TRH on
two occasions 12 hours apart prior to the study.

longation of natural infecundity and through our studies of
nursing-induced prolactin secretion, we have identified the role
of the duration, frequency and intensity of the nursing stimulus
in the release of prolactin. It supports the contention that basal
PRL levels are elevated above the normal range in women who practice nursing on demand. Furthermore, we have shown a positive
correlation exists between the plasma PRL concentration and endo-
metrial biopsy findings in women who develop uterine bleeding
while breastfeeding (19).

    That prolactin may influence ovarian steroidogenic activity
has been reported from this laboratory (19) and by Seppala et al.
(20).

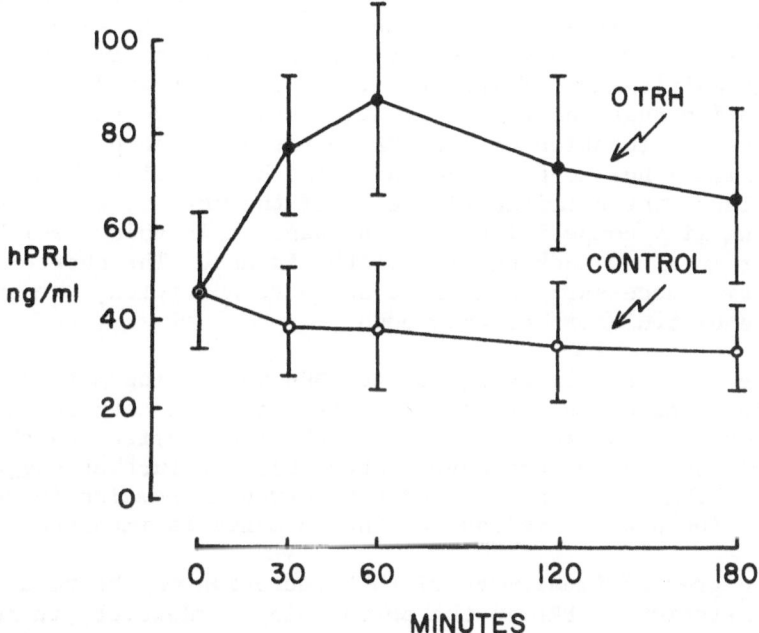

Figure 8. The plasma prolactin (mean ± S.E.) response is shown
following either 5 mg TRH (n=6) or placebo (n=6) given at time 0
in a group of nursing women between the 5th-35th postpartum day.
The rise following TRH was significant (p < 0.05).
(Reprinted from J. Clin. Endocrinol. Metab. 43: 762, 1976)

In this regard, elevated PRL concentrations appear to influence luteal progesterone production. The condition is totally reversed with the use of a dopamine agonist, 2-Brom-α- ergocryptine (20).

We have also shown that the episodic secretion of gonado-tropins in nursing women early in the puerperium appears to be altered compared to the secretion of gonadotropins observed in non-nursing menstruating women. However, as the duration of the post-partum period is extended, the frequency of nursing declines and a gradual resumption of the episodic tonic gonadotropin secretion of good amplitude occurs with an eventual restoration of cyclic gonadotropin secretion. These results appear to imply a relation-ship between PRL and gonadotropin secretion; however, Lu et al. (21) have suggested that the neurogenic reflex controlling LH secretion may be separate from that controlling PRL secretion. Further work in this area is currently under way.

An evaluation of the fluid intake of the four nursing infants in our study lends support to the hypothesis that the frequency and intensity of the nursing stimulus determines the PRL response and perhaps even the degree to which LH secretion will be impaired. While the overall weight gain was similar in each infant after each feeding, the length of the feeding and the PRL response to sucking differed markedly. Rather than denying the importance of PRL in the maintenance of lactation, we believe this data supports the contention that the volume of milk available to the child (which may represent a function of the PRL secreted at the previous feed-ing) determines how long and how hard the baby will suck at the breast. Thus, the nutritional status of the mother, while not influencing milk composition, may influence milk volume which in turn determines the sucking time of the infant. The shorter the suckling time necessary to acquire adequate nutrition, the greater the chance of ovulatory breakthrough.

Since gonadotropin responses to LHRH in nursing mothers were exaggerated over those obtained in bottle-feeding mothers, we believe that PRL may indeed exert an inhibitory effect on the release of LHRH, as others have stated (6). It further suggests that the synthesis and storage of gonadotropins remains intact during nursing but the release of the hormones is impaired.

The degree of impairment of LHRH secretion may be related to the concentration of PRL in the portal blood. However, it remains unresolved as to how much LHRH is necessary to release gonado-tropins (22). A dual effect of PRL must also be considered in view of the work of Bonnar (9). Basal FSH secretion recovers as quickly in nursing mothers as it does in non-nursing mothers but the ovarian response to this appears impaired.

In considering the natural mechanisms of infecundity in post-

partum women, we now know that oral and intravenous TRH can provoke
the secretion of prolactin on a dose response curve independent of
that seen for TSH (14,23,24). Furthermore, the chronic administration of oral TRH can improve the volume of milk production in women
suffering from impaired PRL secretion (10). In this study, the
administration of oral TRH improved milk volume but had a transi-
ent effect on the secretion of PRL. However, it appeared to have
an influence on the volume of milk production in a woman who had
initiated lactation by autostimulation of her own breasts. The
level of PRL in the plasma of this woman before and after the
administration of oral TRH was significantly elevated. The limitations of the study did not allow an evaluation of the 24 hour
secretory pattern of PRL before and during oral TRH ingestion,
although the work of others has suggested that PRL values are
chronically elevated (16).

The significance of this work relates to the ultimate identification of the hypothalamic factors controlling both the secretion
of PRL and LH. Exploitation of these mechanisms when fully defined
will make it possible for physicians to prolong the period of
lactational infertility and in doing so enhance the chances of the
nursing infant's survival by keeping it at the breast. At the
same time, attention must be paid to maternal nutrition since this
appears to be the single most important factor determining the
volume of milk production.

Supported by Grant No. AID/csd-2956 and AID/pha-C-1146 from the
Agency for International Development, Washington, D. C.

References

1. Tyson, J. E. Nursing and prolactin secretion: principal
   determinants in the mediation of puerperal infertility. In:
   Crosignani, P. G. and C. Robyn (eds.), Prolactin and Human
   Reproduction, Academic Press, New York and London, 1976.

2. Tyson, J. E. Neuroendocrine control of lactational infertility.
   J. Biosoc. Sci., 1976, in press.

3. Voogt, J. L. and Carr, L. A. Plasma prolactin levels and
   hypothalamic catecholamine synthesis during suckling.
   Neuroendocrinol. 16: 108, 1974.

4. Voogt, J. L. and Carr., L. A. Potentiation of suckling-
   induced release of prolactin by inhibition of brain catecholamine synthesis. Endocrinology 97: 891, 1975.

5. Andreassen, B. and Tyson, J. E. Role of the hypothalamic-

pituitary-ovarian axis in puerperal infertility. <u>J. Clin</u>. <u>Endocrinol. Metab</u>. <u>42</u>: 1114, 1976.

6. Maneckjee, R., Srinath, B. K. and Moudgal, N. R. Prolactin suppresses release of luteinizing hormone during lactation in the monkey. <u>Nature</u> <u>262</u>: 507, 1976.

7. McNatty, K. P., Sawers, R. S. and McNeilly, A. S. A possible role for prolactin in control of steroid secretion by the human Graafian follicle. <u>Nature</u> <u>250</u>: 653, 1974.

8. Rolland, R., De Jong, F. H., Schellekens, L. A. and Lequin, R. M. The role of prolactin in the restoration of ovarian function during the early postpartum period in the human female. II. A study during inhibition of lactation by bromergocryptine. <u>Clin. Endocrinol</u>. <u>4</u>: 27, 1975.

9. Bonnar, J., Franklin, M., Nott, P. N. and McNeilly, A. S. Effect of breastfeeding on pituitary-ovarian function after childbirth. <u>Br. Med. J</u>. <u>4</u>: 82, 1975.

10. Tyson, J. E., Perez, A., and Zanartu, J. Human lactational response to oral thyrotropin releasing hormone. <u>J. Clin</u>. <u>Endocrinol. Metab</u>. <u>43</u>: 760, 1976.

11. Hwang, P., Guyda, H. and Friesen, H. A radioimmunoassay for human prolactin. <u>Proc. Nat. Acad. Sci</u>. <u>68</u>: 1902, 1971.

12. Greenwood, F., Hunter, W. and Glover, J. The preparation of I^{131} labeled human growth hormone of high specific radio-activity. <u>Biochem. J</u>. <u>89</u>: 114, 1963.

13. Midgely, A. R. Radioimmunoassay: a method for human chorionic gonadotropin and human luteinizing hormone. <u>Endocrinology</u> <u>79</u>: 10, 1966.

14. Tyson, J. E., Friesen, H. G. and Anderson, M. S. Human lactational and ovarian response to endogenous prolactin release. <u>Science</u> <u>177</u>: 897, 1972.

15. Yen, S.S.C., Tsai, C. C., Naftolin, F., Vandenberg, G. and Ajabor, L. Pulsatile patterns of gonadotropin release in subjects with and without ovarian function. <u>J. Clin</u>. <u>Endocrinol</u>. <u>34</u>: 671, 1972.

16. Zarate, A., Villalobos, H., Canales, E. S., Soria, J., Arcovedo, F. and MacGregor, C. The effect of oral administration of thyrotropin-releasing hormone on lactation. <u>J. Clin</u>.

Endocrinol. Metab. 43: 301, 1976.

17. Tyson, J. E., Khojandi, M., Huth, J., and Andreassen, B.
     The influence of prolactin secretion on human lactation.
     J. Clin. Endocrinol. Metab. 40: 764, 1975.

18. Jeppsson, S., Nilsson, K.O., Rannevik, G. and Wide, L.
     Influence of suckling and of suckling followed by TRH or LH-
     RH on plasma prolactin, TSH, GH and FSH. Acta Endocrinol.
     82: 246, 1976.

19. Tyson, J. E., Freedman, R. S., Perez, A., Zacur, H. A. and
     Zanartu, J. Significance of the secretion of human prolactin
     and gonadotropin for puerperal lactational infertility. In:
     Breastfeeding and the Mother, Elsevier/Excerpta Medica/North-
     Holland and Elsevier North-Holland, Inc., 1976.

20. Seppala, M., Hirvonen, E. and Rant, T. Hyperprolactinemia
     and luteal insufficiency. Lancet 1: 229, 1976.

21. Lu, K. H., Chen, H. T., Huang, H. H., Grandison, L., Marshall,
     S. and Meites, J. Relation between prolactin and gonado-
     trophin secretion in postpartum lactating rats. J. Endocrinol.
     68: 241, 1976.

22. Eskay, R. L., Mical, R. S. and Porter, J. C. Relationship
     between luteinizing hormone releasing hormone concentration
     in hypophyseal portal blood and luteinizing hormone release
     in intact, castrated, and electrochemically-stimulated rats.
     Endocrinology 100: 263, 1977.

23. Gautvick, M., Weintraub, B. D., Graeber, C. T., Maloof, F.,
     Zuckerman, J. E. and Tashijian, A. H. Serum prolactin and
     TSH: effects of nursing and pyroGlu-His-ProNH$_2$ administration
     in postpartum women. J. Clin. Endocrinol. Metab. 37: 135,
     1973.

24. Rabello, M. M., Snyder, P. J. and Utiger, R. D. Effects on
     the pituitary-thyroid axis and prolactin secretion of single
     and repetitive oral doses of thyrotropin-releasing hormone
     (TRH). J. Clin. Endocrinol. Metab. 39: 574, 1974.

IMPACT OF MALNUTRITION ON REPRODUCTIVE ENDOCRINOLOGY

Jo Anne Brasel

Columbia University

New York, New York

INTRODUCTION

The material to be covered in this review of the impact of malnutrition on reproductive endocrinology has been arbitrarily limited. Only data related to the human will be covered; furthermore, malnutrition is taken to mean undernutrition and not obesity, even though the latter may be a more serious public health problem in the United States. Although some information on the effects of specific nutrient deficiencies will be mentioned, the major focus will be on the effects of protein-calorie malnutrition on reproductive function. Finally, some data on anorexia nervosa will also be included, even though there are some important differences between simple food restriction and anorexia nervosa.

The report will begin with a brief review of epidemiologic and clinical observations made in the past, usually during war or other times of undernutrition, which suggest that reproductive endocrine function has been altered. This will be followed by a summary of selected information on reproductive and hormonal changes occurring in the various types of malnutrition. Alterations in those hormones not ordinarily thought to be "reproductive" in nature will be briefly reviewed and that data, which is available on the "reproductive" hormones, will be covered in more detail. Intentionally the majority of the biochemical studies have been taken from recent literature sources since the sophistication of the newer techniques for hormone measurement provide a more accurate assessment of changes in production rates, metabolic clearance, response to stimuli, etc., than the older measures of urinary excretion as a sole measure of endocrine function.

EPIDEMIOLOGICAL AND CLINICAL OBSERVATIONS

There are two major accompaniments of famine and malnutrition which affect the potential reproductive capacity of a population which may have their origins, either directly or indirectly, in alterations of endocrine function. First, the growth and development of children are severely affected, especially those growing the most rapidly, i.e., the young infant and the adolescent. In the latter, pubertal development is delayed; this may be related to failure to achieve the "critical body mass" necessary to trigger adolescence, as has been proposed by Frisch and her colleagues (1-5). The malnutrition need not be severe in order to cause some adolescent delay, as seen in Frisch's study of 30 undernourished Alabama girls and 30 well-nourished controls (Figure 1) (6).

The change in growth rates accompanying war which could affect the time of reaching the "critical mass" is clearly shown in Figure 2, which demonstrates weight gain in boys and girls from 7 to 17 years of age in Stuttgart during the years 1911 to 1953 (7). The detrimental effects of the World Wars on weight gain are evident and must be due, at least in part, to poor nutrition.

Others have pointed to a relationship between body size and the onset of puberty; in 1943 Simmons and Greulich (8) reported the results of 1339 physical examinations of 200 girls 7 to 17 years of age and noted that those who reached menarche at 10 to 11 years of age were taller, heavier, and heavier for their height, than girls reaching menarche at 13 years or older. In the paper by Zacharias and Wurtman (9) nutrition is but one of the factors mentioned which may affect the age of menarche.

Age of menarche has certainly been decreasing over the past century in Western Europe and the U.S. (Figure 3). Although many factors, such as improved public health measures, better general health and fewer chronic debilitating diseases, improved nutrition and an overall increase in the physical size of the population, have probably played some role in this trend, it is difficult to assign weighted values to their relative importance. Johnston et al. (10) disagree with Frisch and feel that an invariant weight at menarche cannot be applied meaningfully to individual girls even though, in my opinion, the data for large population groups is impressive.

The second important accompaniment of famine and malnutrition, which may or may not be endocrine-related, is the fall in birth rate, coupled with an increased rate of abortion, stillbirth, and neonatal deaths. Stein et al. (11) have studied the "Dutch Hunger Winter" of 1944 to 1945 in detail and show a striking parallelism

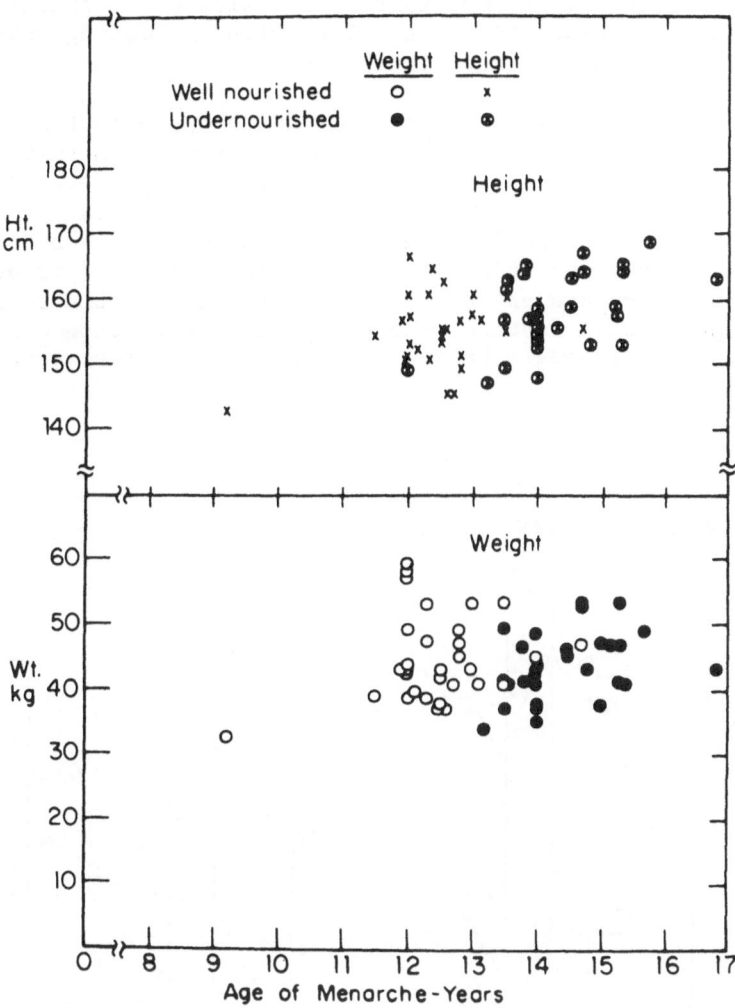

Figure 1. Height and weight at menarche versus chronological age
in well nourished and undernourished Alabama girls. The well
nourished girls fall to the left of the graph, while the undernourished girls fall to the right, suggesting that the achievement
of a certain body size may be more important in the onset of
menses than the chronologic age. (Reprinted with permission from
Frisch, R. E., *Pediatrics* 50:445, 1972.)

between caloric ration at conception and total births, although
the birth rate decrease lags slightly behind the fall in rations.
The birth rate fell more in the manual class than in the non-
manual class which supports the hypothesis that the availability

of food was probably an important factor with other things, such as changes in contraceptive use, alterations in mating habits, etc., being of less, if any, importance.

One indication of endocrinologic disturbance in time of famine is male gynecomastia (12). Other studies have shown that diminished libido, amenorrhea, impotence, fear of death, etc. (13-17), which might affect mating frequency and conception rates, accompany famine and would obviously affect birth rates. It is not clear which effects are nutritional and/or endocrinological in origin versus that which are psychological in origin. In the remainder of the paper I will describe changes with malnutrition which may have some endocrinologic basis and which might affect reproductive functioning.

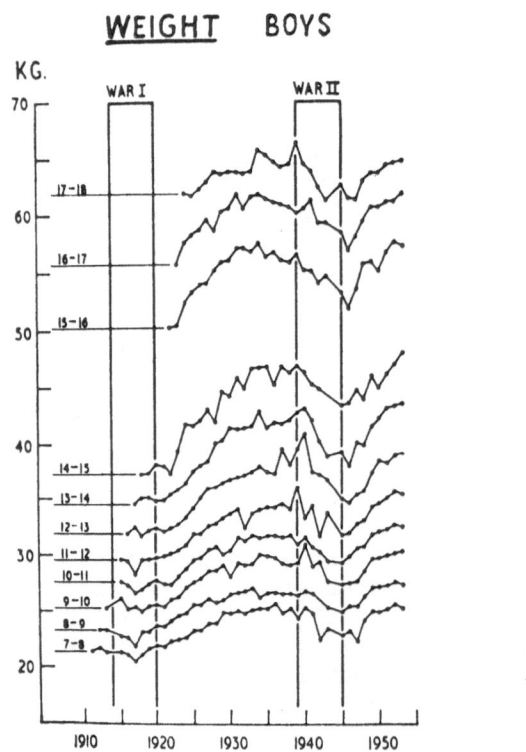
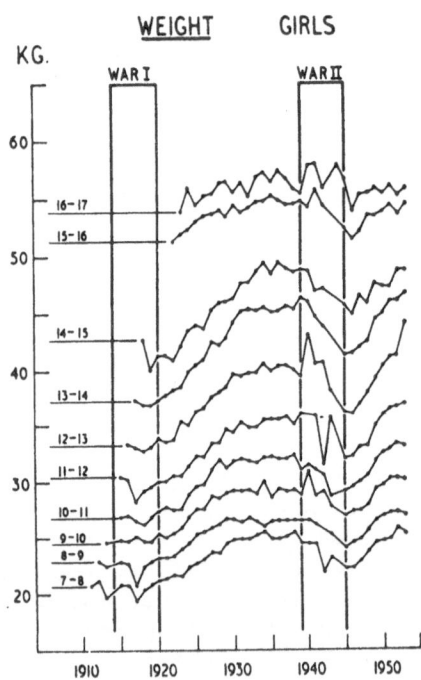

Figure 2. Weights of Stuttgart school children from 1911 to 1953. The general downward trends occurring during the World Wars is clearly seen. (Reprinted with permission from Tanner, J. M., Growth at Adolescence, 2nd ed., 1962, Blackwell Scientific Pub., Oxford.)

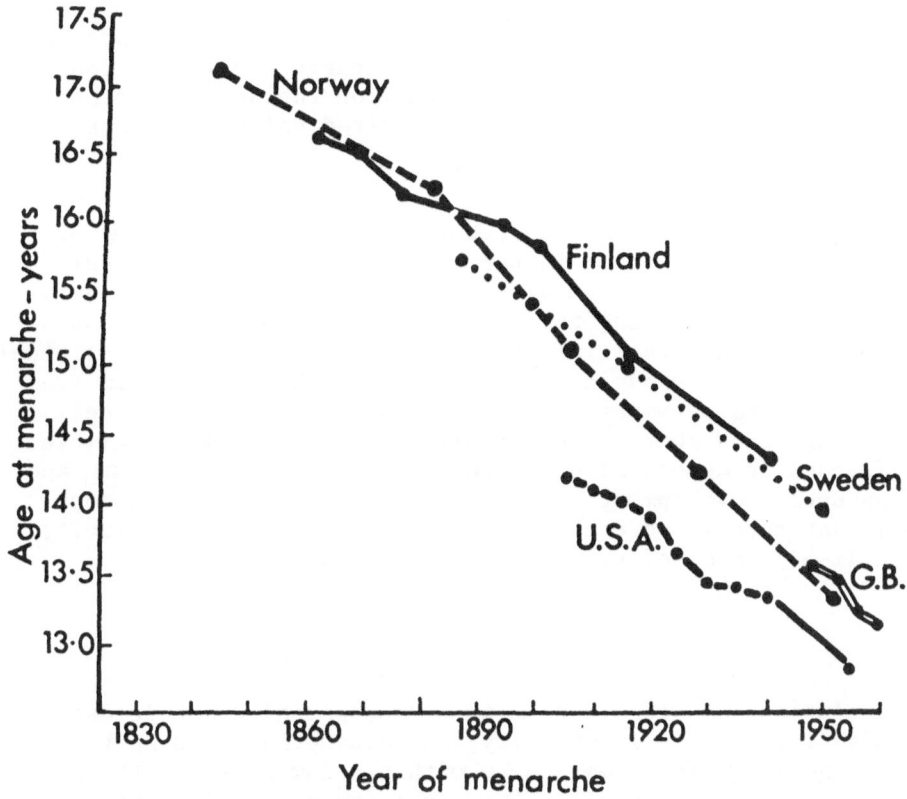

Figure 3. Age at menarche versus year of menarche. (Reprinted with permission from Tanner, J. M., <u>Growth at Adolescence</u>, 2nd ed., 1962, Blackwell Scientific Pub., Oxford.)

SPECIFIC NUTRIENT DEFICIENCIES

Iron

Aksoy et al. (18) have reported five patients, ranging in age from 13 to 25 years, who presented with severe hypochromic, microcytic anemia due to iron deficiency, hepatosplenomegaly or splenomegaly, infantilism and hypogonadism. Growth failure, delayed skeletal maturation and mild biochemical and/or clinical evidence of cirrhosis of the liver were also seen. In all subjects the diets were poor in animal protein and fresh vegetables. One patient had skin lesions compatible with pellagra and in another a kwashiorkor-like syndrome was observed. Therefore it was con-

cluded that the syndrome was due at least in part, to poor dietary
intake since the liver disease, especially, had not been previously reported as an accompaniment to even severe, isolated iron
deficiency. All patients responded to iron therapy from a hema-
tologic point of view although some required splenectomy for
associated hypersplenism.

It is interesting that no details were given regarding dietary treatment or responses in terms of growth rates or sexual
maturation. In the absence of such information one cannot draw
any conclusions regarding the relationship of the severe iron
deficiency to the sexual infantilism. It is a well known clinical
fact that patients whose diets are adequate, but who suffer from
severe congenital anemias, such as thalassemia and sickle cell
disease, in which there is certainly no associated iron deficiency,
also frequently demonstrate developmental delay, poor growth and
late pubertal development. This being the case, it seems more
likely that chronic severe anemia, rather than an iron deficit,
is the likely cause of this disorder in sexual development.

Vitamin B-12

Deficiency of vitamin B-12 in premenopausal women is associated with involuntary infertility, and conception leading to the
birth of normal infants may occur within a few short months of
appropriate therapy (19-24). The mechanism of the infertility is
unknown, but it is interesting that the infertility may precede
by years overt clinical evidence of pernicious anemia. Semen and
sperm abnormalities have been noted in males with pernicious
anemia (25-27). There is one spectacular case in which B-12
therapy led to return to active participation in sheep shearing by
one 73 year old Australian sheep herder and pregnancy in his 37
year old wife (27). In the instances of iron and B-12 deficiency-
induced abnormalities of reproductive function no endocrinologic
studies have been reported.

Zinc

In 1961 Prasad et al. (28) reported a syndrome of dwarfism,
sexual infantilism, hepatosplenomegaly, iron deficiency anemia and
geophagia. Subsequent reports of patients from both Iran and
Egypt (29-31) confirmed the earlier clinical manifestations and
suggested that zinc deficiency, rather than iron deficiency or
protein-calorie deficiency, was the important pathogenic factor
in the syndrome. Initial endocrinologic evaluation (29) suggested
that some degree of anterior pituitary deficiency was present in

these patients. Although the condition is much more common in males, it has also been described in females. Of particular interest was that in most trials zinc replacement brought about the most prompt recovery (29,32), even though sexual development would eventually occur even in untreated cases (33).

In 1971 Coble et al. (34) reported more complete and sophisticated endocrinologic evaluation of a group of 26 boys from the Nile valley; 8 were considered "normal" by local standards even though they were small by Iowa standards, and 18 were "retarded" with the clinical signs and symptoms of "zinc-deficient hypogonadal dwarfism". Routine biochemical tests could not distinguish between the two groups though both had some evidence of hepatic dysfunction felt to be secondary to schistosoma infection. The degree of iron and zinc deficiency were similar; therefore the two groups were different only in their degree of growth failure and sexual development.

Serum TSH and PBI levels were normal. Morning plasma ACTH and cortisol were normal or slightly elevated and responded appropriately to metapyrone and ACTH stimulation; earlier studies (28) had revealed normal urinary cortisol excretion. Therefore no evidence for abnormalities in the pituitary-thyroid or pituitary-adrenal axes were found. In contrast, marked hypoglycemia followed the intravenous administration of insulin in both the "normal" and "retarded" groups. Furthermore only 4 of 18 "retarded" boys and 4 of 8 "normal" boys demonstrated appropriate elevations of serum growth hormone during the insulin-induced hypoglycemia.

Tests of gonadal function were similarly frequently abnormal in both groups. Mean plasma testosterone of these teenaged "retarded" boys was greater than that of prepubertal boys from the U.S., but was less than that of the "normal" group who showed some degree of adolescent development. Approximately 75% of both groups responded normally to the administration of human chorionic gonadotropin by doubling plasma testosterone, suggesting that Leydig cell function was not impaired in most subjects (Figure 4). The response, however, was not as uniform as that seen in boys and men from the West, and the failure of six subjects to respond at all is unexplained. Plasma LH levels were significantly higher in the "normal" group while FSH levels were similar, though both were near the limit of detection for the assay procedure (Figure 5). These authors concluded that in these two groups of Egyptian boys with zinc deficiency and endocrine dysfunction, the growth failure and sexual infantilism could not be attributed solely to endocrine abnormalities. The delayed puberty appears to be related to hypo-gonadotropism; the poor growth hormone response to hypoglycemia is unexplained and the relationship of zinc deficiency to any or all of these abnormalities has not been clarified.

PROTEIN-CALORIE MALNUTRITION

Investigations of endocrine function have been extensive in
subjects with protein-calorie malnutrition, especially in infants
and children with marasmus and kwashiorkor. In the past two to
three years a few reports of alterations in hormones in malnourished
adults have appeared in which modern laboratory techniques have
been employed. Growth hormone, insulin, adrenal function, thyroid
hormones, and the pituitary-gonadal axis have been studied.
Olson's summary of the changes in various enzymes and hormonal
levels in childhood in terms of an adaptive response to limited
dietary intake is a particularly good review of the overall
picture (35).

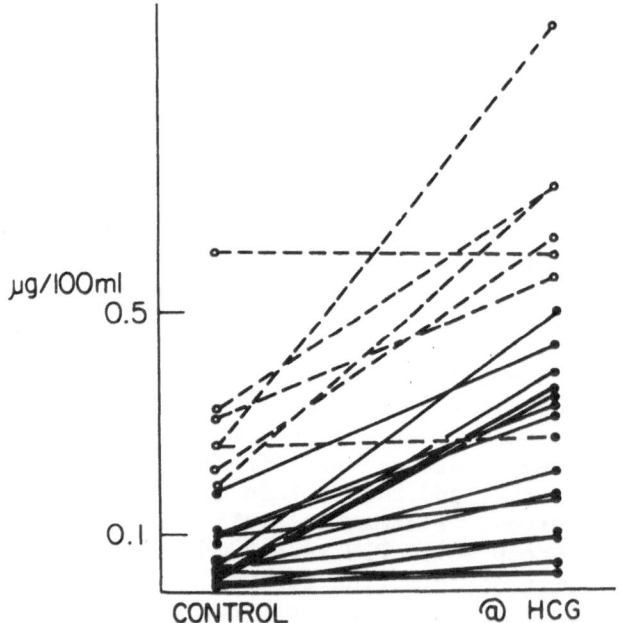

Figure 4. Plasma testosterone in "normal" (dashed lines) and
"retarded" (solid lines) Egyptian boys before and after human
chorionic gonadotropin administration. See text for details.
(Reprinted with permission from Coble, Y.D. et al., J. Clin.
Endocrinol. Metab. 32:361, 1971.)

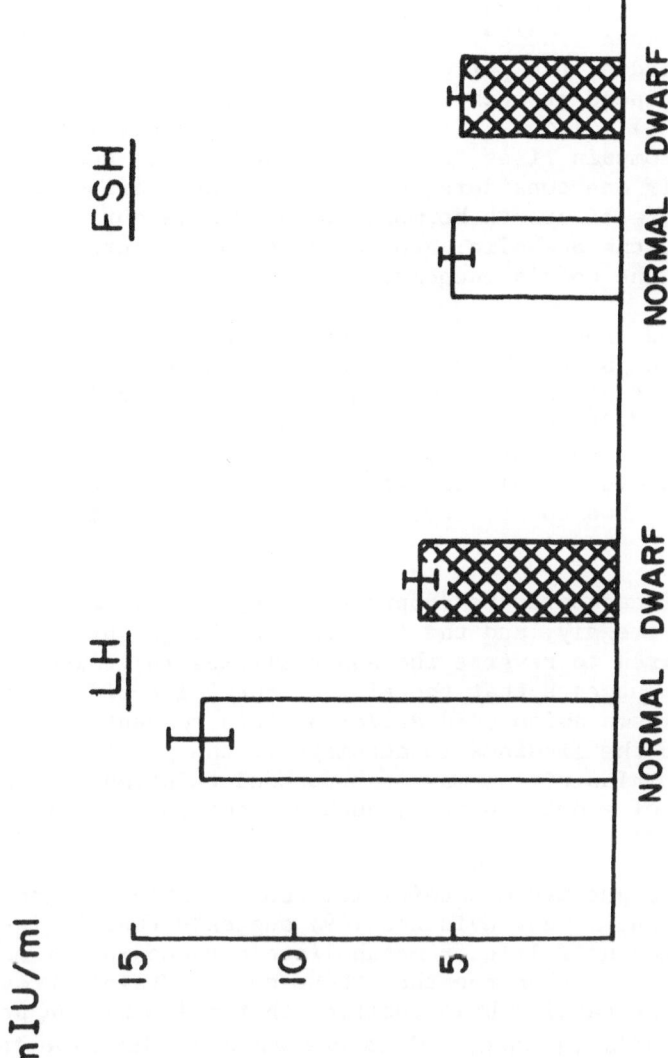

Figure 5. Plasma LH and FSH in "normal" and "retarded" Egyptian boys. (Reprinted with permission from Coble, Y. D., et al., J. Clin. Endocrinol. Metab. 32:361, 1971.)

Growth Hormone

There is no disagreement that basal growth hormone levels are
elevated in kwashiorkor (36-43) (Figure 6). In addition, most
observers agree that it is also elevated in marasmus (Figure 7),
but a few exceptions have been reported (44-45) which may relate
to differences in the patient populations and the conditions under
which they have been studied. In the face of elevated growth
hormone, somatomedin, the peripheral effector of many of the
growth hormone-dependent anabolic actions, especially on bone, is
reduced (Figure 8) (41,46). As growth hormone levels fall with
treatment, somatomedin rises to normal values. This could certainly be adaptive if one considers that the glucose sparing and fat
mobilizing effects of growth hormone are desirable during times of
famine; however, the anabolic, growth-promoting effects are disadvantageous to the body's economy.

The elevated growth hormone is unsuppressible by carbohydrate
infusions, by a high carbohydrate diet over a three day period, or
by the infusion of albumin to bring plasma proteins within normal
limits acutely (37-39, 41-43, 47, 48). However, with a protein
containing diet for as short a period as three days, the growth
hormone levels begin to fall significantly but do not reach normal
levels until some two to four weeks of appropriate dietary therapy
(37,38,41).

The lack of carbohydrate suppressibility is similar to the
situation in acromegaly, and the fact that prolonged protein ingestion is required to reverse the abnormalities in growth hormone
and somatomedin suggests that the site of control resides elsewhere than in plasma amino acid and/or protein concentrations.
Also analgous to the findings in acromegaly, the patients with
protein-calorie malnutrition may over-respond to stimuli used to
provoke release of growth hormone, such as arginine infusion
(Figure 9) (40,42).

Although the precise mechanism for the elevation of growth
hormone is unknown, recent evidence (49) suggests that it is not
due to a prolonged half-life or metabolic clearance in the malnourished subjects. Taken together these data certainly provide
no support for the earlier held position that malnutrition produces
a hypopituitary-like picture, unless one wants to describe the
depressed somatomedin levels in those terms. It should be pointed
out, as an addendum, that other recent studies of short term
starvation in normal adult men and women, after equilibration on
standard or altered diets containing disproportionate amounts of
carbohydrate, fat or protein do not demonstrate precisely the
changes in growth hormone secretion noted after prolonged protein-
calorie malnutrition (50,51). More investigations will be neces-

sary to provide an integrated picture of growth hormone alterations occurring under differing conditions of limited dietary intake.

Insulin

Protein-calorie malnutrition is characterized by hypoglycemia, especially after fasting; glucose intolerance or a flat glucose tolerance curve; hypoinsulinemia, especially following insulino-genic stimuli; and sensitivity to exogenous insulin (39,40,43,52-

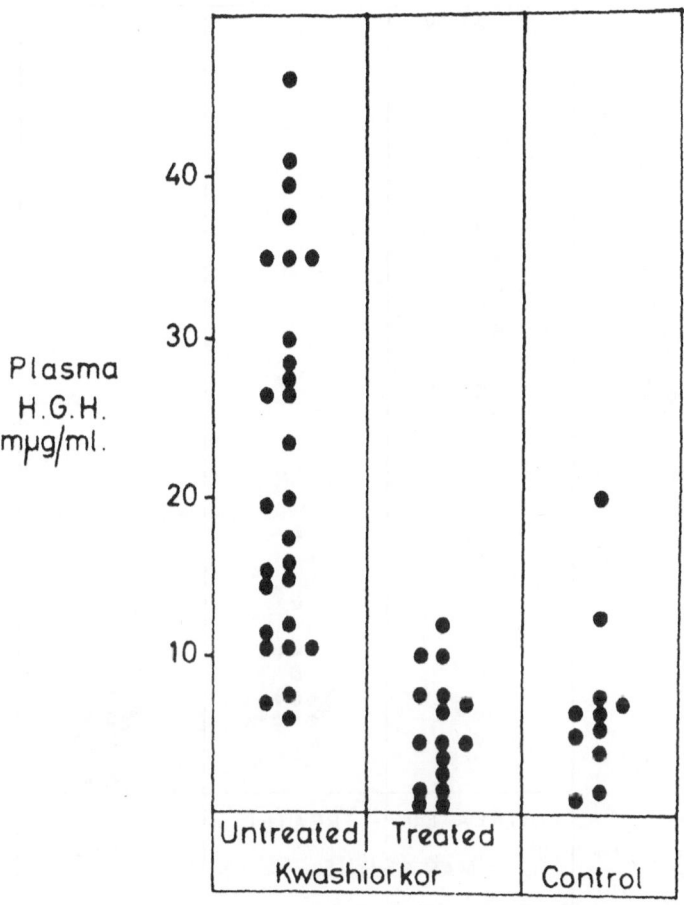

Figure 6. Plasma growth hormone levels in children with kwashi-orkor before and after nutritional rehabilitation and in normal control children. (Reprinted with permission from Pimstone, B.L. et al., Lancet 2: 779, 1966.)

63). These findings can also be seen in growth hormone deficiency, but, as noted above, growth hormone is actually elevated in malnutrition. The degree of insulinopenia following an IV glucose load is proportional to the severity of the malnutrition, to the levels of serum albumin and alanine on admission and to the extent of glucose intolerance and is inversely proportional to basal growth hormone levels (63). In some cases the insulin response to insulinogenic stimuli may not only be blunted, as mentioned above,

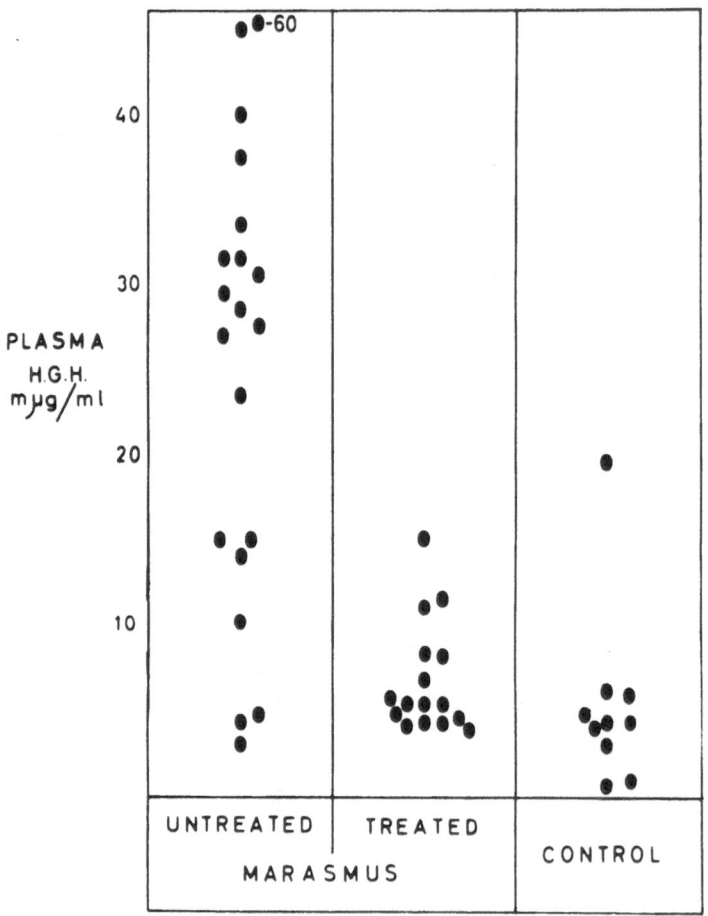

Figure 7. Plasma growth hormone levels in children with marasmus before and after nutritional rehabilitation and in normal control children. (Reprinted with permission from Pimstone, B. L. et al., Amer. J. Clin. Nutr. 21: 482, 1968).

but may reach the peak value later than in normal control subjects (40,56,62). This type of response has also been noted after total

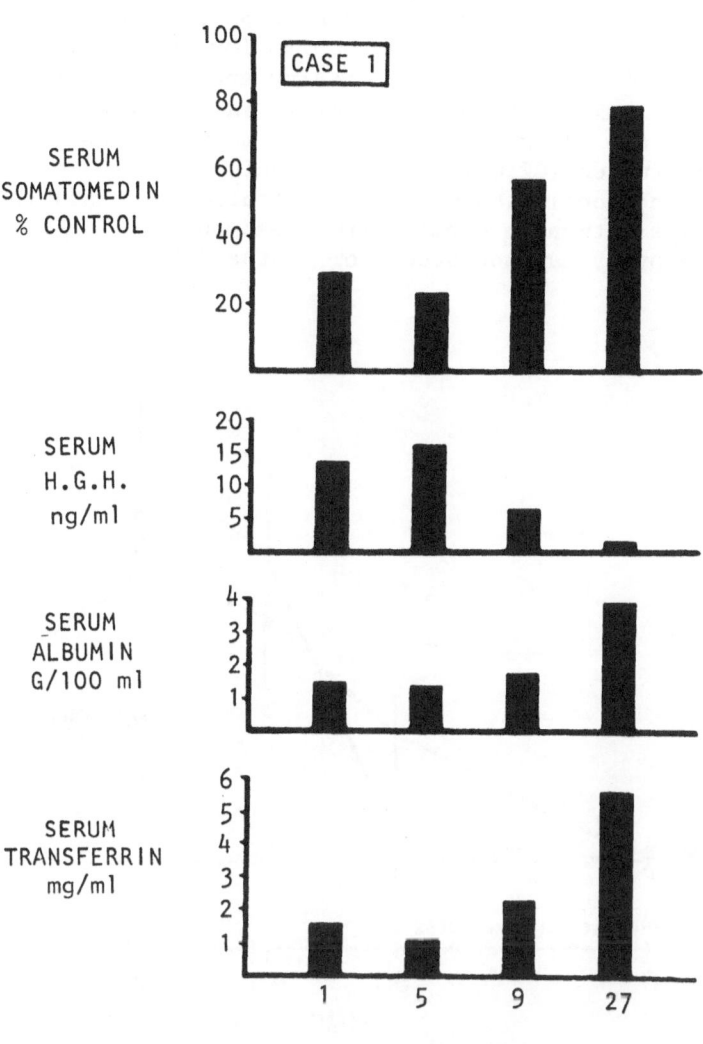

DAYS AFTER ADMISSION

Figure 8. Somatomedin, growth hormone, albumin and transferrin levels in a child with kwashiorkor during the course of nutritional rehabilitation. Growth hormone levels fall to within normal levels while the other variables rise to reach normal as recovery occurs. (Reprinted with permission from Pimstone, B. L. et al., in: Gardner, L. I. and Amacher, P., eds., Endocrine Aspects of Malnutrition, The Kroc Foundation, Santa Ynez, California, 1973.)

starvation or during restricted carbohydrate intake in adults
(64,65).

The reduced insulin release may serve an adaptive role since
in times of energy deficit the actions of insulin to move free
fatty acids into fat tissue or amino acids into muscle would be
disadvantageous. The precise mechanism for the defects in insulin
release are unknown, but body potassium and chromium deficits,
defective gut insulinotropic factor(s), and disordered insulin
transport by the pancreas have all been mentioned and are supported
by several studies (62,66). However, actual pancreatic damage or
decreased functional mass has not been ruled out. All these
abnormalities return to normal with treatment, but in some cases
complete recovery may not occur for months (62).

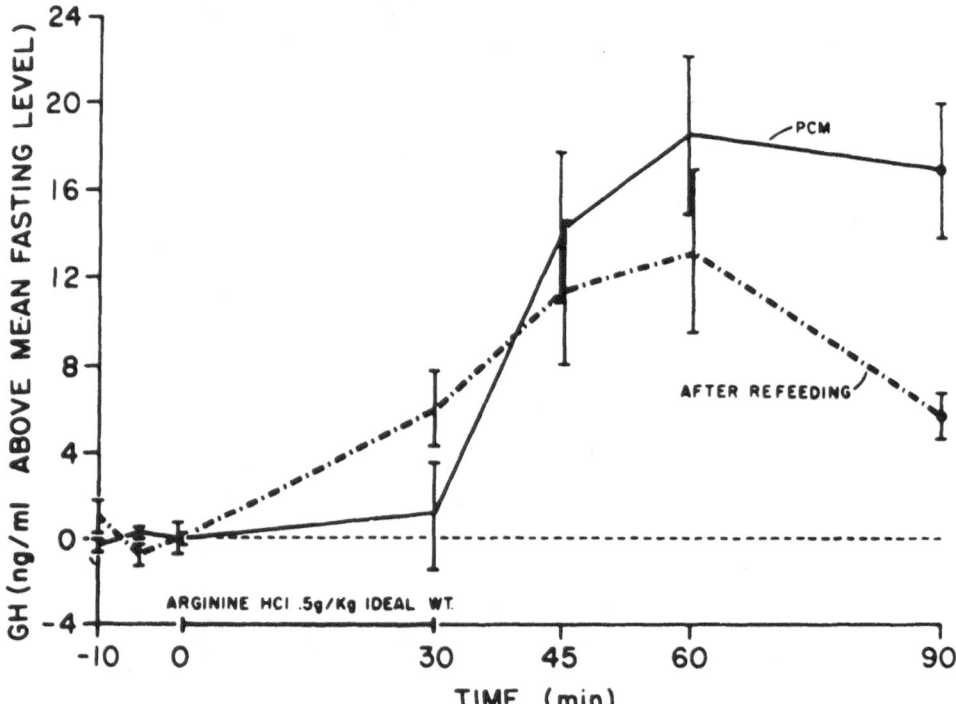

Figure 9. Rise in growth hormone levels above the fasting value
in adult patients with protein-calorie malnutrition before and
after nutritional rehabilitation in response to an intravenous
infusion of arginine. In the malnourished state higher levels of
growth hormone are achieved and are sustained for longer periods.
(Reprinted with permission from Smith, S. R. et al., J. Clin.
Endocrinol. Metab. 39: 53, 1974.)

Adrenal Function

Earlier studies of adrenal function which relied on the urinary excretion of glucocorticoid metabolites, the 17-OHCS, led to the belief that hypoadrenalism accompanied chronic malnutrition. Two recent investigations, utilizing newer methodologies, reveal that the hypothalamic-pituitary-adrenal axis is not only intact and responds appropriately to various types of stimulation including stress, but also may be in a state of slight hyperfunction. The first study (67) was of 10 adults with chronic protein-calorie malnutrition associated with edema and hypoalbuminemia. Both total plasma cortisol and plasma free cortisol, the metabolically active form, were increased; however, the 17-OHCS excretion was diminished, though the urinary total free cortisol was normal. Plasma cortisol metabolic clearance and production rates were decreased. Adrenal responsiveness to exogenous ACTH or metapyrone were normal, but exogenous decadron failed to produce the expected degree of suppression of cortisol production. The authors concluded that the pituitary-adrenal axis was intact, but that ACTH was autonomously controlled by unknown factors, perhaps the chronic stress of the malnutrition, and failed to show the expected reduction in the face of either increased endogenous or exogenous glucocorticoids.

The second study (68) was undertaken in 35 malnourished children; the results are similar. Plasma free cortisol levels were increased and rose promptly in the presence of acute infection. Additionally, corticosteroid binding globulin was diminished, even in those subjects without edema. In both studies dietary therapy was followed by a return toward normal of all abnormalities, which began within a short time of refeeding.

Thyroid Hormones

Of all the endocrine systems studied in patients with malnutrition, there is probably more confusion about the functional status of the thyroid than any of the others. In the extensive literature on the subject, investigators have variously concluded that hypothyroidism, euthyroidism, or hyperthyroidism exists. Some of the confusion is slowly being clarified by recent, sophisticated techniques for determining thyroid hormone metabolism. This summary will focus on the current state of the art and the best guess of what occurs during protein-calorie-malnutrition.

Most of the studies which led to the conclusion that hypothyroidism existed were based on the findings of low BMR values and decreased PBI or total thyroxine levels. There are other obvious reasons for a diminished BMR in severely wasted patients than hypothyroidism. In patients with reduced plasma proteins,

the thyroid binding globulins may also decrease. Thus the free
or metabolically active form of the hormone may remain unchanged,
may decrease or increase, but those alterations could be masked by
changes in the binding globulins (69-71).

Recent work has focused on the measurement of, not only total
thyroxine, but also free thyroxine, total triiodothyronine, and
free triiodothyronine, the latter two probably being more important
in the cellular actions of thyroid hormone. Additionally reverse
triiodothyronine, an alternate, inactive metabolite of thyroxine,
has been measured. In these studies total thyroxine and free
thyroxine have been found to be normal, decreased or increased
(70-74); the possible reasons for these discrepancies will be discussed below.

These studies, by-in-large, are in agreement that total and
free triiodothyronine are decreased (70-74). Marked decreases in
the triiodothyronines can occur with as little as two to four
weeks of caloric restriction in adult obese volunteers (75,76).
A growing consensus is emerging that defective deiodination of
thyroxine to triiodothyronine or increased formation of the inactive reverse triiodothyronine is occurring (70-74). The end
result in either case would be decreased active hormone at the
cellular level.

The changes in thyroxine could be explained by a block in its
metabolism leading to an increased level, an excessive metabolism
to reverse triiodothyronine leading to a decreased level, or some
balance of the two processes leading to no change.

Measurements of thyroid stimulating hormone (TSH) assuming an
intact pituitary, might provide some clue as to whether hypothyroidism is actually present. However, the results are equivocal
again with normal, decreased or increased levels being reported
(70,73-75). Alternatively the hypothalamus could be faulty, and
in fact several studies have attempted to get at this question.
In one, brief fasts (12 to 36 hours) led to diminished TSH release
following administration of synthetic thyrotropin releasing hormone
(TRH) in 9 normal adult men (77). In another study, an exaggerated
release of TSH following administration of TRH was seen in several
children with elevated basal TSH levels in association with
protein-calorie malnutrition (78). This response is reminiscent
of that seen in subjects with primary hypothyroidism.

The many questions regarding thyroid function in malnutrition
remain largely unanswered, but taken on balance, the evidence seems
to point more to some degree of hypothyroidism, at least at a cellular level. It is interesting to point out that all these abnormalities may not be due to the decreased nutritional intake

per se since growth hormone in high levels can cause alterations
in binding of the hormones to their binding proteins and excessive
cortisol or decadron, a synthetic glucocorticoid, can alter binding as well and additionally favor the formation of reverse triiodothyronine from thyroxine (69,79).

Gonadal Function

As noted earlier, amenorrhea, impotence and infertility could
have their origins in either endocrinologic or psychologic factors.
Considering the focus of this conference, it was particularly
disappointing to find that very few studies of gonadal function,
unassociated with psychiatric disease, such as anorexia nervosa,
have been carried out. Smith et al. (80) studied 28 men with
severe protein-calorie malnutrition in Calcutta. They ranged in
age from 25 to 51 years. Hypoalbuminemia and edema were not consistent findings although marked wasting was present in all. All
subjects had clinical evidence of hypogonadism, including diminished body hair and beard growth and diminished libido resulting
in abstention from intercourse; impotence per se is not remarked
upon. Some had soft and/or small testes and one patient had
gynecomastia on admission. Total and free plasma testosterone
were reduced, and rose to normal levels with refeeding. In most
plasma LH and FSH were high at the time of malnutrition and
decreased during refeeding to reach normal values. Human chorionic gonadotropin for three days produced subnormal testosterone
responses in both the malnourished and recovered state (Figure 10).
However, after refeeding, the expected decline in FSH followed the
stimulation.

They concluded that the hypogonadism of chronic malnutrition
is primarily on the basis of testicular failure, probably residing
in the Leydig cells. Since the LH and FSH levels were usually high
on admission, the hypothalamic-pituitary axis appeared to be
responding appropriately to the primary gonadal failure. Additionally, reversal of the malnutrition did not result in complete
recovery of these abnormalities though many of the men developed
more body hair and experienced erections and nocturnal emissions.

In another study (81), obese adult men and women, ranging in
age from 20 to 50 years, were food restricted and the metabolism
of dehydroepiandrosterone sulfate was investigated. Urinary excretion of this compound fell significantly, especially with fasting, while plasma levels rose. Radioactive isotope dilution
studies confirmed that the metabolic clearance and production rates
of this steroid were reduced and the half-life commensurately
increased. These findings are similar to those noted previously

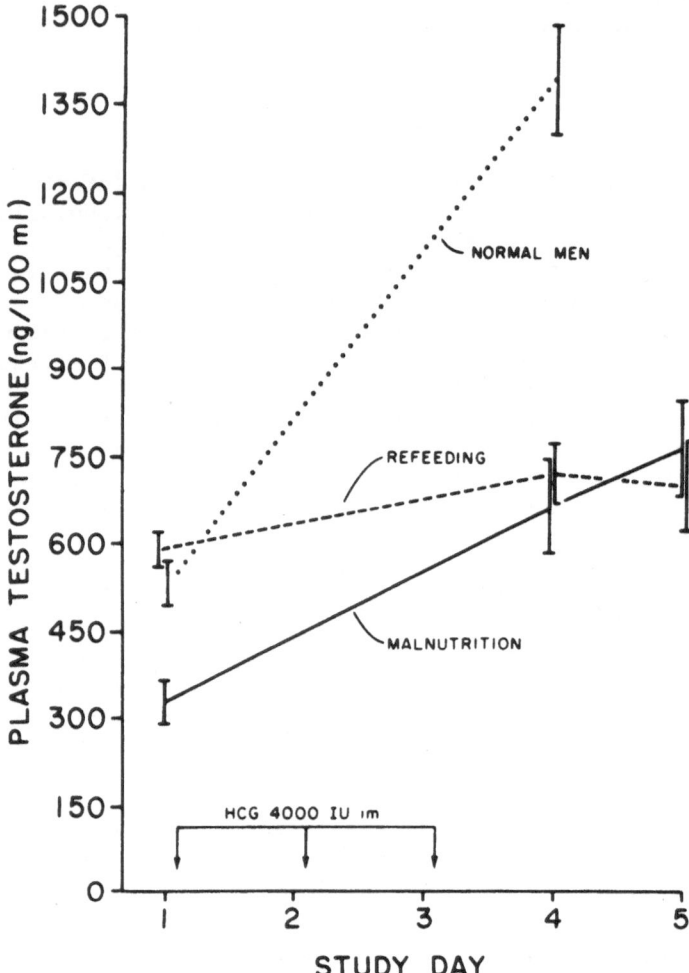

Figure 10. Plasma testosterone in adult men with protein-calorie malnutrition before and after nutritional rehabilitation and in normal men in response to human chorionic gonadotropin stimulation. Basal levels are reduced in the malnourished state and return to normal levels with refeeding; however, the abnormal response to gonadotropin stimulation persists even after normal weight for height has been achieved. (Reprinted with permission from Smith, S. R. et al., J. Clin. Endocrinol. Metab. 41: 60, 1975.)

in cortisol metabolism. However, since the action(s) of this hormone are unknown, the relevance of these findings are uncertain.

In another study (82) six obese men, ranging in age from 24 to 70, were fasted for periods of 27 to 190 days. Serial measurements of plasma testosterone, LH and FSH were made and no significant changes were noted during the starvation periods.

Vigersky et al. (83) compared pituitary LH and FSH release to gonadotropin releasing hormone stimulation in patients with either anorexia nervosa or simple weight loss to normal controls. Basal LH levels were reduced only in the anorexia patients; basal FSH levels in the simple weight loss group were intermediate between the low levels of the anorexia patients and the higher levels of the normal women. The integrated releasing hormone-induced LH responses were the same in the three groups, while the FSH integrated response was greater in the underweight groups. There was also a delay in the time of peak LH and FSH response in the underweight groups, especially in those with anorexia nervosa.

In another study by Warren et al. (84) patients with anorexia nervosa and self-inflicted weight loss, who may or may not have had anorexia, were studied as a group; it is, therefore, difficult to determine if any of the women had simple under-nutrition. As a group, their LH and FSH responses to gonadotropin releasing hormone were diminished and returned toward normal with weight gain. The FSH response returned to normal in a linear fashion in relation to weight gain, while the LH response was exponential, revealing a sudden increase in responsiveness when patients reached a level of 85% of ideal body weight. There was no apparent relationship of the response to the level of plasma estrogens.

These results of studies of gonadal function in patients with various types of weight loss are so scanty and diverse that it seems unjustified to even attempt to summarize the results. Therefore, what should have been the most important part of this report is left up in the air, and the only judgment I can make is that further investigation is sorely needed.

ANOREXIA NERVOSA

The interrelationships of psychologic disturbance, hypothalamic abnormality, endocrine deficiencies and malnutrition in anorexia nervosa have been the topic of numerous papers. One of the best, comparing the findings in anorexia nervosa and malnutrition, was written by Warren and Vande Wiele (85); it is particularly useful since the endocrine measures in the anorexia patients were by-in-large sensitive and up to date. Another paper of extensive and sophisticated endocrinologic investigations of a small number of patients with anorexia nervosa was compiled by Mecklenburg et al. (86.) These descriptions of the condition (85-87) have drawn attention to the clinical signs and symptoms which are compatible with malnutrition, hypothyroidism, hypoadrenalism, hypopituitarism and hypothalamic disease; these include lassitude and weakness, constipation, cold sensitivy and hypothermia, emaciation, lanugo, coarse, dry hyperpigmented skin, slow pulse, decreased systolic blood pressure and pulse pressure, postural hypotension, and delayed water excretion.

Amenorrhea has been particularly commented on and is pertinent to the concerns at this conference. It is considered a major hallmark of anorexia nervosa; in contrast to the situation in simple starvation (11,88,89), it frequently precedes other overt signs of the disease and may persist for long periods after ideal body weight has been achieved.

The biochemical and endocrine alterations in anorexia and their reversal to normal with refeeding and return to a normal body weight (85-87, 90-92) suggest that many may be primarily related to malnutrition. Some of the more pertinent comparisons between anorexia and malnutrition will be made here. Fasting hypoglycemia and insulin sensitivity have been reported in both conditions; flat glucose tolerance curves and curves suggestive of diabetes mellitus can be seen in both conditions. Elevated basal growth hormone levels with overresponse to stimuli are seen in both and at least one anorexia patient with high growth hormone and low somatomedin levels has been reported (90). In both conditions decreased excretion of adrenal glucocorticoid metabolites and pro-longed metabolic clearance of cortisol associated with normal to elevated plasma levels of cortisol, have been reported; likewise, the response to ACTH and metapyrone stimulation are usually normal.

Thyroid function has usually been considered normal in anorexia, as judged by PBI or thyroxine levels, TSH levels and TSH responses to thyrotropin releasing factor. However, an occasional low thyroxine level has been reported and more recent studies of triiodothyronine metabolism (93,94) suggest that triiodothyronine levels may, in fact, be diminished secondary to defective peripheral conversion of thyroxine to the metabolically more active triiodo-thyronine. This has been suggested to occur in several recent reports of thyroid hormone metabolism in malnutrition (72-76). That hypothyroidism may be a more prominent part of anorexia nervosa than previously thought is suggested by Bradlow et al., (95) who reported low plasma levels of triiodothyronine and an abnormally low urinary androsterone/etiocholanolone ratio, which is characteristic of hypothyroidism and which could be corrected by triiodothyronine therapy in their anorexia patients.

Since the amenorrhea of anorexia does not disappear with refeeding and return to a normal body weight, investigations of the
sex hormones in this condition have been extensive (85-87, 90-92,
96,100). The results suggest failure of peripheral gonadal function secondary to inadequate gonadotropin stimulation, which, in

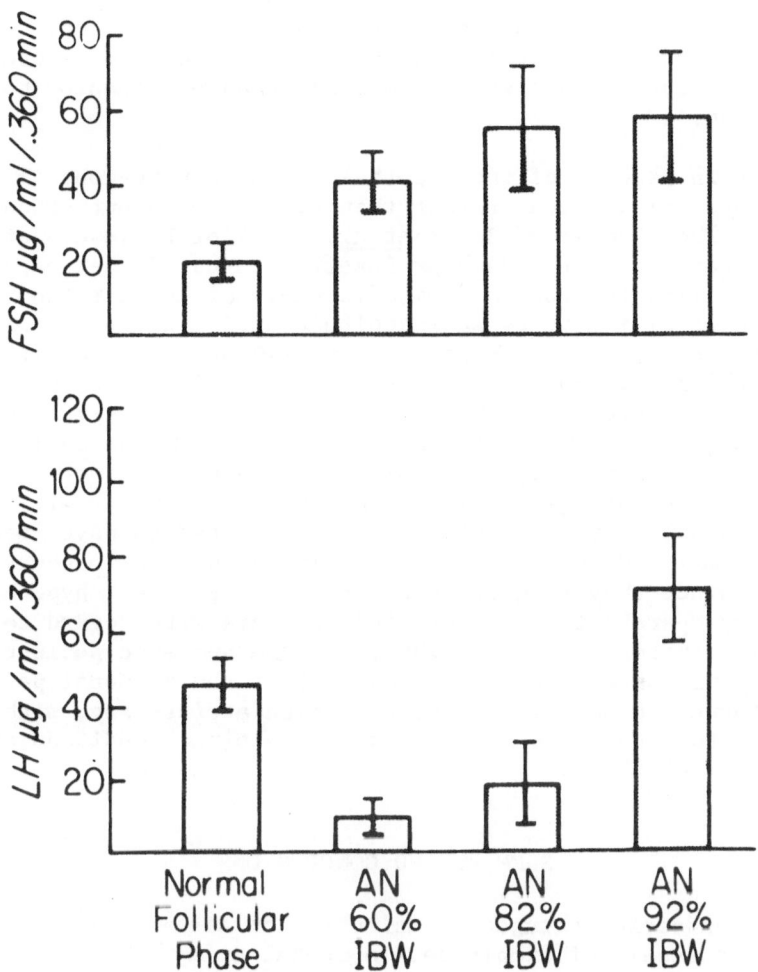

Figure 11. Plasma FSH and LH responses to gonadotropin releasing
hormone, expressed as the integrated response above basal levels,
in normal women during the follicular phase and in patients with
anorexia nervosa at various levels of ideal body weight.
(Reprinted with permission from Sherman, B. M., et al., J. Clin.
Endocrinol. Metab. 41: 135, 1975.)

turn, appears to be secondary to failure of hypothalamic releasing
factor stimulation of the pituitary. Thus, urinary and plasma
levels of LH and FSH are uniformly low when body weight is moderately reduced. Urinary and plasma levels of estrogens in females
and testosterone, in the few males with the condition who have
been studied (101) are likewise decreased. If gonadotropin
releasing hormone is administered, LH and FSH release is evoked
(Figure 11) and in most studies the decreased response, when body
weight is moderatly reduced, returns to normal or may even exceed
the normal response as normal body weight is approached. LH is
seemingly more reduced than FSH; FSH returns to normal more quickly
and is more apt to overrespond to gonadotropin releasing hormone
stimulation.

        Certain aspects of the hypothalamic-pituitary-gonadal axis
are prepubertal in type, rather than of an adolescent or adult
pattern. The studies of Boyar et al. (102) of LH levels at 20
minute intervals over a 24 hour interval revealed that anorexia
patients failed to show the episodic peaks of LH secretion occurring with equal frequency and magnitude during sleep and wakeful-
ness characteristic of the normal sexually developed adult;
rather, their pattern was a low LH which oscillated around a
constant mean which is characteristic of the prepubertal child.
In one patient who gained weight with treatment, the adult pattern
developed. Additionally, prepubertal children will not release LH
and/or ovulate when given clomiphene citrate; neither will anorexia
patients until they have sufficiently recovered to have reached a
nearly normal body weight (98-103). These observations are of
interest since they suggest that the "critical mass" hypothesis of
Frisch may operate in patients with anorexia with regard to
hormonal secretory patterns (104); yet the anorexic patient may
fail to menstruate even though body weight and hormonal patterns
have returned to normal. Thus, the psychiatrists say, with some
tenacity, that anorexia nervosa is not solely a condition of self-
imposed malnutrition.

                        SUMMARY AND CONCLUSIONS

        The endocrine changes in malnutrition are many and varied.
Some are a result of simple developmental delay which accompanies
malnutrition in the growing child; others are a result of complex
alterations in the usual endocrine relationships, which often
seem to be an attempt to adapt to the protein-calorie deficits.
Those of chief concern here are the least well studied and leave
many questions to be answered. From a very pragmatic perspective
one is left with the undeniable fact that overpopulation is one
of the major problems of the countries where malnutrition is most
common. Therefore, whatever the alterations in reproductive

endocrine functioning secondary to malnutrition, nature seems to have made certain that they were at least compatible with survival of the species.

References

1. Frisch, R. E., and Revelle, R. The Height and Weight of Adolescent Boys and Girls at the Time of Peak Velocity of Growth in Height and Weight: Longitudinal Data, Hum. Biol. 41: 536, 1969.

2. Frisch, R. E., and Revelle, R. Height and Weight at Menarche and a Hypothesis of Critical Body Mass and Adolescent Events, Science 169: 397, 1970.

3. Frisch, R. E., and Revelle, R. Height and Weight at Menarche and a Hypothesis of Menarche, Arch. Dis. Child. 46: 695, 1971.

4. Frisch, R. E., and Revelle, R. The Height and Weight of Girls and Boys at the Time of Initiation of the Adolescent Growth Spurt in Height and Weight and the Relationship of Menarche, Hum. Biol. 43: 140, 1971.

5. Frisch, R. E. and McArthur, J. W. Menstrual Cycles as a Determinant of Minimum Weight for Height Necessary for Their Maintenance or Onset, Science 185: 949, 1974.

6. Frisch, R. E. Weight at Menarche: Similarity for Well-Nourished and Undernourished Girls at Differing Ages, and Evidence for Historical Constancy, Pediatrics 50: 445, 1972.

7. Harrison, G. A., Weiner, J. S., Tanner, J. M., and Barnicot, N. A. Human Biology: An Introduction to Human Evolution, Variation and Growth, p. 349, Oxford University Press, New York, 1964.

8. Simmons, K. S. and Gruelich, W. W. Menarcheal Age and the Height, Weight and Skeletal Age of Girls Age 7-17 Years, J. Pediat. 22: 518, 1943.

9. Zacharias, L. and Wurtman, R. J. Age at Menarche: Genetic and Environmental Influences, New Eng. J. Med. 280: 868, 1969.

10. Johnston, F. E., Roche, A. F., Schell, L. M., and Wettenhall, N. B. Critical Weight at Menarche: Critique of a Hypothesis, Am. J. Dis. Child. 129: 19, 1975.

11. Stein, Z., Susser, M., Saenger, G., and Marolla, F. Famine
     and Human Development, The Dutch Hunger Winter of 1944-1945.
     Chapter 9, Fertility, pp. 71-86, Oxford University Press,
     New York, 1975.

12. Klatskin, G., Slater, W. T., and Humm, F. D. Gynecomastia
     due to Malnutrition: I. Clinical Observations, Am. J. Med.
     Sci. 21: 19, 1947.

13. Peraita, M. Deficiency Neuropathies Observed in Madrid Dur-
     ing the Civil War (1936-9), Brit. Med. J. 2: 784, 1946.

14. Valaoras, V. G. Some Effects of Famine on the Population of
     Greece, A Vital Statistics During the Famine, Milbank Mem.
     Fund. Quart. 24: 215, 1946.

15. Antonov, A. N. Children Born During the Seige of Leningrad
     in 1942, J. Pediat. 30: 250, 1947.

16. Smith, C. A. Effects of Wartime Starvation in Holland on
     Pregnancy and its Products, Amer. J. Obstet. Gynec. 53:
     599, 1947.

17. Keys, A., Brozek, J., Henschel, A., Mickelsen, O., and
     Taylor, H. L. The Biology of Human Starvation, v. I.,
     Chapter 11: Morphology of the Endocrine Glands, pp. 209-218
     and Chapter 35: Sexual Function, pp. 749-763, The University
     of Minnesota Press, Minneapolis, 1950.

18. Aksoy, M., Erdem, S., and Baserer, G. On the Pathogenesis
     of the Hepatosplenomegaly in Chronic Iron Deficiency Anemia,
     Acta hepato-splenol. 16: 241, 1968.

19. Adams, J. F. Pregnancy and Addisonian Pernicious Anaemia,
     Scot. Med. J. 3: 21, 1958.

20. Jackson, I., Doig, W. B., and McDonald, G. Pernicious
     Anemia as a Cause of Infertility, Lancet 2: 1159, 1967.

21. Armstrong, B. K., Davis, R. E., Martin, J. D., and Woodliff,
     H. J. Pregnancy and Untreated Addisonian Pernicious Anaemia,
     Brit. Med. J. 4: 158, 1968.

22. Hall, M., and Davidson, R.J.L. Prophylactic Folic Acid in
     Women with Pernicious Anaemia Pregnant after Periods of
     Infertility, J. Clin. Path. 21: 599, 1968.

23. Girdwood, R. H., Eastwood, M. A., Finlayson, N.D.C., and
     Graham, G. S. Pernicious Anaemia as a Cause of Infertility

in Twins, Lancet 1: 528, 1971.

24. Mahmood, A. Pernicious Anaemia as a Cause of Infertility, Lancet 1: 753, 1971.

25. Watson, A. A. Seminal Vitamin B-12 and Sterility, Lancet 2: 644, 1962.

26. Sharp, A. A., and Witts, L. J. Seminal Vitamin B-12 and Sterility, Lancet 2: 779, 1962.

27. Furnass, S. B. Seminal Vitamin B-12 and Sterility, Lancet 1: 59, 1963.

28. Prasad, A. S., Halsted, J. A., and Nadini, M. Syndrome of Iron Deficiency Anemia, Hepatosplenomegaly, Hypogonadism, Dwarfism, and Geophagia, Amer. J. Med. 31: 532, 1961.

29. Sandstead, H. H., Prasad, A. S., Schulert, A. R., Farid, Z., Miale, A., Bassilly, S., and Darby, W. J. Human Zinc Deficiency, Endocrine Manifestations and Response to Treatment, Amer. J. Clin. Nutr. 20: 422, 1967.

30. Eminians, J., Reinhold, J. G., Kfoury, G. A., Amirhakimi, G. H., Sharif, H., and Ziai, M. Zinc Nutrition of Children in Fars Province of Iran, Amer. J. Clin. Nutr. 20: 734, 1967.

31. Prasad, A. S., and Oberlead, D. Zinc: Human Nutrition and Metabolic Effects, Ann. Int. Med. 73: 631, 1970.

32. Carter, J. P., Grivetti, L. E., Davis, J. T., Nasiff, S., Mansour, A., Mousa, W. A., Atta, A-E-D, Patwardhan, V. N., Moneim, M. A., Abdou, I. A., and Darby, W. J. Growth and Sexual Development of Adolescent Egyptian Village Boys, Effects of Zinc, Iron, and Placebo Supplementation, Amer. J. Clin. Nutr. 22: 59, 1969.

33. Coble, Y. D., Schulert, A. R., and Farid, Z. Growth and Sexual Development of Male Subjects in an Egyptian Oasis, Amer. J. Clin. Nutr. 22: 59, 1969.

34. Coble, Y. D., Bardin, C. W., Ross, G. T., and Darby, W. J. Studies of Endocrine Function in Boys with Retarded Growth, Delayed Sexual Maturation and Zinc Deficiency, J. Clin. Endocrinol. Metab. 32: 361, 1971.

35. Olson, R. E. Introductory Remarks: Nutrient, Hormone, Enzyme Interactions, Amer. J. Clin. Nutr. 28: 626, 1975.

36. Pimstone, B. L., Wittman, W., Hansen, J. D.L., and Murray, P. Growth Hormone and Kwashiorkor. Role of protein in growth hormone homeostasis, Lancet 2: 779, 1966.

37. Pimstone, B. L., Barbezat, G., Hansen, J. D. L., and Murray, P. Growth Hormone and Protein-Calorie Malnutrition. Impaired suppression during induced hyperglycemia, Lancet 2: 1333, 1967.

38. Pimstone, B. L., Barbezat, G., Hansen, J.D.L., and Murray, P. Studies on Growth Hormone Secretion in Protein-Calorie Malnutrition, Amer. J. Clin. Nutr. 21: 482, 1968.

39. Hadden, D. R. Glucose, Free Fatty Acid, and Insulin Interrelations in Kwashiorkor and Marasmus, Lancet 2: 589, 1967.

40. Parra, A., Garza, C., Garza, Y., Saravia, J. L., Hazelwood, C. F., and Nichols, B. L. Changes in Growth Hormone, Insulin, and Thyroxine Values and in Energy Metabolism of Marasmic Infants, J. Pediat. 82: 133, 1973.

41. Pimstone, B. L., Becker, D.J., and Hansen, J.D.L. Human Growth Hormone and Sulphation Factor in Protein-Calorie Malnutrition. In: Endocrine Aspects of Malnutrition, Gardner, L. I., and Amacher, P., eds., pp. 73-90. The Kroc Foundation, Santa Ynez, California, 1973.

42. Smith, S. R., Edgar, P. J., Pozefsky, T., Chhetri, M. K., and Prout, T. E. Growth Hormone in Adults with Protein-Calorie Malnutrition, J. Clin. Endocrinol. Metab. 39: 53, 1974.

43. Parra, A., Klish, W., Cuellar, A., Serrano, P. A., Garcia, G., Argote, R. M., Canseco, L., and Nichols, B. L. Energy Metabolism and Hormonal Profile in Children with Edematous Protein-Calorie Malnutrition, J. Pediat. 87: 307, 1975.

44. Monckeberg, F., Donoso, G., Oxman, S., Pak, N., and Meneghello, J. Human Growth Hormone in Infant Malnutrition, Pediatrics 31: 58, 1963.

46. Grant, D. B., Hambley, J., Becker, D., and Pimstone, B. L. Reduced Serum Sulphation Factor Activity in Patients with Protein-Calorie Malnutrition, Arch. Dis. Child. 48: 596, 1973.

47. Becker, D. J., Pimstone, B. L., Hansen, J.D.L., and Hendricks, S. Serum Albumin and Growth Hormone Relationships in Kwarshiorkor and the Nephrotic Syndrome, J. Lab. Clin. Med. 78: 865, 1971.

48. Pimstone, B. L., Becker, D. J., and Hansen, J.D.L. Human
     Growth Hormone in Protein-Calorie Malnutrition. In: Growth
     and Growth Hormone, Proceedings of the Second International
     Symposium on Growth Hormone, Pecile, A., and Muller, E. E.,
     eds., pp. 389-401, Excerpta Medica Foundation, Amsterdam,
     1972.

49. Pimstone, B. L., Becker, D., Kronheim, S. Disappearance of
     Plasma Growth Hormone in Acromegaly and Protein-Calorie Mal-
     nutrition after Somatostatin, J. Clin. Endocrin. Metab. 40:
     168, 1975.

50. Merimee, T. J., and Fineberg, S. E. Growth Hormone Secretion
     in Starvation: A Reassessment, J. Clin. Endocrinol. Metab.
     39: 385, 1974.

51. Merimee, T. J., Pulkkinen, A. J., and Burton, C. E. Diet-
     Induced Alterations of hGH Secretion in Man, J. Clin.
     Endocrinol. Metab. 42: 931, 1976.

52. Sloane, D., Taitz, L. S., and Gilchrist, G. S. Aspects of
     Carbohydrate Metabolism in Kwashiorkor. With special refer-
     ence to spontaneous hypoglycemia, Brit. Med. J. 1: 32, 1961.

53. Baig, H. A., and Edozien, J. A. Carbohydrate Metabolism in
     Kwashiorkor, Lancet 2: 662, 1965.

54. Graham, G. G., Cordano, A., Blizzard, R. M., and Cheek, D. B.
     Infantile Malnutrition: Changes in Body Composition during
     Rehabilitation, Pediat. Res. 3: 579, 1969.

55. Becker, D. J., Pimstone, B. L., Hansen, J.D.L., and Hendricks,
     S. Insulin Secretion in Protein-Calorie Malnutrition.
     I. Quantitative abnormalities and response to treatment,
     Diabetes 20: 542, 1971.

56. Becker, D. J., Pimstone, B. L., Hansen, J.D.L., MacHutchon,
     B. and Drysdale, A. Patterns of Insulin Response to Glucose
     in Protein-Calorie Malnutrition, Amer. J. Clin. Nutr. 25:
     499, 1972.

57. Milner, R.D.G. Insulin Secretion in Human Protein-Calorie
     Malnutrition, Proc. Nutr. Soc. 31: 219, 1972.

58. James, W.P.T., and Coore, H. G. Persistent Impairment of
     Insulin Secretion and Glucose Tolerance after Malnutrition,
     Amer. J. Clin. Nutr. 23: 386, 1970.

59. Parra, A., Garza, C., Klish, W., Garcia, G., Argote, R. M.,
     Canesco, L., Cuellar, A., and Nichols, B. L. Insulin-Growth
     Hormone Adaptations in Marasmus and Kwashiorkor as Seen in
     Mexico. In: Endocrine Aspects of Malnutrition, Gardner, L.I.,
     and Amacher, P., eds., pp. 31-43. The Kroc Foundation, Santa
     Ynez, California, 1973.

60. Robinson, H., Cocks, T., Kerr, D., and Picou, D. Fasting and
     Postprandial Levels of Plasma Insulin and Growth Hormone in
     Malnourished Jamaican Children, During Catch-up Growth and
     After Complete Recovery. Ibid. pp. 45-72.

61. Jayarao, K. S., and Raghuramulu, N. Growth Hormone and
     Insulin Secretion in Protein-Calorie Malnutrition, As Seen
     in India. Ibid. pp. 91-98.

62. Pimstone, B. L., Becker, D., Weinkove, C., and Mann, M.
     Insulin Secretion in Protein-Calorie Malnutrition. Ibid.
     pp. 289-305.

63. Becker, D. J., Pimstone, B. L., and Hansen, J.D.L. The
     Relation between Insulin Secretion, Glucose Tolerance, Growth
     Hormone, and Serum Proteins in Protein-Calorie Malnutrition,
     Pediat. Res. 9: 35, 1975.

64. Unger, R. H., Eisentraut, A. M., and Madison, L. L. The
     effects of Total Starvation upon the Levels of Circulating
     Glucagon and Insulin in Man, J. Clin. Invest. 42: 1031, 1963.

65. Hales, C. N., and Randle, P. J. Effects of Low-Carbohydrate
     Diet and Diabetes Mellitus on Plasma Concentrations of
     Glucose, Non-Esterified Fatty Acids, and Insulin During Oral
     Glucose Tolerance Tests, Lancet 1: 790, 1963.

66. Hopkins, L. L., Ransome-Kuti, O., and Majaj, A. S. Improve-
     ment of Impaired Carbohydrate Metabolism by Chromium (III)
     in Malnourished Infants, Amer. J. Clin. Nutr. 21: 203, 1968.

67. Smith, S. R., Bledsoe, T., and Chhetri, M. K. Cortisol
     Metabolism and the Pituitary-Adrenal Axis in Adults with
     Protein-Calorie Malnutrition, J. Clin. Endocrinol. Metab.
     40: 43, 1975.

68. Samuel, A. M., Kadival, G. V., Patel, B. D., and Desai, A. G.
     Adresocorticosteroids and Corticosteroid Binding Globulins
     in Protein Calorie Malnutrition, Amer. J. Clin. Nutr. 29:
     889, 1976.

69. Ingenbleek, Y., DeNayer, Ph., and DeVisscher, M.

Thyroxine-Binding Globulin in Infant Protein-Calorie Malnutrition, J. Clin. Endocrinol. Metab. 39: 178, 1974.

70. Bermudez, F., Surks, M. I., and Oppenheimer, J. H. High Incidence of Decreased Serum Triiodothyronine Concentration in Patients with Nonthyroid Disease, J. Clin. Endocrinol. Metab. 41: 27, 1975.

71. Pain, R. W., and Phillips, P. J. Thyroid-Hormone Levels in Protein-Calorie Malnutrition, Lancet 1: 202, 1976.

72. Chopra, I. J., Chopra, U., Smith, S. R., Reza, M., and Solomon, D. H. Reciprocal Changes in Serum Concentrations of 3, 3', 5'-Triiodothyronine (Reverse T-3) and 3,3',5-Triiodothyronine (T-3) in Systemic Illnesses, J. Clin. Endocrinol. Metab. 41: 1043, 1975.

73. Ingenbleek, Y., and Beckers, C. Triiodothyronine and Thyroid-Stimulating Hormone in Protein-Calorie Malnutrition in Infants, Lancet 2: 845, 1975.

74. Chopra, I. J., and Smith, S. R. Circulating Thyroid Hormones and Thyrotropin in Adult Patients with Protein-Calorie Malnutrition, J. Clin. Endocrinol. Metab. 40: 221, 1975.

75. Portnay, G. I., O'Brian, J. T., Bush, J., Vagenakis, A. G., Azizi, F., Arky, R. A., Ingbar, S. H., and Braverman, L. E. The Effect of Starvation on the Concentration and Binding of Thyroxine and Triiodothyronine in Serum and on the Response to TRH, J. Clin. Endocrinol. Metab. 39: 191, 1974.

76. Spaulding, S. W., Chopra, I. J., Sherwin, R. S., and Lyall, S. S. Effect of Caloric Restriction and Dietary Composition on Serum T-3 and Reverse T-3 in Man, J. Clin. Endocrinol. Metab. 42: 197, 1976.

77. Vinik, A. I., Kalk, W. J., McLaren, H., Hendricks, S., and Pimstone, B. L. Fasting Blunts the TSH Response to Synthetic Thyrotropin-Releasing Hormone (TRH), J. Clin. Endocrinol. Metab. 40: 509, 1975.

78. Pimstone, B., Becker, D., and Hendricks, S. TSH Response to Synthetic Thyrotropin-Releasing Hormone in Human Protein-Calorie Malnutrition, J. Clin. Endocrinol. Metab. 36: 779, 1973.

79. Chopra, I. J., Williams, D. E., Orgiazzi, J., and Solomon, D. H. Opposite Effects of Dexamethasone on Serum Concentrations of 3,3',5'-Triiodothyronine (Reverse T-3) and 3,3',5-

Triiodothyronine (T-3), _J. Clin. Endocrinol. Metab_. 41: 911, 1975.

80. Smith, S. R., Chhetri, M. K., Johanson, A. J., Radfar, N., and Migeon, C. J. The Pituitary-Gonadal Axis in Men with Protein-Calorie Malnutrition, _J. Clin. Endocrinol. Metab_. 41: 60, 1975.

81. Hendrikx, A., Heyns, W., and DeMoor, P. Influence of a Low-Calorie Diet and Fasting on the Metabolism of Dehydroepi-androsterone Sulfate in Adult Obese Subjects, _J. Clin. Endocrinol. Metab_. 28: 1525, 1968.

82. Suryanarayana, B. V., Kent, J. R., Meister, L., and Parlow, A. F. Pituitary-Gonadal Axis during Prolonged Total Starvation in Obese Men, _Amer. J. Clin. Nutr_. 22: 767, 1969.

83. Vigersky, R. A., Loriaux, D. L., Andersen, A. E., Mecklenburg, R. S., and Vaitukaitis, J. L. Delayed Pituitary Hormone Response to LRF and TRF in Patients with Anorexia Nervosa and with Secondary Amenorrhea Associated with Simple Weight Loss, _J. Clin. Endocrinol. Metab_. 43: 893, 1976.

84. Warren, M. P., Jewelewicz, R., Dyrenfurth, I., Ans, R., Khalaf, S., and VandeWiele, R. L. The Significance of Weight Loss in the Evaluation of Pituitary Response to LH-RH in Women with Secondary Amenorrhea, _J. Clin. Endocrinol. Metab_. 40: 601, 1975.

85. Warren, M. P., and Vande Wiele, R. L. Clinical and Metabolic Features of Anorexia Nervosa, _Amer. J. Obstet. Gynecol_. 117: 435, 1973.

86. Mecklenburg, R. S., Loriaux, D. L., Thompson, R. H., Andersen, A. E., and Lipsett, M. B. Hypothalamic Dysfunction in Patients with Anorexia Nervosa, _Medicine_ 53: 147, 1974.

87. Russell, G. F. M. Anorexia Nervosa, _Proc. Royal Soc. Med_. 58: 811, 1965.

88. Sydenham, A. Amenorrhea at the Stanley Camp, Hong Kong, during Internment, _Brit. Med. J_. 2: 159, 1946.

89. Zuriram, S., Gomez-Mont, F., and Laguna, J. Endocrine Disturbances and Their Dietetic Background in Undernourished in Mexico, _Ann. Intern. Med_. 42: 1259, 1955.

90. Frankel, R. J., and Jenkins, J. S. Hypothalamic-Pituitary Functions in Anorexia Nervosa, _Acta Endocrinol_. 78: 209, 1975.

91. Garfinkel, P. E., Brown, G. M., Stancer, H. C., and Moldofsky, H. Hypothalamic-Pituitary Function in Anorexia Nervosa, Arch. Gen. Psychiatry 32: 739, 1975.

92. Travaglini, P., Beck-Peccoz, P., Ferrari, C., Ambrosi, B., Paracchi, A., Severgnini, A., Spada, A., and Faglia, G. Some Aspects of Hypothalamic-Pituitary Function in Patients with Anorexia Nervosa, Acta Endocrinol. 81: 252, 1976.

93. Miyai, K., Yamamoto, T., Azukizawa, M., Ishibashi, K., and Kumahara, Y. Serum Thyroid Hormones and Thyrotropin in Anorexia Nervosa, J. Clin. Endocrinol. Metab. 40: 334, 1975.

94. Moshang, T., Parks, J. S., Baker, L., Vaidya, V., Utiger, R. D., Bongiovanni, A. M., and Snyder, P. J. Low Serum Tri-iodothyronine in Patients with Anorexia Nervosa, J. Clin. Endocrinol. Metab. 40: 470, 1975.

95. Bradlow, H. L., Boyar, R. M., O'Connor, J., Zumoff, B., and Hellman, L. Hypothyroid-Like Alterations in Testosterone Metabolism in Anorexia Nervosa, J. Clin. Endocrinol. Metab. 43: 571, 1976.

96. Russell, G.F.M., Loriane, J. A., Bell, E. T., and Harkness, R. A. Gonadotropin and Oestrogen Excretion in Patients with Anorexia Nervosa, J. Psychosomatic Res. 9: 79, 1965.

97. Bell, E. T., Harkness, R. A., Loraine, J. A., and Russell, G.F.M. Hormone Assay Studies in Patients with Anorexia Nervosa, Acta Endocrinol. 51: 140, 1966.

98. Beumont, P.J.V., Carr, P. J., and Gelder, M. G. Plasma Levels of Lutenizing Hormone and of Immunoreactive Oestrogens (Oestradiol) in Anorexia Nervosa: Response to Clomiphene Citrate, Psychological Med. 3: 495, 1973.

99. Sherman, B. M., Halmi, K. A., and Zamudio, R. LH and FSH Response to Gonadotropin-Releasing Hormone in Anorexia Nervosa: Effect of Nutritional Rehabilitation, J. Clin. Endocrinol. Metab. 41: 135, 1975.

100. Beumont, P.J.V., George, G.C.W., Pimstone, B. L., and Vinik, A. I. Body Weight and the Pituitary Response to Hypothalamic Releasing Hormones in Patients with Anorexia Nervosa, J. Clin. Endocrinol. Metab. 43: 487, 1976.

101. Beumont, P.J.V., Beardwood, C. J., and Russell, G.F.M. The Occurrence of the Syndrome of Anorexia Nervosa in Male Subjects, Psychological Med. 2: 216, 1972.

102. Boyar, R. M., Katz, J., Finkelstein, J. W., Kapen, S., Weiner, H., Weitzman, E. D., and Hellman, L. Anorexia Nervosa, Immaturity of the 24-Hour Lutenizing Hormone Secretory Pattern, New Engl. J. Med. 291: 861, 1974.

103. Marshall, J. C., and Fraser, T. R. Amenorrhoea in Anorexia Nervosa: Assessment and Treatment with Clomiphene Citrate, Brit. Med. J. 4: 590, 1971.

104. Johanson, A. Critical Body Weight in Anorexia Nervosa, New Engl. J. Med. 291: 904, 1974.

THE EFFECT OF ORAL CONTRACEPTIVES ON MICRONUTRIENTS

Ananda S. Prasad, K. Y. Lei, and Kamran S. Moghissi

Wayne State University School of Medicine, Detroit, Michigan; Veterans Administration Hospital, Allen Park, Michigan

INTRODUCTION

Estrogens and oral contraceptive agents (OCA) are widely used as prophylactic and therapeutic agents in gynecological practice. It is estimated that one out of six women of childbearing age in the United States currently use OCA. These potent pharmacological agents affect many aspects of human metabolism. Alterations in the levels of minerals and vitamins in the plasma as a result of OCA administration has been noted and reviewed by many authors (1,2, 3). Most of these studies, however, were performed in a small number of subjects and as such were limited in scope. The purpose of this paper is to document the effects of OCA on minerals and vitamin metabolism in a large number of subjects representing different socioeconomic groups. Some of our data have been presented in detail elsewhere (4,5,6); as such, only pertinent information will be reviewed in this paper.

METHODS

Study Groups

In this study female subjects between the ages of 18 to 45 years were divided into 8 groups in a factorial arrangement with two socioeconomic levels and four different hormonal states (Tables 1 and 2). The criteria of Myrianthopoulos and French (7) with an income adjustment was utilized in determining the division between the higher (A) and lower (B) socioeconomic classes.

Table 1

Number of Subjects in the Clinical and Biochemical Studies
by Contraceptive Group and Social Class

| | Socioeconomic Class | |
Group	A (Higher)	B (Lower)
None	128	98
Pill 1 (Noriny1)	35	111
Pill 2 (Ovra1)	44	124
Resume Pill (RP)	78	105

Table 2

Number of Subjects in the 24-Hour Dietary Recall Study
by Contraceptive Group and Social Class

| | Socioeconomic Class | |
Group	A (Higher)	B (Lower)
None	49	49
Pill 1 (Noriny1)	30	46
Pill 2 (Ovra1)	25	49
Resume Pill (RP)	42	47

Subjects who were not taking OCA belonged to A-none or B-none
groups. A-1 and B-1 groups consisted of those subjects who used
"Noriny1" (1 mg norethindrone and 50 ùg mestranol) for 3 months
or more. A-2 and B-2 groups of subjects received "Ovral" (which
contained 0.5 mg of norgestrel and 5 ug of ethinly estradiol) for
3 months or more. A-RP and B-RP groups consisted of women who
resumed OCA within 5 weeks after pregnancy during lactation.

Subjects were divided further in each group into "supplemented"
and "non-supplemented" subgroups according to whether or not they
were taking vitamin and/or mineral supplementations by their own
admission.

Records of physical examinations by the physician and nutritional histories were recorded in each case on a form similar to those used in ICNND surveys (8).

Laboratory Techniques

Hemoglobin, hematocrit, cell indices and peripheral blood smear were examined according to routine methods (9). Plasma total protein and serum iron were determined by Technicon Auto-Analyzer methods (10). Cellulose acetate electrophoresis technique was used for plasma protein fractionation (11). Plasma copper, zinc, magnesium and calcium were assayed by atomic absorption spectrophotometry (12). Erythrocyte zinc and magnesium were also determined (12).

Plasma vitamin A and carotene were determined by the modified Carr-Price method (13) and plasma vitamin C was assayed by a modified method of Roe and Keuther (13). Grab samples of urine were collected from subjects for thiamin and riboflavin determinations. Urinary thiamin and riboflavin were measured fluoremetrically by modified methods of Consolazio et al. (13) and Salter and Morell (13), respectively. Creatinine in the urine was determined by a Technicon Auto-Analyzer using a modified procedure of Folin and Wu (10).

Plasma pyridoxal phosphate (PLP) was determined by a simple enzymatic assay (14). Erythrocyte glutamic oxalacetic transaminase (EGOT) was measured in a hemolysate of red blood cells (15). The cells were washed with 0.85% sodium chloride solution and diluted with saline in the proportion of 0.8 ml saline to 1 ml packed cells. The test was carried out on 0.1 ml of a 1 to 20 hemolysate. For measurement of PLP stimulation, 0.1 ml hemolysate was incubated with 0.1 ml of PLP (0.5 mg per ml) for 20 minutes at $37^\circ C$ prior to the colorimetric determination of EGOT.

Erythrocyte and plasma folic acid were determined by a micro-biological assay using Lactobacillus casei. Serum vitamin B_{12} was measured by a microbiological assay using Lactobacillus leichmanii (16).

Statistical Analysis

Nutritional and biochemical data were analyzed statistically by analysis of variance (Table 3). Missing data were processed by the procedure of least squares analysis of variance (17). Means were ranked by the Duncan's New Multiple Range Test (17). Clinical data were statistically analyzed by chi-square (17).

Table 3

Treatment Comparisons in Analysis of Variance

Treatment	Degree of Freedom
P_1 = None vs. Norinyl, Ovral and RP	1
P_2 = RP vs. Norinyl and Ovral	1
P_3 = Norinyl vs. Ovral	1
I = Income	1
S = Supplement	1
Interactions	10
I x P_1	1
I x P_2	1
I x P_3	1
S x P_1	1
S x P_2	1
S x P_3	1
I x S	1
I x S x P_1	1
I x S x P_2	1
I x S x P_3	1

RESULTS

Physical Findings

The prevalence of dry skin, easily pluckable hair, angular lesion of the mouth, caries and debris of teeth, marginal redness, swelling and bleeding of the gums, filiform papillary atrophy, fungiform papillary hypertrophy of the tongue and glossitis, and scaling of skin were more frequently observed in the B groups than in A groups (6). In the A groups some of the above clinical signs were more common in the non-supplemented groups of subjects. In the A groups, higher prevalences of angular lesions of the mouth, caries and debris of the teeth, marginal redness, swelling and bleeding of the gums were seen in the OCA users than in the controls. The prevalences of the easily pluckable hair, angular lesions of the mouth and debris or calculus of the teeth were more frequently observed in the B-1 group as compared to the B-none group. Higher prevalence of angular lesions of the mouth was seen in the B-RP group as compared to the B-none group.

Dietary Intake

In general, the intake of calories, protein, calcium, magnesium, iron, copper and zinc for OCA subjects did not differ from the controls (4,5,6). The consumption of protein, calcium, magnesium, iron, copper and zinc was found to be higher in group A than in group B subjects. The caloric, protein, calcium, magnesium, iron, copper and zinc intakes of the A-RP group was higher than the A-none, A-1 and A-2 groups.

As expected, the supplemented group consumed greater amounts of calcium, iron, magnesium and copper. However, for magnesium and copper, this supplementation effect was seen only in the A groups.

In general, the OCA subjects' intake of vitamin A, C, B_6 and folic acid did not differ from the controls (4,5,6). However, the intake of thiamin and riboflavin in A-1 and A-2 appeared to be lower than the A-none subjects. The A-RP group of subjects had higher intake of vitamin B_6 and folic acid than A-1 and A-2 subjects. As expected, the subjects from the supplementation groups had higher intake of vitamin A, C, B_6, thiamin, riboflavin and folic acid than the non-supplemented groups, and the A groups had higher intake of vitamin C, B_6, riboflavin and folic acid than B groups. Dietary intake of vitamin A, C, B_6, folic acid and riboflavin of the supplemented groups were higher than the non-supplemented groups in A but not in B.

Laboratory Findings

Hemoglobin, hematocrit and RBC count were not affected by OCA but serum iron was increased in both A and B groups taking "Norinyl" but no effect of "Ovral" was seen. Total iron binding capacity (TIBC) was increased as a result of OCA administration in A and B groups (Table 4).

In group A-RP, a decrease in hemoglobin, hematocrit, RBC count and serum iron was observed. TIBC was increased in both A-RP and B-RP groups. In general, the TIBC values were higher in the B groups as compared to the A groups and in the non-supplemented groups as compared to the supplemented groups.

Table 5 shows the results of copper and zinc analysis. Plasma copper was increased in A and B groups as a result of OCA administration. No socioeconomic effect on plasma copper was observed. Plasma copper was also increased in both A-RP and B-RP groups.

Plasma zinc decreased as a result of OCA administration in A and B groups. An increase in the RBC zinc was observed due to administration of "Norinyl" in both A and B groups. A decrease in plasma zinc and an increase in RBC zinc was observed in A-RP group only. Although no socioeconomic effect was observed on plasma zinc level, A groups showed higher RBC zinc as compared to B groups.

With respect to plasma calcium and magnesium and RBC magnesium, no significant effect of OCA administration was observed.

Although there was no effect of OCA administration on plasma total protein, serum albumin was decreased due to intake of OCA in both groups (4,5). Serum albumin was significantly lower in A-RP as compared to A-none, A-1 and A-2 groups.

Plasma vitamin A levels were increased due to OCA administration in both A and B groups of subjects (Table 6). Supplemented subjects had higher levels of plasma vitamin A. No socioeconomic effect was observed. Plasma carotene levels were decreased due to OCA administration and group A subjects had higher levels of plasma carotene. Plasma ascorbate was not affected by OCA administration. Group A subjects had higher plasma ascorbate levels as compared to group B. Supplemented subjects had higher plasma ascorbate levels as compared to non-supplemented subjects.

Urinary excretion of both vitamins was decreased in subjects using OCA in A and A-RP groups (5). Group A subjects had higher excretion of thiamin and riboflavin as compared to group B subjects. Supplementation effect was observed in group A only.

Table 4(a)

Levels of Hemoglobin, Hematocrit, Red Blood Cell Count

Groups	Hemoglobin, g/100 ml			Hematocrit, %			Red blood cell count, 10^6 x mm^3		
	S	NS	Avg	S	NS	Avg	S	NS	Avg
A-None	13.66 ±1.86	13.14 ±1.48	13.45 ±1.73	41.01 ±4.27	40.54 ±3.03	40.82 ±3.80	4.644 ±1.163	4.632 ±0.690	4.640 ±1.001
A-1	13.66 ±1.52	13.09 ±1.47	13.22 ±1.48	40.38 ±3.66	41.33 ±4.06	41.11 ±3.94	4.389 ±0.652	4.676 ±1.132	4.591 ±1.010
A-2	13.30 ±2.22	13.05 ±1.13	13.10 ±1.40	41.00 ±4.80	41.47 ±3.72	41.37 ±3.92	4.656 ±1.125	4.590 ±0.891	4.603 ±0.927
A-RP	12.01 ±1.39	12.39 ±1.85	12.08 ±1.48	36.27 ±4.00	38.67 ±5.47	36.73 ±4.39	4.125 ±0.834	4.347 ±0.781	4.161 ±0.825
B-None	13.30 ±1.50	12.80 ±1.68	12.93 ±1.64	40.20 ±3.35	39.56 ±4.25	39.72 ±4.04	4.984 ±1.594	4.534 ±0.867	4.636 ±1.079
B-1	12.67 ±1.86	12.97 ±1.84	12.92 ±1.84	38.64 ±4.77	40.73 ±4.35	40.40 ±4.46	5.480 ±1.833	5.595 ±1.340	5.572 ±1.433
B-2	12.98 ±1.35	13.49 ±1.47	13.40 ±1.46	40.09 ±3.44	40.65 ±5.32	40.55 ±5.03	4.659 ±0.637	4.804 ±1.001	4.778 ±0.945
B-RP	13.38 ±1.69	13.15 ±1.70	13.23 ±1.69	40.86 ±3.87	40.27 ±3.72	40.47 ±3.76	4.704 ±0.816	4.800 ±0.967	4.764 ±0.914
P values	P_2 0.05; IP_2 0.05			P_2 0.05; IP_2 0.05			I 0.05		

Values are mean ± standard deviation of mean. S = supplemented; NS = nonsupplemented; Avg = average.

Source: Prasad et al., Am. J. Clin. Nutr. 28: 377-384, 1975.

Table 4(b)

Levels of Serum Iron and Total Iron Binding Capacity

Groups	Serum iron, ug/100 ml			Serum total iron binding capacity, ug/100 ml		
	S	NS	Avg	S	NS	Avg
A-None	95.89	81.16	89.68	267.1	271.0	268.7
	±35.99	±24.84	±32.49	±81.0	±68.1	±75.7
A-1	89.00	100.93	98.20	318.4	311.5	312.9
	±30.75	±37.16	±35.73	±81.7	±65.8	±68.0
A-2	84.80	37.42	86.81	317.6	345.4	338.9
	±34.88	±39.86	±38.38	±59.8	±92.1	±85.9
A-RP	50.40	47.75	49.89	305.2	307.0	305.6
	±29.97	±24.99	±28.95	±65.7	±76.9	±67.5
B-None	69.04	69.68	69.38	292.5	312.1	307.3
	±34.43	±34.43	±34.43	±67.6	±86.2	±82.6
B-1	99.52	90.07	91.53	305.6	337.4	332.5
	±19.71	±28.84	±27.77	±70.2	±72.5	±72.7
B-2	74.14	75.53	75.27	305.1	335.4	330.0
	±30.94	±30.02	±30.06	±57.8	±80.6	±77.6
B-RP	73.15	69.40	70.71	304.4	316.0	311.8
	±39.51	±37.73	±38.20	±11.9	±91.6	±99.1
P values	P_1 0.03; P_2 0.001 IP_1 0.001			P_1 0.001; IP_1 0.02; I 0.06; S 0.02		

Values are mean ± standard deviation of mean. S = supplemented; NS = nonsupplemented; Avg = average.

Source: Prasad et al., Am. J. Clin. Nutr. 28: 377-384, 1975.

     Results of PLP, EGOT and percent stimulation of EGOT are pre-
sented in Table 7. In group A plasma PLP level was decreased due
to OCA administration. Supplementation effect was seen mainly in
the A groups. Plasma PLP was found to be lower in the A-RP group
than in the A-1 and A-2 groups.

     EGOT activities were found to be lower in the RP and OCA
groups. This reduction in activities due to OCA was greater in
the B groups as compared to A groups. Supplementation effect was
seen in both groups. The percent stimulation of EGOT was found to
be greater in the OCA and RP groups. No socioeconomic or supplementation effect was seen so far as the EGOT stimulation test
was concerned.

Table 5

Plasma Copper and Zinc, and Erythrocyte Zinc Levels

Group	Plasma copper ug/100 ml			Plasma zinc ug/100 ml			Erythrocyte zinc, ug/g hemoglobin		
	S	NS	Avg	S	NS	Avg	S	NS	Avg
A-None	138.8 ±102.3	126.8 ±38.0	133.8 ±82.3	117.35 ±21.98	119.04 ±16.08	118.04 ±19.74	39.26 ±5.87	40.05 ±7.89	39.58 ±6.73
A-1	230.5 ±73.0	244.9 ±51.1	241.6 ±55.9	109.00 ±21.67	112.89 ±15.97	112.00 ±17.16	36.14 ±7.89	43.08 ±10.05	41.28 ±9.89
A-2	221.6 ±52.9	227.8 ±49.1	226.3 ±49.4	120.40 ±16.05	114.06 ±17.32	115.54 ±17.07	40.84 ±7.22	38.86 ±6.73	39.25 ±6.76
A-RP	245.0 ±63.3	209.3 ±54.9	238.9 ±63.2	108.08 ±21.95	102.53 ±12.25	107.01 ±20.49	45.21 ±10.83	47.98 ±12.64	45.66 ±11.10
B-None	143.8 ±35.0	141.7 ±33.6	142.2 ±33.8	117.68 ±20.89	119.36 ±26.40	118.93 ±25.02	37.71 ±10.95	36.61 ±7.11	36.85 ±7.94
B-1	251.5 ±93.8	222.8 ±57.8	227.5 ±65.2	111.77 ±12.45	113.27 ±16.95	113.04 ±16.29	42.53 ±12.49	41.05 ±7.26	41.34 ±8.38
B-2	211.7 ±232.1	232.1 ±86.2	228.5 ±80.6	112.43 ±22.72	116.56 ±24.81	115.83 ±24.42	37.00 ±6.87	36.97 ±6.89	36.98 ±6.85
B-RP	217.8 ±64.1	231.2 ±63.4	226.4 ±63.6	115.22 ±19.78	115.28 ±40.41	115.26 ±34.38	42.48 ±6.93	41.55 ±9.63	41.86 ±8.78
P values	P_1 0.001			P_1 0.003			P_1 0.001; P_2 0.001; I 0.01; S 0.01; IS 0.002		

Values are mean ± standard deviation of mean.   S = supplemented; NS = nonsupplemented;
Avg. = average.
Source: Prasad et al., Am. J. Clin. Nutr. 28: 385-391, 1975.

Table 6

Levels of Plasma Vitamin A and Carotene Ascorbic Acid in OCA Users

Group	Vitamin A, ug/100 ml			Carotene, ug/100 ml			Ascorbic acid, mg/100 ml		
	S	NS	Avg	S	NS	Avg	S	NS	Avg
A-None	50.94 ±15.75	50.01 ±13.54	50.57 ±14.85	88.87 ±29.99	78.32 ±32.46	84.51 ±31.35	1.34 ±0.57	0.90 ±0.37	1.15 ±0.54
A-1	67.56 ±26.09	60.55 ±24.19	62.15 ±24.42	55.33 ±14.82	69.03 ±19.33	65.90 ±19.11	0.89 ±0.63	0.73 ±0.35	0.77 ±0.43
A-2	67.25 ±19.19	61.57 ±17.31	62.86 ±17.68	61.68 ±20.52	60.97 ±22.34	61.13 ±21.71	1.01 ±0.46	0.76 ±0.37	0.82 ±0.40
A-RP	59.92 ±21.74	64.78 ±15.81	60.86 ±20.73	88.07 ±94.89	60.76 ±23.30	82.82 ±86.41	1.11 ±0.56	0.93 ±0.43	1.08 ±0.54
B-None	52.43 ±17.55	43.32 ±17.57	45.51 ±17.56	61.45 ±24.24	65.63 ±56.34	64.50 ±50.32	0.64 ±0.30	0.75 ±0.45	0.71 ±0.39
B-1	55.18 ±17.91	56.62 ±15.72	56.40 ±16.00	53.01 ±11.74	63.99 ±20.17	62.31 ±19.49	0.78 ±0.42	0.73 ±0.40	0.74 ±0.40
B-2	63.55 ±21.57	56.84 ±19.73	58.06 ±20.15	51.06 ±17.31	57.54 ±18.91	56.35 ±18.73	0.73 ±0.38	0.69 ±0.37	0.70 ±0.37
B-RP	66.19 ±16.84	60.44 ±19.10	62.53 ±18.43	53.00 ±18.89	56.56 ±18.06	55.28 ±18.35	0.72 ±0.44	0.69 ±0.35	0.70 ±0.39
P values	P1 0.001; S 0.06			P1 0.01; I 0.001			I 0.001; S 0.001; IS 0.001		

Values are mean ± standard deviation of mean.   S = Supplemented;   NS = Nonsupplemented; Avg = average.

Source: Prasad et al., Am. J. Clin. Nutr. 28: 385-391, 1975.

Table 7

Levels of PLP and EGOT and Per Cent Stimulation of EGOT (Mean±S.D.)

Group	Supple-mented	Non-Suppl.	Average	Total Subjects
Plasma PLP (ng./ml.)				
A-None	27.3±15.2	12.6±7.3	18.5±13.1	25
A-1	9.5± 5.7	10.6±4.6	10.3± 4.9	14
A-2	11.7± 8.6	7.8±2.8	9.0± 6.3	16
A-RP	6.2± 5.1	6.6±3.0	6.3± 4.8	65
B-none	9.3± 4.3	11.3±5.7	10.9± 5.5	29
B-1	6.1± 3.0	11.9±6.3	11.2± 6.3	25
B-2	7.6± 5.0	10.1±4.0	9.9± 1.1	51
B-RP	12.3±10.3	8.0±3.7	10.0± 7.7	37

P values P_1 0.001; P_2 0.001; S 0.05; I x P_2 0.001; I x P_1 0.01; S x P 0.01; I x S 0.025; I x S x P_1 0.01; I x S x P_2 0.025

		EGOT (RF units*)		
A-None	4.01± 1.86	2.83±1.02	3.61± 1.71	82
A-1	2.43± 1.97	3.70±2.57	3.41± 2.43	13
A-2	3.37± 0.06	3.21±1.61	3.25± 1.40	13
A-RP	3.87± 2.16	3.35±1.81	3.57± 1.81	7
B-none	4.55± 2.16	4.08±1.75	4.20± 1.83	33
B-1	3.79± 2.79	2.85±1.08	3.04± 1.57	40
B-2	3.34± 2.18	2.67±1.29	2.79± 1.48	39
B-RP	3.50± 2.51	3.82±2.63	3.73± 2.57	41

P values P_1 0.05; P_2 0.06; I x P_1 0.02

		% Stimulation of EGOT		
A-None	132 ± 76	163 ± 91	143 ± 82	81
A-1	252 ± 115	188 ± 174	203 ± 160	13
A-2	162 ± 40	166 ± 136	165 ± 119	13
A-RP	117 ± 33	200 ± 139	164 ± 109	7
B-none	104 ± 52	129 ± 87	123 ± 80	33
B-1	186 ± 145	156 ± 74	162 ± 92	39
B-2	154 ± 124	204 ± 124	196 ± 126	37
B-RP	167 ± 138	165 ± 138	165 ± 131	41

P values P_1 0.01

* Raitman-Frankel units per milliliter of plasma on a basis of
  45 percent hematocrit.

Source: Prasad et al., Am. J. Obstet. Gynecol. 125: 1063-1069, 1976.

Table 8

Levels of Erythrocyte and Serum Folic Acid and Serum B_{12} (Mean$\pm$S.D.)

Group	Supple-mented	Non-Suppl.	Average	Total Subjects
	Erythrocyte folic acid (ng./ml.)			
A-none	318$\pm$170	246$\pm$107	295$\pm$150	102
A-1	204$\pm$ 77	175$\pm$ 56	185$\pm$ 64	28
A-2	253$\pm$119	197$\pm$107	208$\pm$110	36
A-RP	457$\pm$313	260$\pm$165	430$\pm$304	88
B-none	230$\pm$ 81	181$\pm$ 73	192$\pm$ 77	63
B-1	222$\pm$160	200$\pm$ 91	204$\pm$107	55
B-2	199$\pm$ 83	172$\pm$ 65	176$\pm$ 69	106
B-RP	263$\pm$214	234$\pm$160	244$\pm$180	82
P values	P_2 0.001; I 0.001; S 0.001; I x P_2 0.01			
	Serum folic acid (ng./ml.)			
A-none	6.59$\pm$4.67	5.84$\pm$3.77	6.30$\pm$4.33	107
A-1	4.47$\pm$1.19	4.71$\pm$2.50	4.62$\pm$2.04	18
A-2	4.92$\pm$3.11	4.47$\pm$3.15	4.55$\pm$3.09	27
A-RP	7.72$\pm$5.86	5.89$\pm$5.23	7.50$\pm$5.79	83
B-none	4.20$\pm$1.93	3.34$\pm$1.24	3.53$\pm$1.45	54
B-1	4.41$\pm$3.48	4.02$\pm$1.64	4.09$\pm$2.01	49
B-2	4.79$\pm$2.18	3.84 1.30	3.96$\pm$1.45	79
B-RP	6.43$\pm$6.78	3.86$\pm$1.89	4.73$\pm$4.33	72
P values	P_2 0.025			
	Serum B_{12} (pg./ml.)			
A-none	469$\pm$172	446$\pm$176	457$\pm$172	28
A-1	350$\pm$127	290$\pm$102	315$\pm$113	17
A-2	590$\pm$433	461 256	482$\pm$279	19
A-RP	435$\pm$173	679$\pm$642	464$\pm$273	60
B-none	416$\pm$ 72	521$\pm$232	499$\pm$212	38
B-1	385$\pm$125	378$\pm$221	380$\pm$204	22
B-2	487$\pm$201	478$\pm$279	479$\pm$259	67
B-RP	452$\pm$274	478$\pm$246	466$\pm$255	36
P value	P_3 0.01			

Source: Prasad et al., *Am. J. Obstet. Gynecol.* **125**: 1063-1069, 1976.

Table 9

Duncan's New Multiple Range Test* for Erythrocyte and
Serum Folic Acid in OCA Users (P < 0.05)

				Groups				
Folic acid	A-RP	A-none	B-RP	A-2	B-1	B-none	A-1	B-3
Erythrocyte (ng./ml.)	430	295	244	208	204	192	185	176

Folic acid	A-RP	A-none	B-RP	A-1	A-2	B-1	B-2	B-none
Serum (ng./ml.)	7.50	6.30	4.73	4.62	4.55	4.09	3.96	3.53

* Any two means not underscored by the same line are significantly
different. Any two means underscored by the same line are not
significantly different.

Source: Prasad et al., Am. J. Obstet. Gynecol. 125: 1063-1069, 1976.

Table 8 shows the results of erythrocyte and serum folate and
B_{12}. Both plasma and red cell folate levels were higher in group
A than in group B. Supplementation effect was seen in both groups.
Erythrocyte and serum folate in the RP groups were higher than in
the OCA groups.

The Duncan's New Multiple Range test indicated that the A-RP
subjects had higher red cell and serum folate than A-none subjects
(Table 9). Erythrocyte folate in A-1 and A-2 groups was decreased
in comparison to subjects in A-none and A-RP groups. Serum folate
in A-2 group only was decreased when compared to A-none and A-RP
groups.

Serum vitamin B_{12} in A-1 and B-1 groups were lower than A-2
and B-2 groups. No other significant differences were found with
respect to serum vitamin B_{12} levels.

DISCUSSION

It is obvious that subjects in group B showed higher frequency of clinical signs, indicative of malnutrition. Although group A supplemented subjects had less prevalence of abnormal clinical findings related to nutrition, this was not observed in group B. This may mean that group B subjects either received inadequate supplements or falsely reported taking nutritional supplements.

In the higher socioeconomic group greater frequencies of abnormal clinical signs, indicative of malnutrition, were observed in OCA users as compared to controls. However, this was not observed in the lower socioeconomic group on OCA except for angular lesions of the mouth and debris or calculus of the teeth. An increase in prevalences of dental caries in OCA users of the higher socioeconomic group was also observed. In rats injected with OCA, elevated incidences of carious lesions proportional to increased doses of OCA have been reported by Liu and Lin (18). Furthermore, these authors postulated that the increased dental caries activity of OCA treated rats may be caused by a decrease in plasma zinc concentration, since such a reduction has been observed in human subjects (4,19) and rats (20,21) receiving OCA.

Increased levels of serum iron and TIBC due to OCA, as observed in our study, is consistent with the reports of other investigators who showed an increase in transferrin level due to OCA administration. Subjects resuming OCA after pregnancy in both groups appeared to be iron deficient as determined by serum iron and TIBC levels. We believe that changes in RP groups are a result of pregnancy and parturition and not due to OCA inasmuch as the subjects received OCA for a short period of time. The hemoglobin, hematocrit and red cell count were, however, decreased in only A-RP group and the explanation for a lack of similar finding in the B group is not apparent. In general, however, hypochromasia was present in group B suggesting that iron deficiency was perhaps a complicating factor in that group.

The effect of OCA on plasma copper was similar to what has been reported (22,23,24). It is believed that this effect is mainly due to increased levels of ceruloplasmin in the plasma, which have been observed in OCA users and in pregnancy (23,25).

With respect to effect of OCA on plasma zinc, conflicting data have been reported in the literature (23,25,27). A significant decrease in plasma zinc as a result of OCA administration was reported by Halsted et al. (26), Briggs and Briggs (25), and Schenker et al. (23). O'Leary and Spellacy (27), however, reported an increase in the mean plasma zinc levels due to OCA. Their subjects received OCA for only 19 days and the range of normal

values were very wide (95 to 175 ug%). In addition, only 16 OCA
users were used in their study. It is possible that small sample
size and probable contamination problems in sample preparation may
have contributed to their conflicting results.

Our studies indicate a significant decrease in plasma zinc
level but an increase in erythrocyte zinc content as a result of
OCA administration. It is well known that estrogens increase
plasma levels of several proteins such as ceruloplasmin, transferrin, thyroxine binding globulin and cortisol binding protein
(22,25,28). Inasmuch as over 80% of zinc in the red cells is
bound to carbonic anhydrase apoenzyme, our data would suggest that
synthesis or turnover of this protein may have been enhanced due
to OCA. A similar effect was observed in RP groups, suggesting
that some estrogen effect due to pregnancy may have been present
in these subjects. Further studies are indicated to document a
specific effect of estrogen on carbonic anhydrase turnover rate.

The mechanisms responsible for a decrease in plasma zinc
remain to be elucidated. Several possibilities exist. Decreased
absorption, or increased excretion due to OCA may be responsible
for such effect in the plasma. A redistribution of zinc between
plasma and red cell pool should also be considered as another possible explanation. We have observed a decrease in serum albumin
in OCA users. This protein is a major carrier for zinc (29); thus
a decrease in plasma zinc may be related to a decrease in serum
albumin levels. Another possibility is that serum albumin may
have decreased in subjects using OCA due to a zinc deficient state
per se as reported by Ronaghy et al. (30). At this stage, however,
one cannot establish zinc deficiency in such subjects by plasma
zinc level alone.

Gal et al. (31) reported a significant increase in vitamin A
level in the serum of patients using OCA as compared to their
controls. Serum carotene level, on the other hand, showed a
decrease in oral contraceptive groups in comparison to the controls
when the serum sample was obtained between 18 to 21 days of the
menstrual cycle. Our results are similar to those of Gal et al.
(31). Yeung and Gillis (32), however, reported that although
plasma vitamin A level may be increased as a result of the use of
oral contraceptive agents, in experimental animals, the liver
content of vitamin A is decreased. Laurell (33) has reported that
a specific α-globulin responsible for binding vitamin A may be
increased in the plasma thus accounting for an increase in plasma
vitamin A level. These results suggest that OCA effects mobil-
ization and redistribution of tissue vitamin A stores and indeed
the possibility that the vitamin A requirement may actually be
increased due to OCA, must be considered. Lowered levels of
plasma carotene in OCA groups remains essentially unexplained.

Decreased ascorbic acid levels in platelets and leukocytes of women using OCA have been reported by some investigators (34,35). Rivers and Devine (36) observed a decrease in plasma ascorbic acid level in four women using OCA. The lower levels and higher rate of metabolism of ascorbic acid in the plasma, leukocytes and platelets of women taking OCA may relate to their increased serum copper levels. Estrogens and OCA increase serum levels of copper and ceruloplasmin, the protein which transports copper. Ceruloplasmin catalyzes the oxidation of ascorbic acid in vitro; thus, it may participate in lowering ascorbic acid level in the plasma and tissues (37). In experimental animals, the lowered plasma ascorbic acid level is believed to be due to estrogens (38).

We were unable to document any change in plasma ascorbate level due to OCA. Further studies are needed in order to determine whether or not ascorbate level in the tissues is being affected in OCA users.

Most investigators believe that the requirement for vitamin B_6 is increased by estrogens (39,40,41). The estrogen effects in vitamin B_6 metabolism appear to occur in two ways. Firstly, estrogen increases circulating levels of cortisol which in turn increases the activity of tryptophan oxygenase (42). This enzyme is rate limiting in the pathway by which tryptophan is converted to niacin. Some of the enzymes in this pathway require vitamin B_6 as co-enzymes, so that the requirement of vitamin B_6 is enhanced. Secondly, the metabolic products of estrogen and estrogen sulfate interfere with the binding of B_6 co-enzymes to B_6 dependent enzymes, thus further increasing the requirement of B_6 for metabolic purposes.

The reduction in PLP level due to OCA was seen only in the upper socioeconomic group of subjects in this study. The subjects in the lower socioeconomic group did not show this effect. The fact that the reduction in EGOT activities due to OCA was greater in the lower than the upper socioeconomic group of subjects tended to support this hypothesis. The activity of EGOT is dependent on the concentration of the coenzyme, pyridoxal phosphate (PLP). Addition of PLP to the assay mixture increases the activity of the EGOT. The activation is related inversely to the concentration of PLP in the red cells and so may serve as an additional indicator of vitamin B_6 status of the subjects. The percent stimulation of EGOT was higher in the OCA and RP subjects in both socioeconomic groups in our study, suggesting a relative deficiency of the vitamin in these subjects. This may indicate that the EGOT stimulation test is a more sensitive index of alterations in vitamin B_6 status than plasma PLP or EGOT.

Folic acid metabolism is altered by orally administered

estrogen but the nature and significance of this alteration is not clear. Several isolated cases of OCA users evidencing clinical signs of folate deficiency have been described (43,44,45,46). In all these cases, the dietary intake has been adequate to good and generally the women were considered to be healthy. Masked malabsorption or occult malabsorption has been implicated as the underlying cause for the folic acid deficiency and severe megaloblastic anemia in some cases.

Conflicting data have been published with respect to serum folate levels in OCA users. However, the majority of reports indicate a decrease in serum folate at least in some of the subjects using OCA (47,48,49). Reduction of red cell folate and elevation of FIGLU excretion following histidine loading has been observed in OCA users (50). These abnormalities are corrected following folic acid supplementation.

Streiff (51) and Necheles and Snyder (52) suggested an oral estrogen induced impairment in the hydrolyzation of the complex folic acid polyglutamate which leads to poor absorption of dietary folate. Later studies of Stephens et al. (53) and Shojania et al. (54), however, indicated that the absorption of the polyglutamate form of folic acid may not be impaired but that folate metabolism is significantly altered in OCA users. According to Stephens et al. (53), the absorption of the polyglutamic acid was similar to that of monoglutamic folic acid in OCA users provided that these subjects were saturated with folic acid prior to the study. These results suggest an alteration in the rate of folic acid uptake or metabolism by the tissues. In experimental animals, oral sex hormones increase the activities of intestinal enzymes involved in folate metabolism, suggesting that estrogens may increase the rate of metabolism of folic acid and its metabolites by the intestine. The most significant result of the modified folic acid metabolism of women taking OCA may be the possible depletion of body stores of folic acid. Since many of the women discontinue OCA to conceive, Pritchard et al. (55) have suggested that the women becoming pregnant soon after discontinuing the pill, may have a high chance of developing folic acid deficiency during pregnancy.

Recently, a protein which binds unreduced folates and dihydrofolate (FH) has been identified in leukocyte lysates and serum from some women taking OCA (56). It has been suggested that with inadequate or marginal intake of folate, the hormonal induction of this protein may contribute to megaloblastosis by sequestering dihydrofolate, and intermediary folate co-enzyme in DNA-thymine synthesis.

In the lower socioeconomic group, both the plasma and red cell folate were lower than the upper socioeconomic group of subjects,

indicating that this population may be marginally deficient in
folic acid. Our results show a definite lowering effect of OCA on
red cell and serum folate in subjects of upper socioeconomic level.
This was not seen in the lower socioeconomic group.

In our study, groups of subjects resuming the pill after pregnancy (A-RP and B-RP) demonstrated mainly the effects of pregnancy
inasmuch as they resumed OCA within 5 weeks postpartum and their
blood was sampled at first visit after starting the pill. Our
data indicate that the A-RP group was relatively deficient in
vitamin B_6 but adequate in folic acid, suggesting that nutritional
intake of B_6 was inadequate in this group.

Impairment of glucose tolerance was an important abnormality
found in some OCA users which may be related to vitamin B_6 deficiency. Increased resistance to insulin by peripheral tissues, such
as parametrial adipose tissues and diaphragm muscle, in vitro and
in vivo was found to be responsible for the impairment of glucose
tolerance in experimental animals treated with OCA (57,58).
Murikami (59) suggested that xanthurenic acid is capable of complex-
ing with insulin thereby reducing its biological activity. A
significant reduction in biological activity of the insulin in the
complex was observed by means of rat diaphragm and epididymal fat
pad bioassays (59), and a 50% reduction in the hypoglycemic effect
of the insulin complex was observed when injected into dogs and
rabbits (60,61). Indeed, a small group of women whose carbohydrate
tolerance had become impaired while taking OCA improved after
vitamin B_6 administration (62). Several investigators have suggested that large doses of vitamin B_6 should be added to OCA
indiscriminately. However, Adams et al. (63) indicated that the
administration of co-enzyme may increase apo-enzyme synthesis and
this may enhance the plasma amino acid lowering effect of OCA,
which may have an untoward effect in communities where protein
malnutrition exists. At present, it would appear that the idea of
supplementation of B_6 should be approached cautiously since the
long term effect of such therapy is uncertain.

In this study, changes due to OCA with respect to thiamin,
riboflavin, folate and PLP, were seen mainly in subjects of upper
socioeconomic level only. The subjects in the lower socioeconomic
level did not show this effect. This may have been due to the
fact that subjects in lower socioeconomic groups were already
marginally deficient with respect to these micronutrients, as
suggested by our data, and as such further small alterations due
to OCA may not have been detected in this study. Although an
effect of OCA on the levels of thiamin, riboflavin, B_6 and folate
was observed in subjects of the upper socioeconomic group, the
clinical significance of this observation is not clear. Further
studies are needed in order to define the clinical significance of
these changes.

SUMMARY

Clinical, biochemical, and nutritional data were collected
from a large population of women using oral contraceptive agents
(OCA). Subjects on OCA used either "Norinyl" (1 mg norethindrone
and 50 ug mestranol) or "Ovral" (0.5 mg norgestrel and 5 ug of
ethinly estradiol). A higher prevalence of abnormal clinical signs
related to malnutrition was observed in the lower (B) as compared
to the higher (A) socioeconomic groups, and also in the non-
supplemented (NS) groups as compared to the supplemented (S) groups
in the B subjects. In the A groups, a higher prevalence of abnormal
clinical signs was seen in OCA users than in the controls.

In general, the intake of OCA subjects for calories, protein,
calcium, magnesium, iron, copper, and zinc did not differ from the
controls. The intake of the above nutrients in group A subjects
was higher than that of group B except for calories. The subjects
who took supplements had higher intakes of calcium, iron, magnesium
and copper.

As a rule, the OCA subjects' intake of Vitamin A, C, B_6 and
folic acid did not differ from that of the controls. As expected,
subjects from the supplemented (S) groups had higher intake of
vitamin A, C, B_6, thiamin, riboflavin, and folic acid, and A groups
had higher intake of vitamin C, B_6, riboflavin and folic acid.
In group A higher intake of vitamin B_6 and folic acid was observed
in subjects resuming the pill as compared to the subjects using
OCA.

No effect of OCA was seen on hemoglobin, hematocrit and
erythrocyte count. Serum iron was increased due to "Norinyl".
Total iron binding capacity (TIBC) was increased as a result of
OCA administration. TIBC values were higher in group B as compared
to group A and in the non-supplemented as compared to the supplemented groups. Plasma copper was increased and plasma zinc was
decreased as a result of OCA administration. An increase in
erythrocyte zinc was observed due to "Norinyl". No effect of OCA
on plasma calcium, magnesium and erythrocyte magnesium was observed.
Although no effect of OCA on plasma total protein was found, serum
albumin was decreased.

Increased plasma vitamin A and decreased carotene levels were
observed in OCA users. In general, OCA had little or no effect on
plasma ascorbic acid. Urinary excretion of both thiamin and riboflavin in group A subjects using OCA were lower than the controls.
Plasma PLP, red cell and serum folate were lower in OCA subjects
in group A as compared to the controls. Reduction in EGOT activity
and elevation in the EGOT stimulation test were observed in OCA
subjects in both groups (A and B). These observations suggest a
relative deficient state with respect to B_6 and folic acid in OCA

users. No significant effect on serum vitamin B_{12} was observed as a result of OCA administration.

Supported by Contract #NIH=NICHD-NO1-HD-2-2786,
Center for Population Research, N.I.C.H.D.

ACKNOWLEDGEMENTS

We gratefully acknowledge the technical help of Elizabeth Bowersox, Kay Lord, Elizabeth DuMouchelle, Daria Koniuch, Jim Novak and Ray Collins. We are most grateful to Miss Selma Stevens for typing the manuscript. PLP and EGOT determinations were performed in the laboratory of Dr. Paul Gyorgy and Dr. Catherine Rose, Philadelphia, and serum B_{12} and folate determinations were done in the laboratory of Dr. Jack Smith, Dr. Jeff Lawrence, and Dr. Grace Goldsmith. We wish to express our most sincere appreciation to the above for their help.

References

1. Theuer, R. C. Effect of Oral Contraceptive Agents on Vitamin and Mineral Needs: A Review. J. Rep. Med. 8: 13, 1972.

2. Briggs, M. H., Pitchford, A. G., Staniford, M., Barker, H. M., and Taylor, D. Metabolic Effects of Steroid Contraceptives. Steroid Biochemistry and Pharmacology 2: 111, 1970.

3. Anonymous: Oral Contraceptive Agents and Vitamins. Nutrition Reviews 30: 229, 1972.

4. Prasad, A. S., Oberleas, D., Lei, K. Y., Moghissi, K. S., and Stryker, J. C. Effect of Oral Contraceptive Agents on Nutrients: I. Minerals. Am. J. Clin. Nutr. 28: 377-384, 1975.

5. Prasad, A. S., Lei, K. Y., Oberleas, D., Moghissi, K. S., and Stryker, J. C. Effect of Oral Contraceptive Agents on Nutrients: II. Vitamins. Am. J. Clin. Nutr. 28: 385, 1975.

6. Prasad, A. S., Lei, K. Y., Moghissi, K. S., Stryker, J. C., and Oberleas, D. Effect of Oral Contraceptives on Nutrients: III. Vitamins B_6, B_{12} and folic acid. Am. J. Obstet. Gynecol. 125: 1063, 1976.

7. Myrianthopoulos, N., and French, K. An Application of the U.S. Bureau of the Census Socioeconomic Index to a Large, Diversified Patient Population. Soc. Sci. Med. 2: 283, 1968.

8. Interdepartment Committee on Nutrition for National Defense. Manual for Nutrition Surveys, ed. 2, Bethesda, Maryland, National Institutes of Health, 1963.

9. Wintrobe, M. M. Clinical Hematology, Sixth Edition. Philadelphia, Lea & Febiger, 1967.

10. Technicon Auto-Analyzer Methodology. Technicon Instrument Corp., Tarrytown, New York, 10591, 1972.

11. Zip Zone Serum Protein Electrophoresis Procedure. Helena Laboratories, Beaumont, Texas. Procedure 1, 1973.

12. Prasad, A. S. Zinc Metabolism. New York: Charles G. Thomas, 1966, Chapter 2, p. 27.

13. Manual for Nutrition Surveys, 2nd Ed. Interdepartmental Committee on Nutrition for National Defense, National Institutes of Health, Bethesda, Maryland, 1963.

14. Chabner, B. A., and Livingston, D. M. A Simple Enzymatic Assay for Pyridoxal Phosphate. Anal. Biochem. 34: 413-423, 1970.

15. Reitman, S. and Frankel, S. A Colorimetric Method for the Determination Serum Glutamic Oxalacetic and Glutamic Pyruvic Transaminases. Am. J. Clin. Path. 28: 56-63, 1967.

16. Skeggs, H. R. Vitamin B_{12} in The Vitamins, Vol. 7, 277-293, 1967. Edited by Gyorgy, P. and Pearson, W. N. Academic Press, New York and London.

17. Winer, B. J. Statistical Principles in Experimental Design. McGraw-Hill, New York, 1962.

18. Liu, F.T.Y., and Lin S. Effect of the Contraceptive Steroids Norethynodrel and Mestranol on Dental Caries Activity in Young Adult Female Rats. J. Dental Res. 52: 753-757, 1973.

19. Halsted, J. A., Hackley, B. M., and Smith, J. C., Jr. Plasma Zinc and Copper in Pregnancy and after Oral Contraceptives. Lancet 2: 278-279, 1968.

20. McBean, L. D., Smith, J. C., Jr., and Halsted, J. A. Effect of Oral Contraceptive Hormones on Zinc Metabolism in the Rat. Proc. Soc. Exp. Biol. Med. 137: 543-547, 1971.

21. Lei, K. Y., Prasad, A. S., Bowersox, E., and Oberleas, D. Oral Contraceptives, Norethindrone and Mestranol: Effects on Tissue Levels of Minerals. Am. J. Physiol. 231: 98, 1976.

22. Carruthers, M. E., Hobbs, C. B., and Warren, R. L. Raised
     Serum Copper and Ceruloplasmin Levels in Subjects Taking Oral
     Contraceptives. J. Clin. Path. 19: 498, 1966.

23. Schenker, J. G., Hellerstein, S., Jungreis, E., and Polishuk,
     W. Z. Serum Copper and Zinc Levels in Patients Taking Oral
     Contraceptives. Fertility and Sterility 22: 229, 1971.

24. Russ, E. M., and Raymunt, J. Influence of Estrogens on Total
     Serum Copper and Ceruloplasmin. Proc. Soc. Exp. Biol. Med.
     92: 465, 1956.

25. Briggs, M. H. and Briggs, M. Contraceptives and Serum
     Proteins. Brit. Med. J. 3: 521, 1970.

26. Halsted, J. A., Hackley, B. M., and Smith, J. C., Jr. Plasma-
     Zinc and Copper in Pregnancy and after Oral Contraceptives.
     Lancet 2: 278, 1968.

27. O'Leary, J. A. and Spellacy, W. N. Zinc and Copper Levels in
     Pregnant Women and Those Taking Oral Contraceptives.
     Am. J. Obst. & Gynec. 102: 131, 1969.

28. Jacobi, J. M., Powell, L. W., and Gaffney, T. J. Immuno-
     chemical Quantitations of Human Transferrin in Pregnancy and
     During the Administration of Oral Contraceptives. Brit. J.
     Haematol. 17: 503, 1969.

29. Prasad, A. S. and Oberleas, D. Binding of Zinc to Amino
     Acids and Serum Proteins in vitro. J. Lab. Clin. Med. 76:
     416, 1970.

30. Ronaghy, H. A., Reinhold, J. G., Mahloudji, M., Ghavami, P.,
     Fox, M. R. Spivey, and Halsted, J. A. Zinc Supplementation
     of Malnourished Schoolboys in Iran: Increased Growth and
     Other Effects. Am. J. Clin. Nutr. 27: 112, 1974.

31. Gal, I., Parkinson, C., and Craft, I. Effects of Oral Contra-
     ceptives on Human Plasma Vitamin-A Levels. Brit. Med. J. 2:
     436, 1971.

32. Yeung, D. L., and Gillis, C. Oral Contraceptives and Vitamin
     A. Abstracts IX International Congress on Nutrition, 21, 1972.

33. Laurell, C. B., Kullander, S., and Thorell, J. Effect of
     Administration of a Combined Estrogen-Progestin Contraceptive
     on the Level of Individual Plasma Proteins. Scand. J. Clin.
     & Lab. Invest. 21: 337, 1968.

34. Briggs, M. and Briggs, M. Vitamin C. Requirements and Oral Contraceptives. Nature 238, 277, 1972.

35. Kalesh, D. G., Mallikarjuneswara, V. R., and Clemetson, C.A.B. Effect of Estrogen-containing Oral Contraceptives on Platelet and Plasma Ascorbic Acid Concentrations. Contraception 4: 183, 1971.

36. Rivers, J. M. and Devine, M. M. Plasma Ascorbic Acid Concentrations and Oral Contraceptives. Amer. J. Clin. Nutr. 25: 684, 1972.

37. Humoller, F. L., Mockler, M. P., Holthaus, J. M., and Mahler, D. J. Enzymatic Properties of Ceruloplasmin. J. Lab. Clin. Med. 56: 222, 1960.

38. Saroja, N., Mallikarjungswara, V. R., and Clemetson, C.A.B. Effect of Estrogens on Ascorbic Acid in the Plasma and Blood Vessels of Guinea Pigs. Contraception 3: 269, 1971.

39. Luhby, A. L., Reyniak, J. V., Brin, M., Sambour, M., and Brin, H. Abnormal Vitamin B6 Metabolism in Menopausal Women Given Estrogenic Steroids and its Correction by Pyridoxine. Amer. J. Clin. Nutr. 26: 468, 1973.

40. Rose, D. P. The Influence of Oestrogens on Tryptophan Metabolism in Man. Clin. Sci. 31: 265, 1966.

41. Wolf, H., Brown, R. R., Price, J. M., and Madsen, P. O. Studies on Tryptophan Metabolism in Male Subjects Treated with Female Sex Hormones. J. Clin. Endo. 31: 397, 1970.

42. Bulbrook, R. D., Hayward, J. L., Herian, M., Swain, M. D., Tong, D., and Wang, D. Y. Effect of Steroidal Contraceptives on Levels of Plasma Androgen Sulphates and Cortisol. Lancet 1: 628, 1973.

43. Johnson, G. K., Ceenan, J. E., Hensley, G. T., and Soergel, K. H. Small Intestinal Disease, Folate Deficiency Anemia, and Oral Contraceptive Agents. Amer. J. Dig. Dis. 18: 185, 1973.

44. Paton, A. L. Oral Contraceptives and Folate Deficiency. Lancet 1: 418, 1969.

45. Ryser, J. E., Farquet, J. J., and Petite, J. Megaloblastic Anemia Due to Folic Acid Deficiency in a Young Woman on Oral Contraceptives. Acta Haematologica 45: 319, 1971.

46. Salter, W. M. Megaloblastic Anemia and Oral Contraceptives.
     Minn. Med. 55: 554, 1972.

47. Shojania, A. M., Hornady, G., and Barnes, P. H. Oral Contra-
     ceptives and Serum Folate Level. Lancet 1: 1376, 1968.

48. Shojania, A. M., Hornady, G., and Barnes, P. H. Oral Contra-
     ceptives and Folate Metabolism. Lancet 1: 886, 1969.

49. Wertalik, L. F., Metz, E. N., LoBuglio, A. F., and Barcerzak,
     S. P. Decreased Serum B Levels with Oral Contraceptive Use.
     J. Amer. Med. Assoc. 221: 1371, 1972.

50. Luhby, A. L., Shimizu, N., Davis, P., and Cooperman, J. M.
     Folic Acid Deficiency in Users of Oral Contraceptive Agents.
     Fed. Proc. 30: 239, 1971.

51. Streiff, R. R. Folate Deficiency and Oral Contraceptives.
     J. Amer. Med. Assoc. 214: 105, 1970.

52. Necheles, T. F., and Snyder, L. M. Malabsorption of Folate
     Polyglutamates Associated with Oral Contraceptive Therapy.
     New Eng. J. Med. 282: 858, 1970.

53. Stephens, M.E.N., Craft, I., Peters, T. J., and Hoffbrand,
     A. V. Oral Contraceptives and Folate Metabolism. Clin. Sci.
     42: 405, 1972.

54. Shojania, A. M., Hornady, G. J., and Barnes, P. H. The Effect
     of Oral Contraceptives on Folate Metabolism. Amer. J. Obst.
     & Gyn. 111: 782, 1971.

55. Pritchard, J. A., Scott, D. E., and Whalley, P. J. Maternal
     Folate Deficiency and Pregnancy Wastage. Amer. J. Obst. &
     Gyn. 109: 341, 1971.

56. DaCosta, M. and Rothenberg, S. P. Appearance of a Folate
     Binder in Leukocytes and Serum of Women Who are Pregnant or
     Taking Oral Contraceptives. J. Lab. Clin. Med. 83: 207, 1974.

57. Lei, K. Y. and Yang, M. G. Oral Contraceptives, Norethynodrel
     and Mestranol: Effects on Glucose Tolerance, Tissue Uptake of
     Glucose-u-14 and Insulin Sensitivity. Proc.-Soc. Exp. Biol.
     Med. 141: 130-136, 1972.

58. Lei, K. Y., Yang, M. G., Oberleas, D., and Prasad, A. S. Oral
     Contraceptives: Effects on Plasma Insulin Response to Glucose
     and on the Response to Insulin and 2-Deoxyglucose Uptake by
     Peripheral Tissue. Proc. Soc. Exp. Biol. Med. 149: 417-421,
     1975.

59. Murakami, E. Studies on the Xanthurenic Acid - Insulin Complex. I. Preparation and Properties. J. Biochem. 63: 573-577, 1968.

60. Kotake, Y., Sotokawa, T., Murakami, E., Hisatake, A., Abe, M., and Ikeda, Y. Studies on the Xanthurenic Acid - Insulin Complex. II. Physiological Activities. J. Biochem. 63: 578-581, 1968.

61. Kotake, Y., Sotokawa, T., Murakami, E., Hisatake, A., Abe, M., and Ikeda, Y. Physiological Activities of Xanthurenic Acid - 8 Methyl Ether - Insulin Complex. J. Biochem. 64: 895, 1968.

62. Spellacy, W. N., Buhi, W. C., and Biric, S. A. The Effects of Vitamin B_6 on Carbohydrate Metabolism in Women Taking Steroid Contraceptives: Preliminary Report. Contraception 6: 265, 1972.

63. Adams, P. W., Wynn, V., Rose, D. P., Foldard, J., Seed, M., and Strong, R. Effect of Pyridoxine Hydrochloride (Vitamin B_6) upon Depression Associated with Oral Contraception. Lancet 1: 897, 1973.

NUTRITION, FERTILITY AND INFANT MORTALITY

INTRODUCTORY STATEMENT

W. Henry Mosley

The Johns Hopkins University

Baltimore, Maryland

The papers in this section review both historical records as well as recent studies which highlight how malnutrition, specifically maternal malnutrition, may depress reproductive performance in human populations. In these reports attention is focused particularly on nutrition and its effect on the reproductive life span, on fecundibility, and on survival of the offspring.

The paper by Frisch provides the broadest overview of the potential relationship between nutrition and reproductive performance. She suggests that undernutrition has been a major determining factor in holding down the fertility of poor couples in historical populations as well as in developing countries far below the "human maximum." In this context, it is important to note that Frisch uses as her frame of reference for a healthy well-nourished population the Hutterite women whose completed fertility averaged ten to twelve children. This she contrasts with the more commonly observed completed fertility of six to seven children seen in many historical populations as well as in developing countries.

The clearest and best documented relationship of nutrition to a reproductive variable (other than mortality) is the relationship with age at menarche. Frisch summarizes in detail the extensive work in this area and her own hypothesis about fatness as the determinant of this relationship. Unanswered is the question of the nature of the hormonal signals precipitating menarche and how they are altered by nutritional status. Nutrition may also affect menopause, although the data are very deficient on this point.

Frisch enters into more speculative areas in searching for data to support the hypothesis that malnutrition reduces reproductive performance, particularly fecundity, within the childbearing years. While it is clear that severe starvation and famine have a profound effect on reproduction in populations, as the next paper by Stein and Susser shows, the evidence that chronic malnutrition alters fecundity is much less clear. Frisch has proposed, for example, that menstrual cycles stop with the weight loss or energy drain of lactation (see Frisch Figure 1), although there is no direct evidence supporting this view. In fact, the studies by Chowdhury, by Delgado, et al., and by Carael reported elsewhere in this volume provide rather strong evidence against maternal malnutrition (as measured by body weight) being a major determinant of the duration of lactational amenorrhea.

In searching for medical or biological explanations for fertility in nineteenth century Europe being below the Hutterite level, Frisch provides an interesting review of the historical medical literature on this topic. She finds among the numerous clinical descriptions and anecdotal accounts by physicians and other observers reports such as "about a quarter of the working women in mills suffered from either retarded or suppressed menses" and "about half of all married women between the ages of twenty and forty-five years were reported to have diseases of the uterus which included amenorrhea." "Causes" of amenorrhea in these reports range from poor diet, disease, and anaemia, to unsuitable employment, and cold and damp. It is difficult to know how these accounts, many of which are based on physicians' experiences with sick women, can be related to the health conditions and thus the reproductive performance of the general population.

Interpretation of these historical accounts is also difficult because of problems in terminology. For example, in one study cited by Frisch "absolute sterility" is referred to as no children by three years after marriage. In the study cited in Edinburgh in the late 19th century, the level is reported to be 15 percent. This figure, however, is almost uninterpretable unless one knows the age of marriage and cohabitation patterns and contraceptive practice in the early years of marriage. For example, in Bangladesh, a poorly nourished population where there is no contraception but marriage is close to menarche, the first birth may be delayed beyond three years in more than 40 percent of the couples due to adolescent subfecundity, although less than 5 percent of women are ultimately childless at the end of their reproductive years. Given these considerations, it is not appropriate to contrast the Edinburgh experience in the last century with the 2 percent incidence of "absolute sterility" reported for the modern Hutterite wife.

In searching for data on the length of the birth interval, the only data Frisch refers to in her historical review is the report

from a publication in 1851 which notes that the average birth
interval for "working and lower middle class women" was about 20
to 24 months. This is impressively short since it is equivalent
to a marital fertility rate averaging 500 to 600 births per
thousand women per year. This actually suggests that there was
no detrimental effect of malnutrition for these women since this
is virtually the level of Hutterite fertility. Frisch's paper is
useful because it does lead to hypotheses that can be tested. At
the same time, it illustrates many of the problems of attempting
to relate nutritional data to reproductive performance. Human
reproduction is strongly influenced by both social as well as biological factors and, as the conceptual framework presented in the
first chapter illustrates, these factors can act through the same
basic mechanisms to alter the reproductive life span, fecundity,
pregnancy outcome, and lactational amenorrhea.

While it may be true that "hard physical work and poor living
conditions can explain the relatively small completed family size
of the lower socio-economic classes in about 1850-1860 in Britain,"
it is not at all clear from the data available that this is largely
due to biological constraints on the capacity to reproduce. More
data is required not only on factors such as age of marriage,
breast-feeding patterns, and practice of contraception within marriage but also on the suppression of fertility due to involuntary
separation of spouses due to working conditions or diseases, as
well as separation and divorce due to social disorganization and
even the unreported practice of abortion and infanticide. Definitive answers to these questions are not likely to come from
further review of the historical records; thus the search for
evidence on the effects of nutrition on fertility will have to be
from modern day experience in the developing world.

The paper by Stein and Susser is also a review of historical
records but of a much more dramatic event: the 1944-45 Dutch famine
occurring in World War II. This famine was associated, after a
nine month lag, with a sharp decline in fertility. With the liberation of the famine affected cities there was a rapid recovery in
fertility with a rebound phenomena. The primary effect of the
famine was to reduce conception rates; there was no clear evidence
of a rise in fetal deaths. A social class difference in fertility
decline suggested that the upper classes were less subjected to
the effects of food restriction. The dramatic decline in fertility
with the famine as well as the sharp rise following availability of
food suggests that psychological as well as physiological factors
were playing a role in suppressing the conception rate.

While the effects of famine on fertility are dramatic, it is
not clear how these observations are helpful in elucidating how
chronic malnutrition, such as seen in many developing countries,

may affect fertility. This is because a famine represents an
acute social and psychological as well as physiological insult on
a population, whereas many adaptive mechanisms have evolved in
populations with chronic malnutrition.

   The effect of malnutrition on overall mortality, particularly
infant and child mortality, is well established as a major factor
in influencing the dynamics of population growth. This topic is
not reviewed in depth at this Conference. The paper by Lechtig,
et al., does explore in some depth, however, the particular relationship between maternal nutrition and infant mortality. Their
review of the literature as well as the analysis of a recent study
by INCAP in Guatemala provides convincing evidence that maternal
malnutrition has an adverse effect on infant survival. Of
particular interest is the evidence that both the short and long
term nutritional status of the mother are independently related to
infant mortality. The authors note that the general relationship
of low socio-economic status with high infant mortality appears
to work in large measure through maternal malnutrition and illness
which leads to the delivery of poorly viable infants. In their
conclusion they translate these observations into a proposal for
an integrated effort which not only tackles nutrition and health
problems but also the social and economic context in which they
occur.

NUTRITION, FATNESS AND FERTILITY: THE EFFECT OF FOOD INTAKE ON REPRODUCTIVE ABILITY

Rose E. Frisch

Harvard University

Cambridge, Massachusetts

INTRODUCTION

"Tell me what you eat, and I will tell you what you are."
Brillat-Savarin's aphorism (1) can be expanded to: "Tell me what
you eat, and I will also tell you how well you reproduce." Recent
findings that the onset and maintenance of regular menstrual function in the human female are each dependent on the maintenance of
a minimum weight for height, apparently representing a critical
fat storage (2), imply that a particular body composition of relative fatness, (fat/lean ratio, or fat/body weight) may be an
important determinant for human female reproductive ability (3-6).

A woman who loses about 10 to 15 percent of her body weight
loses about a third of her body fat and becomes amenorrheic (2,3).
An excess of body fat also affects menstrual function, since very
obese women are amenorrheic or have irregular cycles (3). Too
little fat, or too much fat therefore is associated with a disruption of female reproductive ability (3,6). This paper will discuss
the limiting effects of undernutrition and high energy requiring
activities, such as hard physical work and lactation on reproductive ability (2,7,8).

Charles Darwin described this common sense relationship
between food supplies and fertility, observing that: 1) domestic
animals, which have regular, plentiful food without working to get
it are more fertile than the corresponding wild animals; 2) "Hard
living retards the period at which animals conceive;" 3) the amount
of food affects the fertility of the same individual (9); and 4)
It is difficult to fatten a cow which is lactating (10). All of
Darwin's dicta apply to human beings, as I will show.

NUTRITION AND VARIATION IN NATURAL FERTILITY

In many historical populations, poor couples living together
to the end of their reproductive lives had only 6 to 7 living
births (11,12). Most poor couples in many developing countries
today also only have 6 to 7 living births during their reproductive
lifespan (13,14). Six children per couple today results in a very
rapid rate of population growth because of decreased mortality
rates, resulting from the introduction of modern public health
procedures. However, 6 or 7 births is far below the human maximum
of 11 or 12 children found among non-contracepting, well nourished
peoples such as the Hutterites (15,16).

The usual explanation of the lower than maximum fertility
observed in both historical and contemporary societies is that it
is due to the use of "folk" methods of contraception, abortion, or
venereal disease, in combination with social customs which can
affect fertility, such as late age of marriage, or a taboo on
intercourse during lactation (11,15,17). Because food intake can
directly affect fecundity, undernutrition is an alternate explanation of the observed sub-maximum fertility (8). Undernutrition,
of course, may also interact with social customs which affect the
degree of exposure to risk of pregnancy in a particular society.

Differences in natural fertility have been recognized and
explained by differences in length of birth intervals (18) or by
variation in general health and food intake without specification
of the mechanism. Carr-Saunders (20) gives many examples from
hunting and fishing societies to show that poor living conditions
limit human fecundity and better conditions increase human fecundity. Recognizing the general principle for all species, he states:

> "... fecundity has been spoken of as if it was fixed at
> a certain strength for each species. As a matter of fact,
> it varies within fairly wide limits - increasing with
> better conditions. In this fact lies the explanation of
> the increase of species under favorable conditions which
> has often been observed, although when conditions are less
> favourable, there is little or no evidence of starvation
> among such species."

Mauldin (21) cites data of Mahalanobis and others which
suggest that low levels of fertility at certain periods of Indian
history may have been due to impaired fecundity because of low
levels of consumption. Gopalan and Naidu (22) relate malnutrition
and relatively low fertility in India. Chen et al. (14) show from
a prospective study that fertility in Bangladesh varied in correlation with the food supply in an essentially non-contracepting
population. Finally, there is evidence that the fertility of the

well nourished, non-contracepting Hutterites increased from 1880
to 1950, in association with an increased standard of living (16).

This paper presents: first, the biological basis for a direct
nutritional effect on fecundity and, hence, fertility; second,
historical data on reproduction growth and food intake in support
of the hypothesis that subfecundity due to undernutrition and hard
living was the main reason why poor married couples in mid-19th
century Britain had 6 or 7 children instead of 10 or 12 (8).

FOOD INTAKE AND THE REPRODUCTIVE LIFESPAN

Undernutrition affects reproductive ability by shortening the
duration of the reproductive lifespan and by reducing its efficiency
(Figure 1) (7,8). The undernourished female has menarche later
and menopause earlier than does a well nourished female. The undernourished female has a high frequency of irregular and anovulatory
cycles, which stop completely (amenorrhea) if undernutrtion is
severe. During pregnancy, an underfed woman has a higher probability of a miscarriage and of a stillbirth (pregnancy wastage).
If she delivers an infant successfully, her lactational amenorrhea
may be longer after parturition than that of a well nourished
woman, resulting in longer birth intervals than that of a well
nourished woman (7,8,14).

In the adult male, severe undernutrition results in loss of
libido, decreased prostate fluid, decreased sperm number, the loss
of sperm mobility, and eventually the cessation of sperm production,
in that order (23,24). Undernutrition also delays the onset of
sexual maturation in boys (25,26), similar to the effect of undernutrition on menarche (8,27). Male fecundity declines with age
(23), similar to the female, and this decline may be more rapid
with undernutrition, as it is in the female (8).

These direct effects of undernutrition result, in turn, from
the physiological basis of reproductive ability (Figures 1 and 2).

The Physiological Basis of Reproductive Ability

The idea that relative fatness is important for female reproductive ability follows from earlier findings that menarche is
closely related to a critical body weight (28,29), which represents
a critical fat/lean ratio, or fat/body weight percentage (4,5).
These findings, both on weight and body composition, are in accord
with the data at puberty for other mammals (30), including pigs
(31,32), cattle (32), and the rat (33-35).

The initial finding from longitudinal growth data of United States girls was that the mean weight at menarche (about 47 kg) did not differ significantly for early and late maturing girls, whereas their mean height at each of these events increased significantly with the age of the event (28,29). These results accounted for the many observations in the literature that early maturers have more weight for height than do late maturers.

Even before taking the next step of the meaning of the critical weight for an individual girl, the idea that menarche is associated with a critical weight for a population explained simply many observations associated with early or late menarche. Observations of earlier menarche are associated with attaining the critical weight more quickly. The most important example is the secular

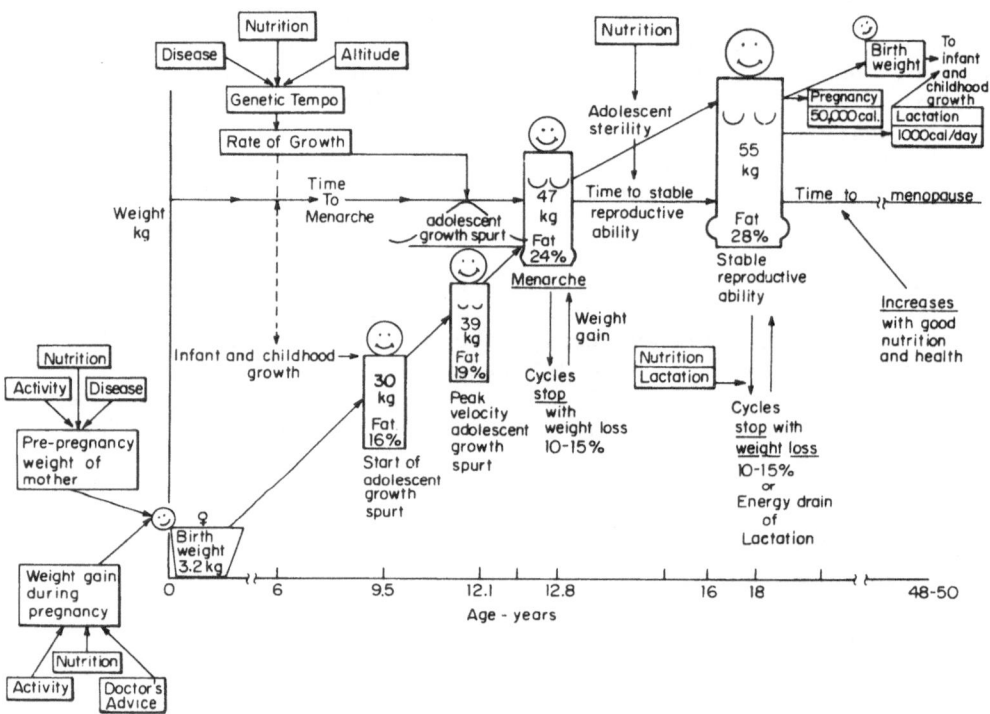

Figure 1. The biological determinants of female reproductive ability. Each reproductive milestone can be affected by environmental factors, as shown. The maintenance of regular ovulatory cycles is related to a minimum level of fat storage and is thus directly affected by undernutrition and energy-draining activities such as lactation. Reprinted from Frisch (7) with permission from Social Biology.

trend to an earlier menarche of about 3 or 4 months per decade in
Europe in the last one hundred years. Our explanation, supported
by historical data, was that children now are bigger sooner (27-29).
Therefore, girls on the average reach 46-47 kg, the mean weight at
menarche of United States and many European populations, more
quickly. According to our hypothesis also, the secular trend
should end when the weight of children of successive cohorts
remains the same because of the attainment of maximum nutrition
and child care, which now may have happened (27-29).

Conversely, a late menarche is associated with body weight
growth that is slower prenatally, postnatally, or both, so that
the average critical weight is reached at a later age: malnutrition
delays menarche (27); twins have later menarche than singletons of
the same population, and high altitude delays menarche (29).

The hypothetical mechanism we suggested, based on Kennedy's

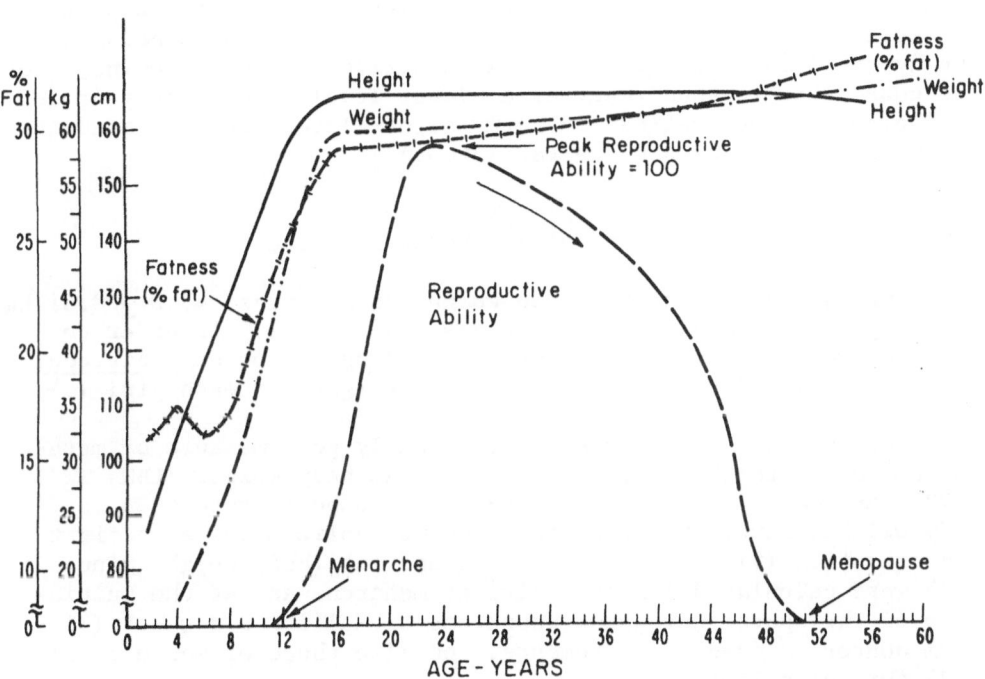

Figure 2. The synchronization of peak female reproductive ability
with the attainment of mature height, weight and relative fatness.
Timing and levels for 1950-1975.

Table 1

Total Water (TW)/Body Weight (BWt) Percent
as an Index of Fatness

	Female	Male
Weight (kg)	65	65
Total Water (liters)	33	40
Lean BWt (kg)(TW/0.72)	46	56
Fat (kg)	19	9
Fat/BWt %	29	14
TW/BWt %	51	62

$$\text{Fat/Body Wt \%} = 100 - \frac{\text{TW/BWt \%}}{0.72}$$

(33) for the rat, was that the critical weight, which later analysis showed to represent a critical fatness level, represents a particular metabolic rate, which would be signaled to the hypothalamus. The hypothalamus then becomes less sensitive to gonadotropins, and the gonadostat is thus reset at a higher level. This early crude mechanism has been refined in terms of our later findings both in the human female (6) and the rat (34,35).

Components of Weight at Menarche

The variability of the mean weight at menarche, 47.8 ± 0.51 kg, was large; the standard deviation was 6.9 kg (29). In order to make the notion of a critical weight meaningful for an individual girl, we analyzed the components of the weight for each girl (5).

Body weight is considered a reasonably good measure of metabolism, but total body water (TW) and lean body weight (LBW = TW/0.72), are more closely correlated with metabolic rate than is body weight, since they represent the metabolic mass, as a first approximation (5). These components and fat (body weight minus LBW) were calculated for each girl at menarche and at the initiation of the spurt, using the equations of Mellits and Cheek (36) from deuterium oxide measurements, and also those of Moore et al. (37) for comparison.

The greatest change in body composition of both early and late maturing girls during the adolescent growth spurt up to menarche

Table 2

Height, Weight, Total Water/Body Weight (TW/BW) Percent,
Lean Body Weight (LBW), Fat, Fat/Body Weight Percent,
and Ratio of LBW to Fat of Girls Grouped by
Height at Menarche

Height Category (cm)	No.		Height (cm)	Weight (kg)	TW/BWt %	LBW (kg)	Fat (kg)	Fat/ Body Weight %	Ratio LBW to Fat
			All Ages of Menarche						
<152.0	25		147.8	40.2	56.3	31.4	8.9	21.8	3.5:1
		SD	3.6	3.5	2.4	1.7	2.0	3.3	
152.1- 158.0	58		155.1	46.9	54.7	35.2	11.6	24.6	3.0:1
		SD	1.8	6.6	4.2	2.4	4.3	5.8	
158.1- 164.0	64		161.0	49.5	54.8	37.5	12.1	23.8	3.1:1
		SD	1.5	6.0	3.7	2.2	3.8	4.6	
>164.1	34		167.4	51.9	55.3	39.7	12.3	23.2	3.2:1
		SD	3.4	5.7	3.2	2.3	3.7	4.4	
All Subjects	181		158.5	47.8	55.1	36.3	11.5	23.5	3.2:1
		SD	6.5	6.9	3.6	3.4	3.9	4.8	

is a 120% increase in body fat, from about 5 kg to 11 kg; lean
body weight (LBW), in contrast, increases only about 44%. The
ratio of LBW to fat thus changes from 5:1 at initiation of the
spurt to 3:1 at menarche. A fall in metabolic rate/kg body weight
would be expected from this change in body composition (4,5,38).

A Fatness Index: Total Water as Percent of Body Weight

Total body water as percent of body weight (TW/BWt %) is a
more important index than the absolute amount of total water
because it is an index of fatness (39) as shown by Table 1. When
girls are grouped by height at menarche rather than by age at
menarche, the shortest, lightest girls and the tallest, heaviest
girls differ in height by about 20 cm and in weight by about 12 kg.
But these two extreme groups have the same relative fatness, as
shown by their similar percentages of total water/body weight,

56.3 $\pm$ 0.5 %, and 55.3 $\pm$ 0.5 %, respectively. Both these values
are similar to the mean for all subjects, 55.1 $\pm$ 0.3 % (Table 2).

Although the shortest, lightest girls at menarche have a
smaller absolute amount of fat, 8.9 $\pm$ 0.4 kg, compared to that of
the tallest, heaviest girls, 12.3 $\pm$ 0.6 kg (the mean for all subjects is 11.5 $\pm$ 0.3 kg), both extreme groups have about 22% of
their body weight as fat at menarche as do all subjects, and the
ratio of lean body weight to fat of both groups is in the range of
3.1, as it is in all subjects (4,5,30,38) (Table 2).

Prediction of Menarche from the Fatness Index

Quartiles of total water/body weight percent are essentially
quartiles of fatness. Of the 169 girls who could be followed from
spurt initiation to menarche, 82% remained in the same quartiles
of total water/body weight percent from initiation to menarche,
compared to only 47% remaining in the same quartiles of weight, and
only 39% remaining in the same quartiles of total body water. This
finding gave a method of prediction of age of menarche from the
height and weight of a premenarcheal girl at each age from 9 to 13
years (40). At each age, prediction of age of menarche was better
for the heavier girls, who are found in the lowest total water/
body weight quartiles (inversely to the weight quartiles) than for
the lighter weight girls. This was because of an exceptional group
of early maturing girls (9.5% of all subjects) who were very short
and light weight at menarche (mean height 148.6 $\pm$ 0.6 cm; mean
weight 40.9 $\pm$ 0.8 kg). Normally at menarche the short girls have
more weight for their height than do tall girls. The small number
of short, light, later maturing girls (4.4% of all subjects) were
also exceptional, since late maturers at menarche are usually
taller than early maturers. Both groups of short girls had less
absolute fat than the average girl at menarche, but their relative
fatness, about 22%, was in the normal range at menarche (40).

The short, light, early girls might be the equivalent of the
meat type now being sought by sheep breeders: fast growing, early
maturers with a small leg joint and not too heavily marbled with
fat (30).

Fatness as a Determinant of Minimal Weights for Menstrual Cycles

The total water/body weight percent data of each of the same
181 girls followed from menarche to the completion of growth at
ages 16-18 years provided a method of determining a minimal weight
for height necessary for the onset of menstrual cycles (menarche)
in primary amenorrhea and for the restoration of menstrual cycles

in cases of secondary amenorrhea, when the amenorrhea is due to undernourishment (2).

Patients with amenorrhea due to weight loss, other possible causes having been excluded, were studied in relation to the weights indicated by the diagonal percentile lines of total water/ body weight percent in Figures 3 and 4. We found that 56.1 percent of total water/body weight percent, the 10th percentile at age 18 years, which is equivalent to about 22% fat of body weight, indicates a minimal weight for height necessary for the restoration and maintenance of menstrual cycles. For example, a 20 year old woman whose height is 160 cm should weigh at least 46.3 kg before menstrual cycles would be expected to resume.

The weights at which menstrual cycles ceased or resumed in post-menarcheal patients ages 16 and older (Figure 4) are about 10 percent heavier than the minimal weights for the same height observed at menarche (Figure 3).

In accord with this finding, the body composition data show that both early and late maturing girls gain an average of 4.5 kg of fat from menarche to age 18 years. Almost all of this gain is achieved by age 16 years, when mean fat is 16.0 ± 0.3 kg, 28 percent of the mean body weight of 57.1 ± 0.6 kg. Reflecting this increase in fatness, the total water/body weight percent decreases from 55.1 ± 0.2 percent at menarche (12.9 ± 0.1 years) to 52.1 ± 0.2 percent (S.D. 3.0) at age 18 years (3).

Because girls are less fat at menarche than when they achieve stable reproductive ability, the minimal weight for height for the onset of menstrual cycles in cases of primary amenorrhea due to undernutrition is indicated by the 10th percentile of fractional body water at menarche, 59.8 percent, which is equivalent to about 17 percent fat of body weight (2) (Figure 3).

The absolute and relative increase in fatness from menarche to age 16 to 18 years is of special interest because this interval coincides with the period of adolescent sterility. During this time there is rapid growth of the uterus and the ovaries (3).

Reproductive Efficiency and Stored Energy

The weight changes associated with the cessation and restoration of menstrual cycles are in the range of 10 to 15 percent of body weight. Weight loss or gain of this magnitude is mainly loss or gain of fat. This finding suggested that a minimum level of stored, easily mobilized energy is necessary for ovulation and menstrual cycles in the human female (2,7). The main function of

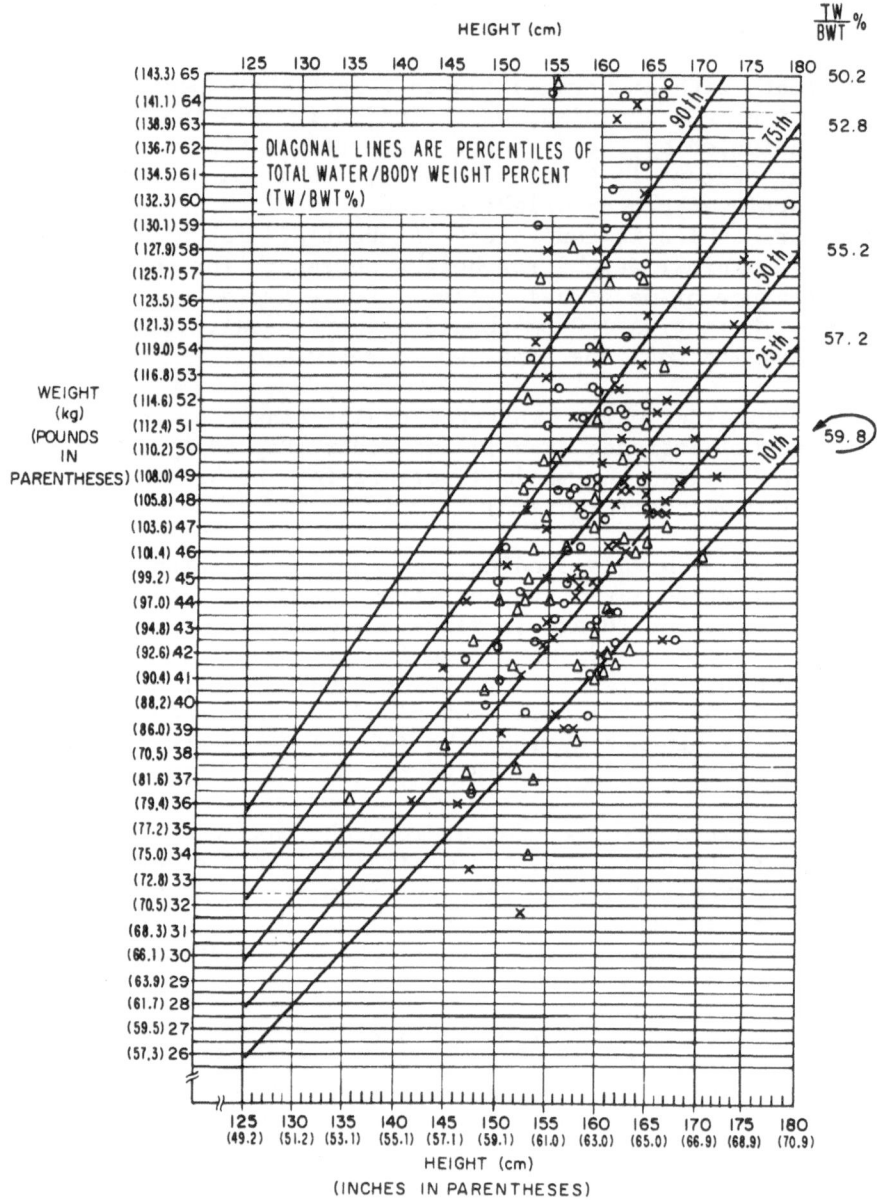

Figure 3. The minimal weight necessary for a particular height for onset of menstrual cycles is indicated on the weight scale by the 10th percentile diagonal line of total water/body weight percent, 59.8% (equivalent to about 17% fat of body weight), as it crosses the vertical height lines. Height growth of girls must be completed or approaching completion. For example, a 15-year old

the 16 kg of fat stored on average by early and late maturing girls by age 18 years may be to provide easily mobilized energy for a pregnancy and for lactation; the 144,000 calories would be sufficient for a pregnancy and 3 months' lactation (38). The human brain, it should be noted, grows most rapidly during the last trimester of pregnancy and the first months after birth (41).

Irrespective of any causal relationship, the weight dependency of menarche in human beings, as in animals, operates as a "compensatory mechanism" for both environmental and genetic variation. The result is a reduction in the variability of body size at sexual maturity, and, therefore, a reduction in the variability of adult body size. As in many other animals, human body size at sexual maturity is close to adult size; weight and height at menarche are 85% and 96% of adult weight and height, respectively. The regulation of female body size has obvious selective advantages for the species since birth weight is correlated with the pregnancy weight of the mother, and infant survival is correlated with birth weight (27,38).

An example of the uniformity of adult weight and height in well fed populations is the similarity of the weights termed "underweight" for height in a large sample of normal American women given by Sargent (42) and the minimal weights for height given by Frisch and McArthur (2) in Figure 4 (Table 3) for the restoration of menstrual cycles.

Different racial groups have different critical weights at menarche (25,38). Matsumoto et al. (43) give 44 kg for the weight of Japanese girls at menarche. These authors also note that the mean weight at menarche did not differ between early and late maturing Japanese girls. We do not know as yet whether the different critical weights at menarche of other racial groups represent the same or different body compositions of fatness (38).

Other factors, such as emotional stress, affect the maintenance or onset of menstrual cycles in human beings. Therefore, menstrual cycles may cease without weight loss and may not resume in some subjects even though the minimum required weight is attained (2).

---

girl whose completed height is 160 cm (63 inches) should weigh at least 41.4 kg (91 lbs.) before menstrual cycles can be expected to start. Symbols are the height and weight at menarche of 181 girls from three longitudinal growth studies (28,29). Reprinted from Frisch and McArthur (2) with permission from Science.

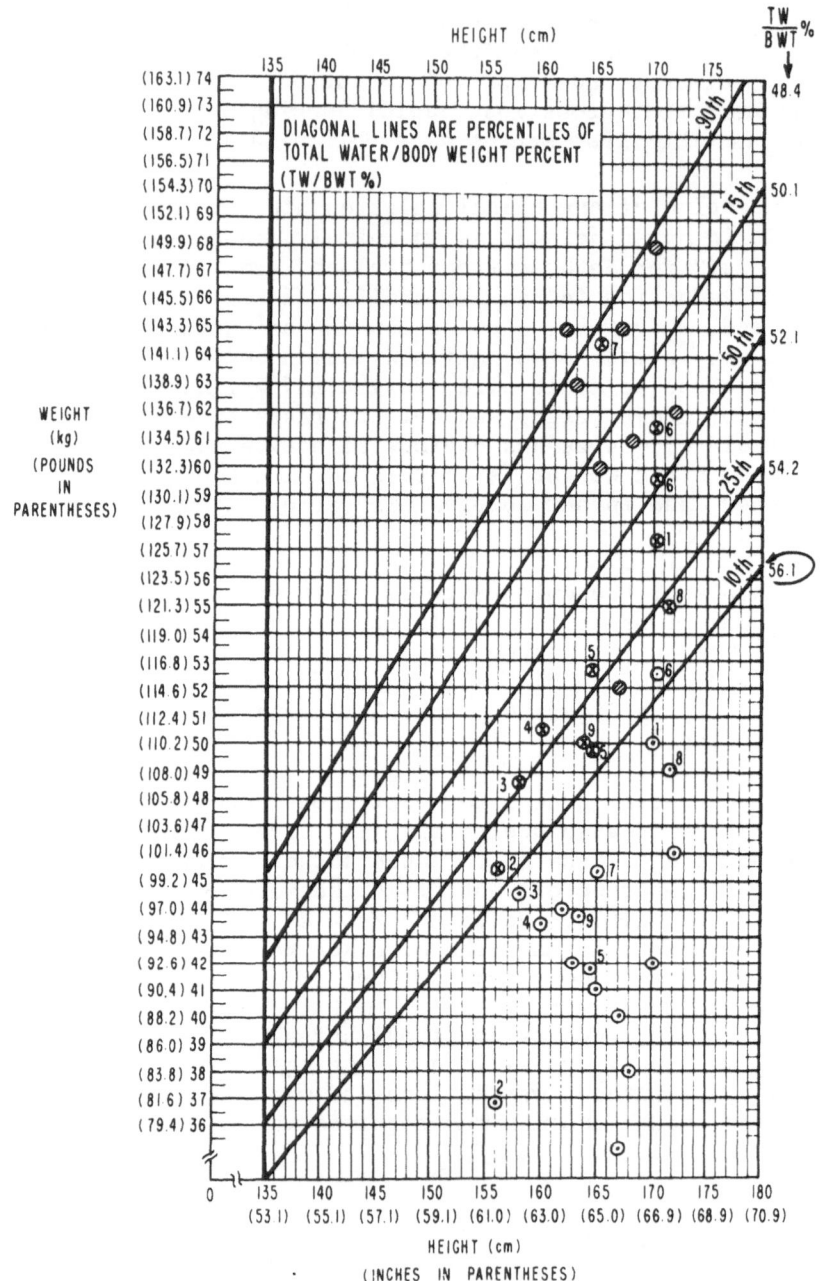

Figure 4. The minimal weight necessary for a particular height
for restoration of menstrual cycles is indicated on the weight
scale by the 10th percentile diagonal line of total water/body

Table 3

Comparison of Minimum Weight for Height for Maintenance of
Menstrual Cycles from Frisch, R. E. and McArthur, J. W.
(Science 185: 949, 1974) and "Underweight", Weight for
Height Classification by Sargent, D. M. (Am. J. Clin.
Nutr. 13: 318, 1963). Also, Frisch and McArthur,
50th Percentile, and Sargent, "Normal",
Weight for Height

Height cm	Frisch-McArthur Minimum Weight kg	Classified "Underweight" by Sargent kg	Frisch-McArthur 50th Percentile kg	Classified "Normal" by Sargent kg
146	39.4	39.2	45.2	46.1
148	40.4	40.0	46.4	47.1
150	41.4	40.9	47.5	48.1
152	42.4	41.8	48.7	49.2
154	43.4	42.7	49.8	50.3
156	44.4	43.7	51.0	51.4
158	45.4	44.6	52.1	52.5
160	46.4	45.6	53.3	53.6
162	47.4	46.6	54.4	54.8
164	48.4	47.6	55.6	56.0
166	49.4	48.6	56.7	57.2
168	50.4	49.7	57.8	58.5
170	51.3	50.8	59.0	59.8
172	52.3	51.9	60.1	61.1
174	53.3	53.0	61.3	62.4
176	54.3	54.2	62.4	63.8
178	55.3	55.4	63.6	65.2
180	56.3	56.6	64.7	66.6

weight percent, 56.1 percent (equivalent to about 22% fat of body
weight) as it crosses the vertical height line. For example, a 20
year old woman whose height is 160 cm should weigh at least 46.3
kg (102 lb.) before menstrual cycles would be expected to resume.
⊙ Weights of patients while amenorrheic. Reprinted from Frisch
and McArthur (2) with permission from Science.

THE VIGOR OR DECREPITUDE OF THE REPRODUCING INDIVIDUAL

The Historical Data

Quantitative interest in the body in relation to nutrition,
growth, and reproductive ability in both sexes was strong in the
nineteenth century, probably inspired by Quetelet's pioneer work
(8). In the earlier Malthusian view, human reproductive power is
an irrepressible force, fulfilling itself regardless of circum-
stance, to be cut down by the positive check of increased mortality,
or held in check by the moral restraint of later marriage (44).
In contrast, the medical and biological literature of 1850-1880
expresses the view that reproductive ability in both sexes is directly related to the state of vigor or decrepitude of the reproducing individuals (8). The individual does not reproduce the
species at any cost. Instead, if the choice is individuation
versus genesis, individuation wins. When food supplies are inadequate, women and men, like other mammals, are less fecund.
When food intake is very low, reproduction stops (8,45).

Reproduction Requires Energy: The Historical View

Medical texts up to about 1885 state that "constitutional"
reasons for sterility are more important and more prevalent than
sterility due to disease of the organs. It therefore is not always
wise to cure sterility: A sterile woman may be deficient in "reproductive energy;" if she did not have children there is a high risk
of miscarriage, or of weakly children, or of the death of the
mother (45).

The degree of "pinquidity" - fatness - was considered important in relation to sterility (2,3). She's too thin to get pregnant
or to menstruate regularly was a common observation, especially in
association with tuberculosis or chlorosis, a virulent anemia
common among working women, which colored them a sickly green. The
prescription was: "recover her flesh" by puddings, roast meats, a
good wine, fresh air and sun (8).

"She's too fat to get pregnant," was also observed (45,46)
(also correctly, since excessive fatness also causes amenorrhea)
(3,6). A light diet and exercise were prescribed (46).

The observation that women often got fatter after menopause
was explained by the fact that a female no longer expended energy
in creating "that most subtle human extract, the ovum" (47).

Curves of Reproductive Ability: Age-specific Fertility

The fertility of women gradually increases with age to a climax and then gradually wanes (Figure 5) (1,15,48), similar to "the fertile career of the domestic hen" (Figure 6), as Dr. Duncan advised the Royal College of Physicians in 1884 (45). Reproductive errors are more frequent at the beginning and end of reproductive life, as is found in all animals (48).

Age specific fertility data for the British female in about 1850 show that the fertile career of the mid-nineteenth century female began with a relatively late menarche at about 15-16 years. It was already observed that a period of relative infertility, now termed adolescent sterility or sub-fecundity (49), followed men-

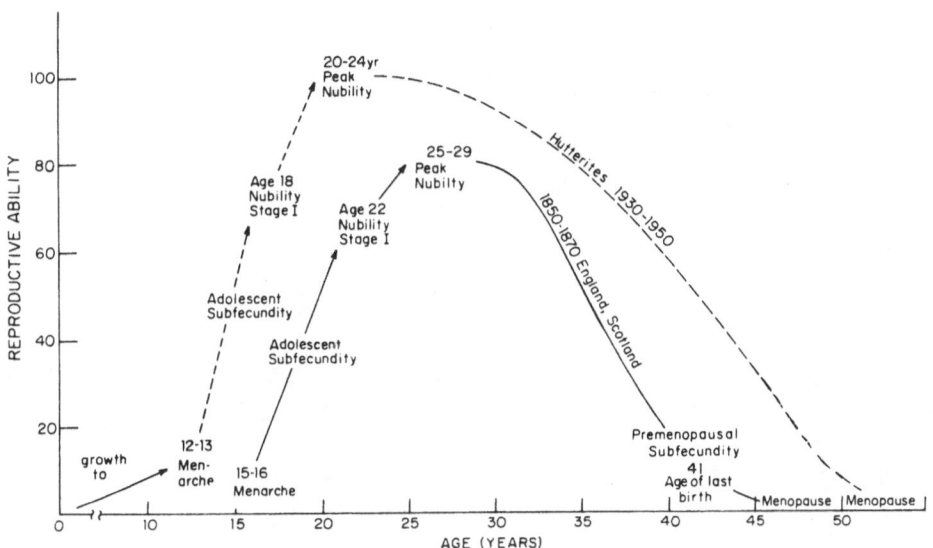

Figure 5. The mid-nineteenth century curve of female reproductive ability (variation of the rate of childbearing with age) compared to that of the well nourished, non-contracepting, modern Hutterites. Hutterite maximum fertility is taken as 100. The ages of menarche and adolescent subfecundity of the Hutterite curve are based on data for contemporary United States girls (3,4,28). The age of menopause is based on data for contemporary United States women (61). The mid-nineteenth century maximum level is scaled and timed according to historical age-specific fertility data (8). The ages of other reproductive events are based on historical data (8). The Hutterite fertility schedule results in about 10 to 12 children, depending on age of marriage; the 1850-1870 fertility schedule in about 6 to 8 children (8,18,48).

arche. This period lasted until the completion of physical growth at about age 22 years when 2) the first stage of nubility, the <u>fitness for procreation</u>, was attained. Then came the rise to the climax: 3) the <u>age of peak nubility</u>, or <u>best fitness for procreation</u>, at ages 25 to 29 years. This was the age of full physical vigor when a woman had the best chance of surviving her first birth. The curve descended gradually to 4) the <u>age of cessation of childbearing</u>, at about 40 years, and then to 5) the <u>cessation of menses</u>, the <u>menopause</u>, at about age 47 years (45,50).

The risk of maternal mortality, infant mortality and congenital deformities decreased from menarche up to the age of nubility (25 to 29 years) and then increased with the increasing age of the mother. A "turning-off" period of <u>pre-menopausal sterility</u> between

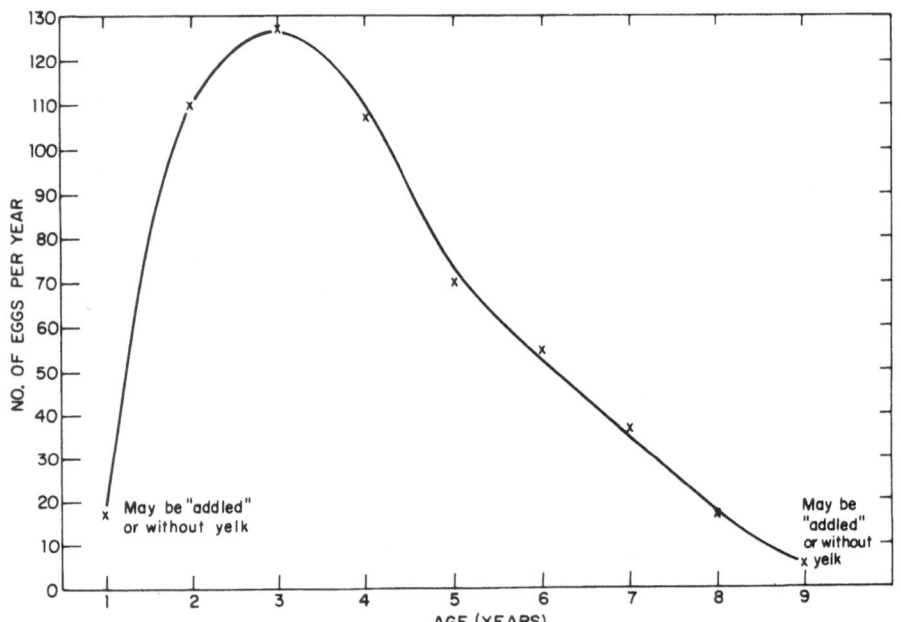

Figure 6. The number of eggs laid annually by a hen in 1865 (45). Dr. J. M. Duncan (45,48) used the 1865 hen's fertile career to illustrate the importance of nutrition on fertility. Severe under-feeding and overfeeding reduce egg laying of the hen to zero, similar to the reduction to zero of the reproductive ability of other animals, including the human female. Reproductive error, as shown by the number of "addled eggs" (45, p. 78), is greater at the beginning and end of the reproductive span for both the hen and other animals, including the human female (pregnancy wastage).

the end of childbearing and the ending of menstrual cycles, at about
age 47 years, was noted, analogous to the "turning-on" period of
adolescent sterility (1,8,48). In the mid-nineteenth century,
these periods were of about equal length, six years (50).

The fertility of women before age 30 years was more than twice
as great as after 30 years (48). Therefore, the age of marriage
could affect subsequent fertility more sharply historically than
in the modern era, when the age-specific fertility curve does not
decline so rapidly (Figure 2) (8).

Reproduction and Physical Growth

Nineteenth century doctors were aware that each reproductive
stage related to physical growth, and the coordinated growth of
the genital organs. If a female, human or cattle, is bred too
young, it is "at the expense" of the completion of normal growth
and may result in both an inferior offspring and the death of the
mother. Duncan studied the age-specific fertility data of Edinburgh
to find the age of reproduction of least risk to the mother. "If
a woman is to multiply and replenish the earth, as married women
ordinarily do, she must survive her first confinement" (48). This
was not easy in 1850-1860, since the mortality of mothers having
their first child was twice as great as that of all subsequent
births combined (48). The recommended age of marriage of 25 years
for the female was based on the survival rates from the fertility
data, and the data on the late completion of normal growth of the
uterus (about 22 years) (7) and the bony pelvis, at about 25 to 30
years (48). The interest in the changes of dimensions of the
pelvis with age is understandable since the head of the baby often
had to be crushed to save the life of the mother (51). Malforma-
tions of the pelvis were common among poor women because of rickets
(52).

Social Class Differences in Age of Menarche

The average age of menarche in mid-nineteenth century Britain
was 15.5 to 16.5 years; menarcheal age differed by social class,
upper class women having menarche 0.5 to 1 year earlier on average
than working-class women (8,26,48,50). Undernutrition and hard
living were the explanations given for the class differences and
for the great variability in age of menarche, which ranged from 10
to 26 years in the working class. A girl who did not have menarche
by age 17 or 18 years was considered in a weak state of health (50).
Girls who had menarche at 11.5 or 12.5 years were considered to be
cases of precocious puberty (53). (The average age of menarche in
the United States is now about 12.5 to 12.8 years). In accord with

Frisch and McArthur (2), the heights, weights, and body compositions of the cases in 1870 of precocious puberty (53) are similar to those observed at menarche now for normal, contemporary girls.

Norwegian data on changes in menarcheal age from about 1830 to 1930 show the disappearance of class differences in age of menarche as the average age became earlier, as would be expected with the gradual equalization of diet and mode of living among the social classes (26).

Traveling English doctors collected menarcheal data for foreign populations for comparison with local data. For example, black slave women in the West Indies, where food was poor and physical work hard, had menarche at 15.5 to 15.8 years, similar to the English working class (54).

Evidence for Subfecundity

About a quarter of the women working in the mills suffered from either "retarded or suppressed" menses. About half of all married women between the ages of 20 and 45 years were reported to have "diseases of the uterus," which included amenorrhea (50,55). Leucorrhea, the "whites," and its cure is a standard topic in medical texts (55). Prolapsed uterus was another common problem among women of all social classes (50,56).

The main causes given for amenorrhea were those which "impair the constitutional tone and impoverish the blood": poor diet, disease, particularly tuberculosis and chlorosis (anemia), unsuitable employment, and cold and damp. Doctors noted that working class women were underweight and amenorrheic because of poverty; upper class women because of their desire to be fashionably thin (55). Stress ("violent fits of passion") was also noted as a cause of amenorrhea (50).

The Incidence of Absolute Sterility

Absolute sterility (no children by three years after marriage) occurred in 15 percent of the 16,301 married women of ages 15 to 44 years in the Edinburgh study (48). Other English surveys show about 10 percent sterility (48). Among upper class marriages, Ansell reports that 8 percent were childless and 7 percent had only one child (57). The modern Hutterite wife has a 2 percent incidence of absolute sterility (58).

The Length of Birth Intervals

Lactation (nursing) was regarded as the regulator of the birth interval in the human female (59). The length of the birth interval in turn determined the ultimate size of the family and the health of the mother and child (48,59). The average birth interval for working class and lower middle class women was about 20 to 24 months (59). This and much higher levels (up to 36 months) is characteristic of underfed women today (14). This time interval included unsuccessful pregnancies, which averaged about 1.5 for each woman (48). It was already observed, however, that the birth interval became longer as the mother became older: fecundity is proportional to the number of years a woman's age is under 50 (Tait's Law) (60). It was also observed that women "low in fecundity" bred at greater intervals at all ages, beginning with the first birth (48,57).

Age of Menopause

The average age of menopause in about 1850 was between 45 and 50 years (45). "Intelligent" women in Manchester and York finished childbearing at 41.7 years and had menopause at 47.5 years (50). These ages are considerably earlier than that of present day Hutterite women, some of whom still have births at ages 45 to 49 years (16,58). The average age of menopause for present day women is now about 50 years or later (61). The mean age of cessation of childbearing for Ansell's upper class women was age 38 years (57). This earlier age than that of lower middle class women may indicate the use of contraception by the better nourished upper class women. An alternate explanation is that the age of marriage of upper class men was so late (age 30) that by the time their wives were age 40 years, frequency of coitus was low (62).

The Average Completed Family Size

The Scottish mothers married at age 25 and living with spouses to the end of their reproductive lives had about 7 to 8 children. The fertility of the Scottish women was higher than that of the English lower socioeconomic class. In St. Georges-in-the-East, a poor part of London, the average number of children "consequent of the prolific marriages" was 5.3 (48).

Upper class spinsters married to bachelors at a mean age of 25 years and living in fruitful wedlock until the end of the childbearing period, had a total of 5.7 children (57).

Male Reproductive Ability

The historical male curve of reproductive ability is more speculative than that of the female, but the time of beginning and the peak are reasonably well estimated from the height data on peak velocity and completion of growth, and the relation to the female ages (4,25,26). Routh gives the age of peak fecundity in males in about 1850 as 31 to 33 years (Figure 7) compared to about age 26 years for the female (63).

Differential Growth Among the Social Classes

The physical growth and development of the poorer economic classes differed significantly from that of the upper classes (64-66) (Figure 8). The growth data show that the well fed and "most favoured" class (I) were taller and attained final height sooner than the ill fed and "least favoured" of the community. Most men of the lower social classes did not complete growth until ages 23 to 25 years; even upper class men were relatively late, 21 to 23

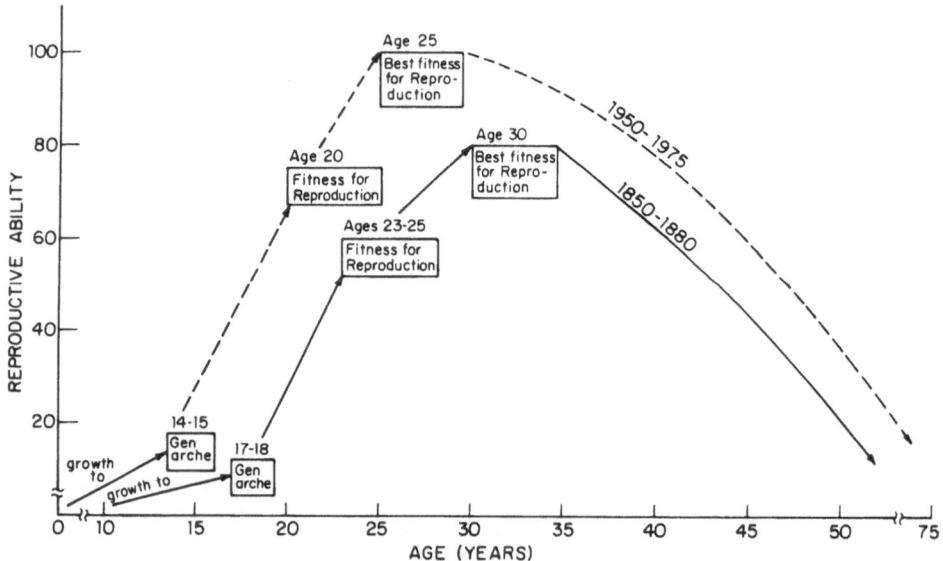

Figure 7. Hypothetical curves of male reproductive ability (pro-creative power) for modern males and males in 1850-1870, based on ages of peak height velocity, completion of height growth and hormonal data for modern males and the relation to ages of menarche of the female in Figure 5. Adapted from Frisch (8).

years (64) compared to the present age of completion, age 18 to 20 years, for well nourished males (4). Women did not complete height growth until about age 20-21 years (64), compared to 16-18 years today (4).

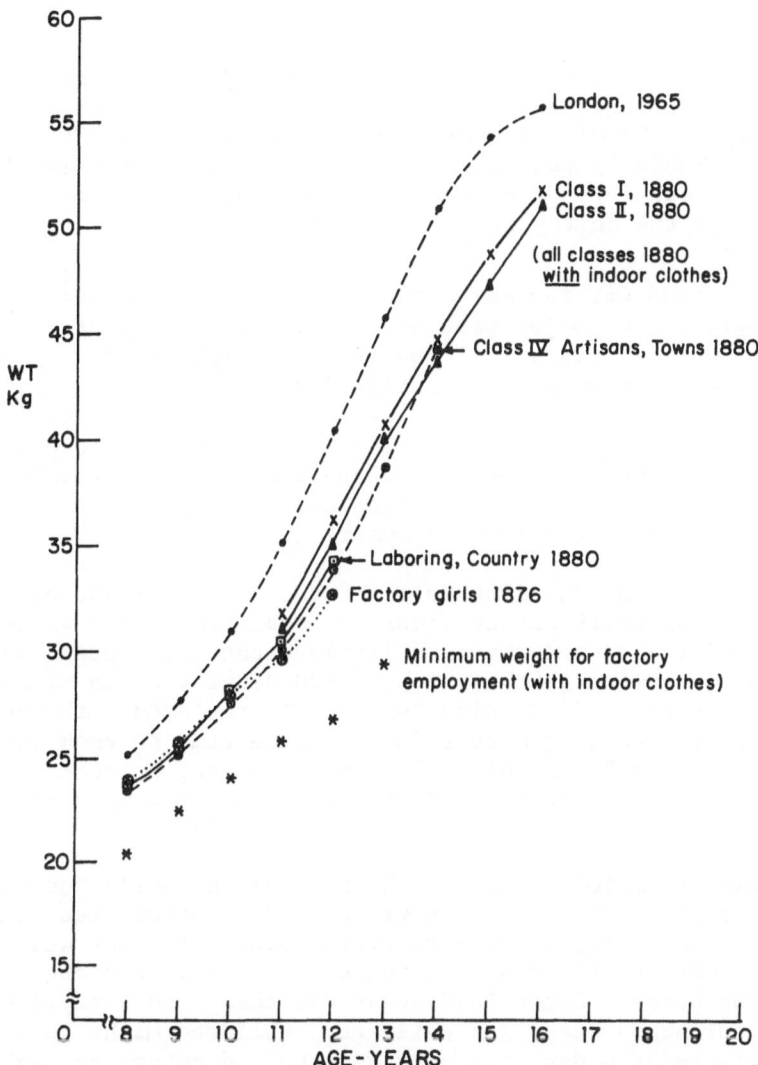

Figure 8. Body weight by age for British girls of different social classes in 1876, in 1880, and in 1965. The 1876 and 1880 weights include indoor clothing and clogs or shoes. The minimum weights for factory employment (1876) (66) also included clothes. From Frisch (8). Reprinted with permission from Science, in press, 1977.

The committee noted the "check which growth receives as we
descend lower and lower in the social scale" (64). Not surprisingly, children who worked in factories had the slowest growth and
hence latest sexual maturation of any of the groups studied
(Figure 8).

Food Intake by Social Class

One of the reasons physical growth differed so markedly by
social class in the 19th century in Britain was that the quantity
and quality of the diet differed by social class (8). The laboring
class diet (Table 4) was judged "inadequate for health and strength"
(67) up to about 1870 when cheap grain and meat began to arrive in
quantity from the United States (68,69).

Wheat bread was the main constituent of the working class
diet, supplying the major part of the calories and most of the
protein of working class families (Table 4) (67). In very poor
families bread was almost the entire diet, supplemented with small
amounts of butter, bacon, cheese and tea (68). Wheat was a symbol
of social status and potatoes were at first resisted, especially by
agricultural workers. However, the potato became increasingly
important in the diet of all working class groups after 1815, when
bread became relatively more expensive (70).

The quality of the diet deteriorated in the middle of the
19th century as white patent flour was substituted for whole wheat
bread, tea for ale, and jam or a little bacon for cheese (68,69).
In Scotland, oatmeal which was cheap and usually eaten with milk,
making a nutritious diet, also began to be replaced with bread and
jam because the working mother did not have time to cook oatmeal.
Broth, another Scotch stable, also took too long to cook. The
economic development of Scotland was therefore accompanied by a
decline in nutrition for the working class (71).

Nutrition varied within the working class family, as well as
between classes. The male breadwinner had a better diet than the
children or the wife, who had the worst diet. If meat was available, most went to the husband; the wife and children ate the
dripping on bread. After 1840 sugar was cheap and treacle became
a common spread on bread for children. Children might have bread
and treacle twice a day, and perhaps a boiled potato or cabbage
smeared with bacon fat. Sunday dinner was the best meal, especially in the towns where fried fish, black pudding or sheeps'
trotters were available. In rural areas milk was used freely for
tea, but in towns the whole supply of milk per family was only one-
fourth to one-half pint daily (67). Working class infants were
often fed on "sops," (bread, water and sugar) especially if the

Table 4

Foods Consumed Weekly by the Laboring Classes in About 1860(a)

	Bread, Flour and Other Farinaceous Foods	Sugar or Treacle	Butter Dripping or Suet	Bacon or Meat	Milk	Cheese	Tea
			Grams				
Agricultural workers in own homes	5,594	208	156	454	907	157	14
Silk weavers Kid glovers Stocking weavers Shoemakers	4,309	227	142	383	510	-	21
Needlewomen	3,515	206	128	425	199	-	21

(a) A person over age 10 or two persons below age 10.

Source: Smith, E. Practical Dietary for families, schools and the laboring classes. London 1865, based on Dr. Smith's Reports to the Privy Council, 1862, 1863. (Pounds and ounces converted to grams).

mother worked away from home. Upper class infants were usually nursed. If a mother could not nurse, a wet nurse who "was and is well-fed" was recommended. Upper class infants were weaned onto milk and other high quality protein foods (67).

The middle and upper socioeconomic classes in Britain ate more meat and other varied foods and less bread than the working class. The adults and older youth ate much as well-off people do today, with perhaps more little meals of bread, butter, and milk. Eggs, vegetables and meat were included daily in the diet.

An important factor in the poor nutrition of the working classes was the lack of facilities for cooking hot foods. Ovens and cast iron ranges were only owned by the upper classes; even cooking pots were too expensive (67) until the invention of the hydraulic press (72). Bakers provided hot pies and tarts in addition to bread. Some rural areas lacked fuel for cooking and a hot meal was eaten only once or twice a week (57). By about 1880 in cities, the pennymeter brought a rise in the use of the gas cooker (72).

Dr. Smith also gave an estimate of the energy output of a worker: he estimated that a person attending a spinning mill walked or ran 1.3 miles per hour (67).

The 19th Century Controversy on the Fall in the Birth Rate

These biological facts and views were involved in the turn of the century controversy on the reasons for the fall in the birth rate in England (8,73-75). The argument was, as today: does low fertility necessarily imply the use of contraception? In the middle of the 19th century, marital fertility did not differ significantly among the social classes or occupations, but the similarity had different causes for the upper and lower classes (8).

The fall in fertility which began in England after 1870 did not affect all classes equally: the fall "affected social strata from the top downwards in a rapidly decreasing degree" (73). Therefore, by the turn of the century fertility differed by social class and occupation (73-75). The rich were probably practicing the prevention of childbearing but among the poor "the practice is almost unknown." Poverty and not "prudential action" was the cause of the relatively low birth rate of the poor. The mass of the population were intermediate in both birth rate and the use of contraceptive practice (75).

The Cost of Contraceptives

The contraceptive devices available before about 1880 were of the ineffective variety and expensive. An effective male device, a reliable condom, was not available in England until about 1880 when new processes of manufacture and vulcanization were used. Effective female devices, diaphrams and pessaries, also became available with the advances in rubber manufacture (8,76). The cost of these devices, however, makes it improbable that they were used by the working classes. Condoms cost 2 to 10 shillings a dozen; rubber pessaries from 2 to 5 shillings each (70). The staple of the diet, a four pound loaf of bread, cost about 7 pence (8).

Less effective methods were equally expensive, relative to the cost of bread. The contraceptive sponge, recommended by A. Besant in her Law of Population (56), cost one shilling each. Soluble quinine pessaries cost 2 shillings a dozen in about 1890 (76).

SUMMARY AND CONCLUSIONS

A short and less efficient reproductive span due to poor nutrition, hard physical work, poor living conditions can explain the relatively small completed family size of the lower socioeconomic classes in about 1850-1860 in Britain.

The relatively late age of menarche and late attainment of adult height of even upper class girls and boys compared to contemporary well fed children (4) suggests that some submaximum fecundity in combination with a late age of marriage may have contributed also to the small completed family size of the upper classes in 1850. A late age of marriage would have placed most of the childbearing years in the period of declining female and male fecundity. The historical decrease of fecundity with age was more rapid because of the partial subfecundity (8).

One cannot disprove the use of coitus-interruptus as the explanation of the observed lower fertility of both the lower and upper classes. However, the physical and reproductive data provide an alternate explanation, especially for the lower socioeconomic classes (8).

Undernutrition, instead of the widespread use of folk contraception, may also be the explanation of the completed family size of 6 to 7 children found in many developing countries today, as has already been suggested (7,14,21,22). If so, the nutrition programs necessary for a vigorous, productive society should be closely integrated with family planning programs, for the well-being of the mother, the child and the society (7,22). The need for family planning programs also may be much greater than realized heretofore.

If subfecundity is the main reason for relatively low observed fertility in the 19th century, a reasonable question is: who was using the many methods of contraception devised during human history (76,77)? The data suggest that only females (and males) who were well nourished, and hence fully fecund, whose reproductive ability exceeded their aspirations for offspring, would have used contraception. This would be a small percent of the population: the relatively well fed aristocracy (76) especially when they used wet nurses; the wet nurses themselves since pregnancy would affect their ability to nurse; and prostitutes whose aspirations of fertility were zero (8).

Questions for Future Research

Finally, the 19th century data raise some fundamental bio- logical questions. The fact that undernourished human beings and animals are less fecund than well nourished populations can be regarded as an ecological adaptation to reduced food supplies of the environment and of obvious advantage to the population. It is a less wasteful mechanism than the regulation of overpopulation by mortality. But, by what mechanism is a slower rate of growth of females and males within a population related to a subsequent shorter and less efficient reproductive span? Why is late menarche in a population usually associated with an earlier menopause, with long lactation intervals, and with higher pregnancy wastage (22)? Are there exceptions in some environments to these associated events? How much is reversible after growth is completed (8)?

Recent experiments with rats on high-fat and low-fat diets suggest that the estrogen levels were higher in the high-fat diet rats (34,35). The well nourished human female and male, particu- larly on diets with a high percentage of calories from fat, also may have higher endocrine levels, which result in high reproductive efficiency (8).

ACKNOWLEDGEMENTS

The preparation of this paper was supported by Biomedical Research Grant 5-S07-2RR-05446-15, NIH. The historical data are from research supported by The Population Council Grant #D74.94C.

References

1. Brillat-Savarin, A. Quoted in Brody, S., <u>Bioenergetics and Growth</u>, New York: Reinhold, 1945.

2. Frisch, R. E. and McArthur, J. W. Menstural Cycles: Fatness as a Determinant of Minimum Weight for Height Necessary for their Maintenance or Onset. <u>Science</u> <u>185</u>: 949, 1974.

3. Frisch, R. E. Fatness of Girls from Menarche to Age 18 Years, with a Nomogram. <u>Human Biol</u>. <u>48</u>: 353, 1976.

4. Frisch, R. E. The Critical Weight at Menarche and the Initiation of the Adolescent Growth Spurt and the Control of Puberty. In: <u>The Control of the Onset of Puberty</u>. Grumbach, M. M., Grave, G., Mayer, F., Wiley, New York, 1974.

5. Frisch, R. E., Revelle, R. and Cook, S. Components of the Critical Weight at Menarche and at Initiation of the Adolescent Spurt: Estimated Total Water, Lean Body Mass and Fat. <u>Human Biol</u>. <u>45</u>: 469, 1973.

6. Frisch, R. E. Food Intake, Fatness and Reproductive Ability. In: <u>Anorexia Nervosa</u>, R. Vigersky (ed.), Raven, New York. In press.

7. Frisch, R. E. Demographic Implications of the Biological Determinants of Female Fecundity. <u>Social Biology</u> <u>22</u>: 17, 1975.

8. Frisch, R. E. Population, Food Intake and Fertility: Historical Evidence for a Direct Effect of Nutrition on Reproductive Ability. <u>Science</u>, in press, 1977.

9. Darwin, C. <u>The Variation of Animals and Plants under Domestication</u>, 1868. New York: D. Appleton & Co., 2nd ed., Vol. 2, 1894.

10. Darwin, C. <u>Origin of Species</u>, ed. 1 facsimile (1859). Harvard University Press, Cambridge, Mass., 1975.

11. Wrigley, E. A. <u>Population and History</u>. Weidenfeld and Nicolson, London, 1969.

12. Glass, D. V. Fertility and Population Growth. <u>J. Roy. Stat. Soc.</u> <u>129</u>: 210, 1966.

13. Brass, W. Population Size and Complex Communities, with a Consideration of World Population. In: Population and Its Problems: A Plain Man's Guide, Parry, H. B. (ed.), Clarendon Press, 1974.

14. Chen, L. C., Ahmed, S., Gesche, M., and Mosley, W. H. A Prospective Study of Birth Interval Dynamics in Rural Bangladesh. Population Studies 28: 277, 1974.

15. Coale, A. J. The Growth and Structure of Human Populations: A Mathematical Investigation. Princeton University Press, Princeton, N. H., 1972.

16. Eaton, J. W. and Mayer, A. J. The Social Biology of Very High Fertility Among the Hutterites: The Demography of a Unique Population. Human Biol. 25: 206, 1953.

17. Dumond, D. E. The Limitation of Human Population: A Natural History. Science 187: 713, 1975.

18. Henry, L. Some Data on Natural Fertility. Eugenics Quarterly 8: 81, 1961.

19. Coale, A. J. The History of the Human Population. Scientific American 231: 40, 1974.

20. Carr-Saunders, A. M. The Population Problem, 1922. Clarendon, Oxford (reprinted by Arno Press, New York, 1974).

21. Mauldin, W. P. The Population of India: Policy, Action, and Research. Economic Digest 3: 14, 1960.

22. Gopalan, C. and Naidu, A. N. Nutrition and Fertility. Lancet 2: 1077, 1972

23. Bishop, M. W. H. Aging and Reproduction in the Male. J. Reprod. Fert., Suppl. 12: 65, 1970.

24. Keys, A., Brožek, J., Henschel, A., Mickelsen, O., Taylor, H. L. The Biology of Human Starvation. University of Minnesota Press, Minneapolis, Vol. 1, 1950.

25. Frisch, R. E. and Revelle, R. Variations in Body Weights and the Age of the Adolescent Growth Spurt among Latin American and Asian Populations in Relation to Calorie Supplies. Human Biol. 41: 536, 1969.

26. Kiil, V. Stature and Growth of Norwegian Men During the Past Two Hundred Years. Skr. norske VidenskAkad. 2: 1, 1939.

27. Frisch, R. E. Weight at Menarche: Similarity for Well-nourished and Under-nourished Girls at Differing Ages, and Evidence for Historical Constancy. Pediat. 50: 445, 1972.

28. Frisch, R. E. and Revelle, R. Height and Weight at Menarche and a Hypothesis of Critical Body Weights and Adolescent Events. Science 169: 397, 1970.

29. Frisch, R. E. and Revelle, R. Height and Weight at Menarche and a Hypothesis of Menarche. Arch. Dis. Childh. 46: 695, 1971.

30. Frisch, R. E. The Physiological Basis of Reproductive Efficiency. In: Meat Animals, Growth and Reproductivity, Lister, D., Rhodes, D. N., Fowler, V. R., and Fuller, M. F. (eds.). New York and London: Plenum Press, 1976.

31. Dickerson, J. W. T., Gresham, G. A., and McCance, R. A. The Effect of Undernutrition and Rehabilitation on the Development of the Reproductive Organs: Pigs. J. Endocrin. 29: 111, 1964.

32. Hammond, Jr., J., Mason, I. L., and Robinson, T. J. (eds.) Hammond's Farm Animals. Arnold, London, ed. 4, 1971.

33. Kennedy, G. C. and Mitra, J. Body Weight and Food Intake as Initiating Factors for Puberty in the Rat. J. Physiol. 166: 408, 1963.

34. Frisch, R. E., Hegsted, D. M., and Yoshinaga, K. Body Weight and Food Intake at Early Estrus of Rats on a High-Fat Diet. Proc. Nat. Acad. Sci. U.S.A. 72: 4172, 1975.

35. Frisch, R. E., Hegsted, D. M. and Yoshinaga, K. Carcass Components at First Estrus of Rats on High-Fat and Low-Fat Diets: Body Water, Protein and Fat. Proc. Nat. Acad. Sci. U.S.A., in press, 1977.

36. Mellits, E. D. and Cheek, D. B. The Assessment of Body Water and Fatness from Infancy to Childhood. Mongr. Soc. Res. Child. Devel. 35: 12, 1970.

37. Moore, F. K., Olesen, H., McMurrey, J. D., Parker, V., Ball, M. R. and Boyden, C. M. The Body Cell Mass and Its Supporting Environment. Philadelphia: Sauders, 1963.

38. Frisch, R. E. Critical Weights, a Critical Body Composition, Menarche, and the Maintenance of Menstual Cycles. In: Biosocial Interrelations in Population Adaptation, Watts, E. S., Johnston, F. E., Lasker, G. W. (eds.), Mouton, The Hague, 1975.

39. Friis-Hansen, B. J. Changes in Body Water Compartments During Growth. <u>Acta Paediat.</u>, <u>Suppl. 110</u>: 1, 1956.

40. Frisch, R. E. A Method of Prediction of Menarche from Height and Weight at Age 9-13 Years. <u>Pediatrics</u> <u>53</u>: 384, 1974.

41. Frisch, R. E. Does Malnutrition Cause Permanent Mental Retardation in Human Beings? <u>Psychiatria, Neurologia, Neurochirurgia</u> <u>74</u>: 463, 1971.

42. Sargent, D. Weight-Height Relationship of Young Men and Women. <u>Am. J. Clin. Nut.</u> <u>13</u>: 318, 1963.

43. Matsumoto, S., Ozawa, M. and Nogami, Y. Menstrual Cycle in Puberty. <u>Gunma J. Med. Sciences</u> <u>12</u>: 119, 1963.

44. Malthus, T. R. <u>An Essay on the Principle of Population.</u> Flew, A. (ed.) ed. 1 facsimile (1798) ed. 2 facsimile (1830), Penguin Books, Baltimore, 1970.

45. Duncan, J. M. <u>On Sterility in Women</u> (Gulstonian Lectures, 1883). Blakiston, Son & Co., Philadelphia, 1884.

46. Hollick, F. <u>Diseases of Woman: Their Causes and Cure Familiarly Explained</u>. T. W. Strong, New York, ed. 49, 1847.

47. Gardner, A. K. <u>The Causes and Curative Treatment of Sterility</u>. DeWitt and Davenport, New York, 1856.

48. Duncan, J. M. <u>Fecundity, Fertility, Sterility, and Allied Topics</u>. Adam & Charles Black, Edinburgh, ed. 2, 1871.

49. Montagu, M.F.A. <u>The Reproductive Development of the Female</u>. Julian Press, Inc., New York, 1957.

50. Whitehead, J. <u>On the Causes and Treatment of Abortion and Sterility</u>. John Churchill, London, 1847.

51. Gardner, A. K. In: <u>A Course of Lectures on Obstetrics</u>. Smith, W. T., Robert M. DeWitt, New York, ed. 3, 1858.

52. McHenry, E. W. <u>Basic Nutrition.</u> J. B. Lippincott Co., Philadelphia, 1963.

53. Harris, R. P. Early Puberty. <u>Am. J. Obstet.</u> <u>3</u>: 611, 1871.

54. Roberton, J. On the Period of Puberty in the Negro. <u>Edinburgh Med. Surg. J.</u> <u>69</u>: 69, 1848.

55. Smith, W. T. Pathology and Treatment of Leucorrhaea.
    John Churchill, London, 1855.

56. Besant, A. The Law of Population: Its Consequences, and Its
    Bearing upon Human Conduct and Morals. Freethought Publishing
    Co., London, ed. 1884.

57. Ansell, Jr., C. On the Rate of Mortality, the Age at Marriage,
    the Number of Children to a Marriage, the Length of a Genera-
    tion and Other Statistics of Families in the Upper and
    Professional Classes. Layton, London, 1874.

58. Sheps, M. C. An Analysis of Reproductive Patterns in an
    American Isolate. Population Studies 19: 65, 1965-1966.

59. Roberton, J. Essays and Notes on the Physiology and Diseases
    of Women and on Practical Midwifery. John Churchill, London,
    1851.

60. Tait, P. G. In: Part VI, Duncan, J. M., Fecundity, Fertility,
    Sterility, and Allied Topics. Adam & Charles Black, Edinburgh,
    ed. 2, 1871.

61. MacMahon, B. and Worcester, J. Age at Menopause. National
    Center for Health Statistics, Series 11, No. 19, Washington,
    D.C., 1966.

62. Anderson, B. A. Male Age and Fertility: Results from Ireland
    Prior to 1911. Population Index 41: 561, 1975.

63. Routh, C. H. F. On Procreative Power. London J. of Med. 2:
    240, 1850.

64. Galton, F. Report of the Fifty-third Meeting of the British
    Association for the Advancement of Science, Anthropometric
    Committee, 1883. John Murray, London, 1884.

65. Roberts, C. A Manual of Anthropometry. John Churchill,
    London, 1878.

66. Roberts, C. The Physical Requirements of Factory Children.
    J. Stat. Soc. London 39: 681, 1876.

67. Smith, E. Practical Dietary for Families, Schools, and the
    Labouring Classes. Walton and Maberly, London, 1865.

68. Burnett, J. In: Our Changing Fare. Barker, T. C., McKenzie,
    J. C., Yudkin, J. (eds.), MacGibbon Kee, London, 1966.

69. Drummond, J. C. and Wilbraham, A. The Englishman's Food, 1939, Jonathan Cape, London, ed. 1958.

70. Salaman, R. N. The History and Social Influence of the Potato. Cambridge University Press, Cambridge, 1949.

71. Campbell, R. H. In: Our Changing Fare. Barker, T. C., McKenzie, J. C., Yudkin, J. (eds.), MacGibbon & Kee, London, 1966.

72. McNamee, B. In: Our Changing Fare. Barker, T. C., McKenzie, J. C., Yudkin, J. (eds.), MacGibbon & Kee, London, 1966.

73. Yule, G. U. The Fall of the Birth-Rate. Cambridge University Press, Cambridge, 1920.

74. Yule, G. U. On the Changes in the Marriage and Birth-rates in England and Wales during the Past Half Century; With an Inquiry as to their Probable Causes. J. Roy. Stat. Soc. 69: 88, 1906.

75. Newsholme, A. and Stevenson, T. H. C. The Decline of Human Fertility in the United Kingdom and Other Countries as Shown by Corrected Birth-rates. J. Roy. Stat. Soc. 69: 34, 1906.

76. Peel, J. The Manufacture and Retailing of Contraceptives in England. Population Studies 17: 113, 1963.

77. Himes, N. E. Charles Knowlton's Revolutionary Influence on the English Birth Rate. New Eng. J. Med. 199: 461, 1928.

FAMINE AND FERTILITY

Zena Stein and Mervyn Susser

Columbia University

New York, New York

INTRODUCTION

This paper will be concerned with "famine" rather than "malnutrition." "Famine," according to the Oxford English Dictionary, is "a period of extreme and general scarcity of food." The starvation is extreme, population-wide, and limited in time. Famine is an acute episode which, if continued for long enough, will terminate in death of the population. People experience a sensation of hunger, gnawing hunger, day and night. There are psychological manifestations (irritability and apathy), anti-social behavior (suspiciousness, aggressiveness, finally cannibalism), illnesses (infections, famine oedema, osteomalacia) and death (which comes sooner to men and to those at the extremes of life than to women and the middle-aged). In the newborn, there is a reduction in mean birth weight and a decrease in viability. There is finally a reduction in fertility that can become absolute. Once food becomes available, recovery in the population is rapid.

If famine is superimposed on a poorly nourished population as in the Sahel, the transition from chronic malnutrition to starvation may be ill defined and present a problem of definition (1). In the Dutch famine of 1944-45 (2,3), which we discuss in this paper, there is no such problem. This society was not at the margin of survival before and after the famine, either in the health and physiological characteristics of the population, or in its values and mores. These conditions made the effects on fertility distinct. At the same time, they should deter us from facile generalizations extrapolated to populations chronically suffering from malnutrition.

Famines have been part of human history since the earliest
times, and are described on Egyptian papyrus and in the Old
Testament. Keys, Brozek et al. (4) have a historical chapter
listing famines by year and place and referencing the historians
who have described them up to 1933. More recently (5), the account
has been brought up to date. Famines were commonly associated with
war, as in the Dutch famine, or equally often, with natural disasters. A natural disaster, the potato blight in Ireland in the
middle of the last century, precipitated the famine that so influenced American history (6,7). In modern times, small scattered
communities and groups like the Australian aborigines and the
Eskimos suffer episodes of acute food deprivation fairly frequently,
and it is not unusual for whole groups to perish at these times.

Although the circumstances leading to famines are well documented, it has been more difficult to document their effects,
including any systematic effect on the birth rate. Notable exceptions are the account by Valaoras (8) of the effect of the famine
in Greece in 1941-42, on births, deaths, and child growth; and that
by Antonov (9) on the effects of the siege of Leningrad in 1942 on
fertility and perinatal morbidity and mortality, and that by Smith
(10) on the Dutch famine of 1944-45.

We will discuss the Dutch famine of 1944-45 (known as the
"Hongerwinter") in some detail, believing it to be the most fully
analyzed in respect to fertility.

THE DUTCH FAMINE OF 1944-45

Historical Background

The Dutch famine was a tragic final episode in the long wartime ordeal of the Netherlands people during World War II. In
September 1944, an ambitious but unsuccessful attempt was made by
the Allies to establish a bridgehead over the Rhine. A dramatic
account of this endeavor (nicknamed "Operation Breadbasket") is
given in "A Bridge Too Far" (11). The Dutch railworkers in the
Nazi occupied territories responded to the call of their government-
in-exile for a strike. For this brave action they paid heavily,
for when the military offensive failed the Nazi command retaliated
by imposing an embargo on the movement of all goods including foodstuffs. No food could be imported into the cities from rural
supply areas. There followed an early and severe winter that froze
the barges in the canals, aggravating the food crisis. There was
a general, severe, and acute deprivation of food (12,13,14). For
six months, from November 1944 to the end of April 1945, the situation continued grave. Then, in the first week of May the Allied

armies crossed the Rhine, liberated the Western Netherlands, and relieved the famine (15,16,17). By the end of May, food relief had reached most of the affected population. Figure 1 shows these time relations, grouping conceptions, gestation and births in relation to the period of the famine.

The main impact of the famine was suffered by the large cities of the West: Amsterdam, Rotterdam, 's-Gravenhage (The Hague), Leiden, Delft, Haarlem and Utrecht (Figure 2). By its nature, the famine affected cities rather than the rural areas which grew their own food. The country south of the Rhine was occupied by the Allied armies and not exposed to the "Hongerwinter." The towns of the East and North were liberated earlier and had easier access to food even before the liberation. The geographic distribution of the famine thus enables us to designate "famine" cities and "control" cities in our design (2).

Data Sources Relating to Fertility (1944-1946)

These stem from three sources. First, we used the birth registrations from the 16 study* cities. Second, we used records from the military induction procedures, covering virtually all 18 year old male survivors living in the Netherlands. Since these were acquired independently from the birth registrations, they served as a supplementary source, and a check on validity. Third, we used the records from five large maternity hospitals. We also refer en passant to conclusions based on a study of death notifications. Each of these sources is described in detail, with the full account of the effects on development of those conceived or born during the famine period in the book: "Famine and Human Development: The Dutch Hunger Winter of 1944-1945" (2).

Data Sources Relating to Diet (1944-1946)

The average calories (as well as proteins, carbohydrates and fats) provided in the daily food rations were estimated from official sources (Figure 3). Rations were uniform across the country up to the period September 1944, and again they were similar after July 1945. The diet in the Western Netherlands was demons-

---

* The famine cities were: Amsterdam, Rotterdam, The Hague, Haarlem, Leiden and Utrecht; the northern control cities were: Groningen, Leeuwaarden, Zwolle, Enschede and Hengelo; the Southern control cities were: Breda, Tilburg, Eindhoven, Heerlen and Maastricht. For two cities (Rotterdam and Hengelo) there was an 18 month gap in the population register; estimates based on the inducted population were substituted.

trably reduced relative to other areas for the defined period of
the Hongerwinter, and not otherwise. Apart from the record of the
rations, the nutritional relief team carried out sample surveys of
the recent diet of many individuals (17). The documentation of
the food intake is therefore remarkably systematic and rich, considering the disasterous circumstances.

THE EFFECTS OF THE FAMINE ON BIRTH RATE

Decline in Births: Comparison by Time and Place

In the famine area, a distinct fall in the number of births
is evident, beginning nine months after the onset of acute starvation (which we consider to be mid-October 1944) (Table 1). Our
study of maternities shows that no great error follows from the

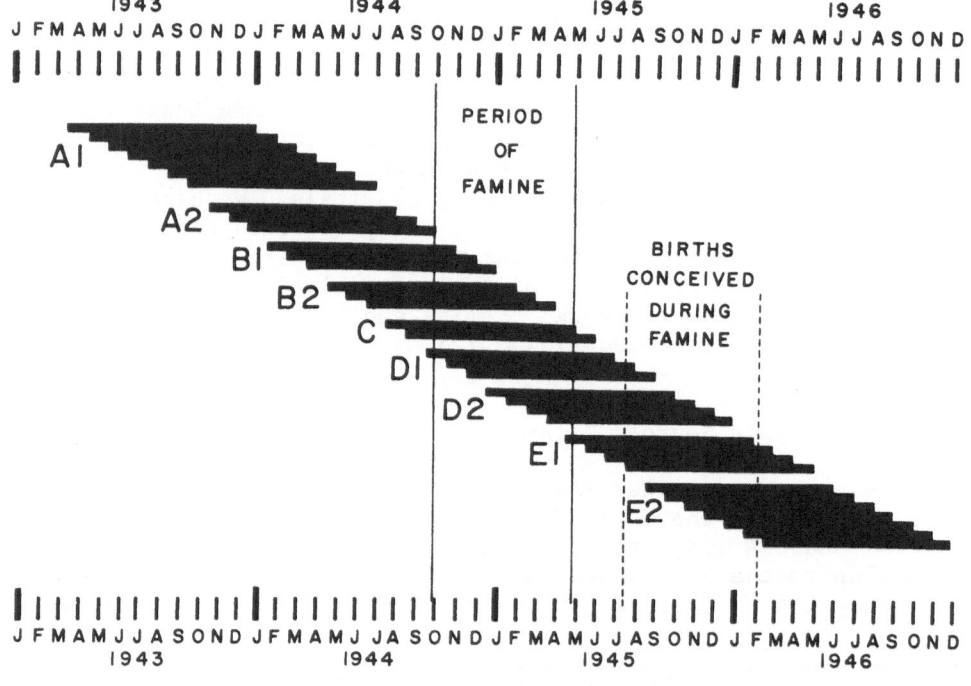

Figure 1. Design of Study. Cohorts by month of conception and
month of birth, in the Netherlands, 1943 through 1946, related to
famine exposure. Solid vertical lines bracket the period of
famine, and broken vertical lines bracket the period of births
conceived during famine.

assumption which we make in assigning dates of conception by usual
length of gestation. Thus, among births conceived early in the
famine during November-December 1944, there was a slight decline
in numbers; among births conceived in January 1945, there was a
moderate decline; among births conceived late in the famine and at
its most severe, from February through April 1945, there was a
marked decline. The famine was relieved on May 7, 1945, and the
number of conceptions must have risen almost immediately. Births

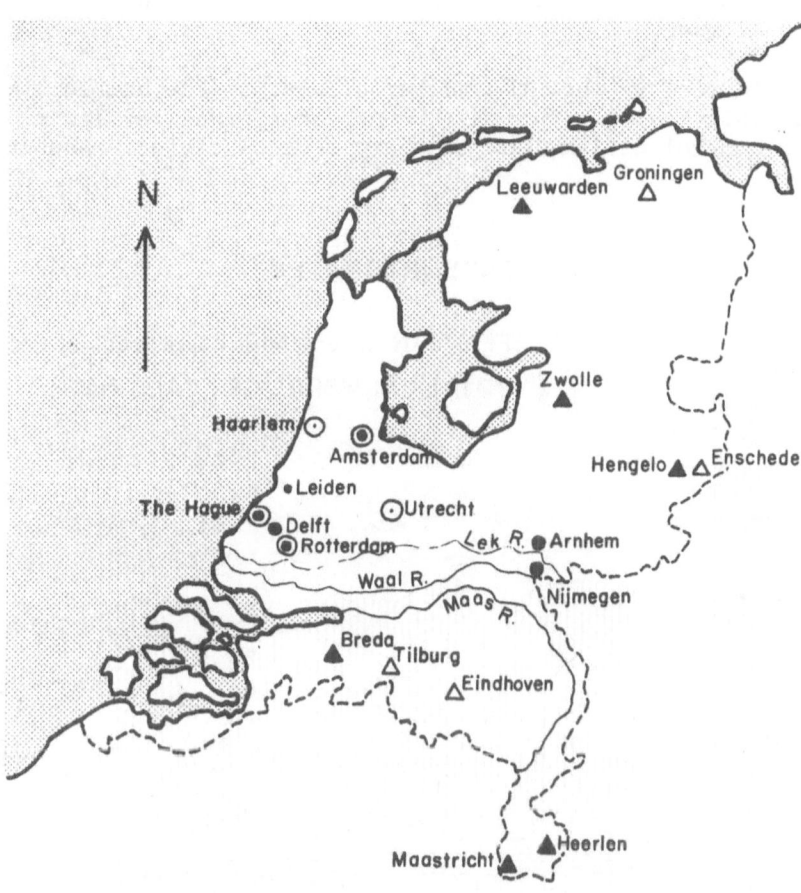

Figure 2. The Netherlands.

- ◉ Famine city above 500,000 population
- ☉ Famine city 100,000 - 500,000 population
- • Famine city 40,000 - 100,000 population
- △ Control city 100,000 - 500,000 population
- ▲ Control city 40,000 - 100,000 population
- ● Eligible to study but omitted

following conceptions in the period as soon as the fourth to eighth
week after the famine (June 1945) had restored numbers to the pre-
famine level and, temporarily, even higher.

The official rations declined to below 1500 calories daily
in September 1944, but not before November does a decrease in subsequent births reflect infertility in the cohort of conceptions.
This asynchromy of onset of famine and infertility suggests that
it took some time to exhaust the nutritional resources of couples.
By contrast, with relief of the famine recovery of fertility was
immediate. It seems that with the provision of nutrients, the
preconditions of fertility (sexual activity and fecundity) were
restored at once.

In Figure 4 we show the number of births (the broken line) and
the mean daily caloric ration (the unbroken line) for famine cities,
northern control cities, and southern control cities, respectively.

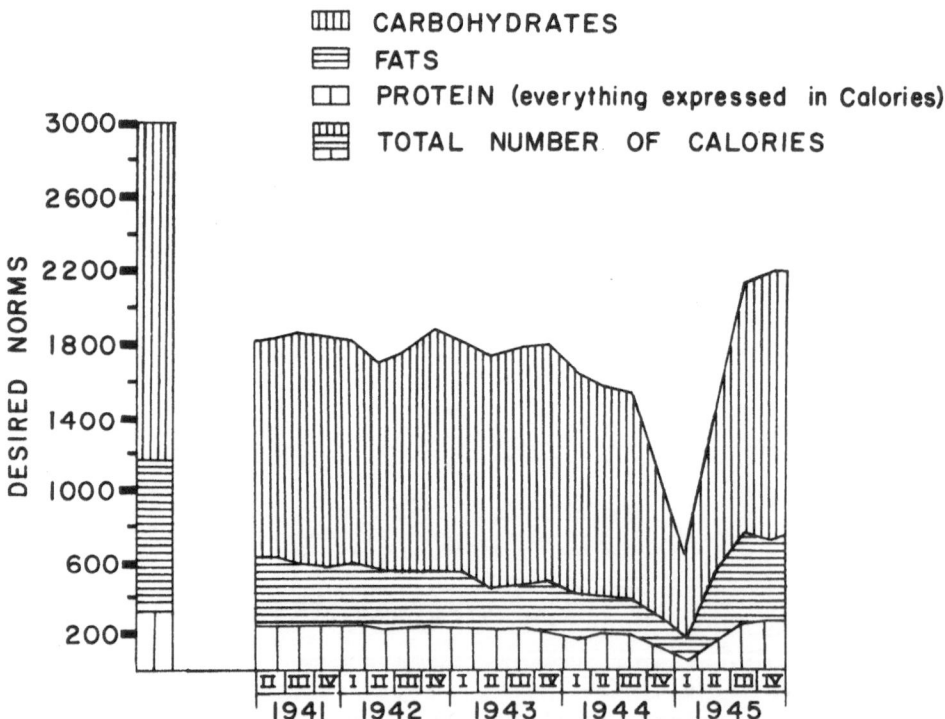

Figure 3. Average quarterly distribution of food rations in
calories, protein, fats and carbohydrates in the Western Netherlands, 1941 through 1945 (Burger, Drummond and Sandstead (1948).

Table 1
Numbers of Conceptions Ending in Live and Still Births
by Place of Birth and Estimated Month of Conception,
and Sex Ratio for Live Births Only

Estimated Mo. of Conception Beginning With	Famine Area		North Control		South Control	
	All Births	Sex Ratio	All Births	Sex Ratio	All Births	Sex Ratio
1943						
Mid April	3916	1.168	781	1.116	903	1.130
Mid May	3793	1.083	674	1.032	940	1.070
Mid June	4044	1.006	795	.894	1039	1.106
Mid July	3805	1.124	749	1.158	954	1.022
Mid Aug.	3989	1.031	820	.975	1028	1.006
Mid Sept.	3935	1.003	678	1.064	963	1.013
Mid Oct.	4034	1.053	780	1.058	987	1.155
Mid Nov.	3938	1.066	748	1.179	1057	1.042
1944						
Mid Dec.	4199	1.063	772	1.077	954	1.065
Mid Jan.	4023	1.078	763	1.090	947	1.119
Mid Feb.	3962	1.033	632	1.027	829	.978
Mid March	3983	.992	683	1.131	928	1.002
Mid Apr.	4182	1.046	774	.826	984	1.039
Mid May	3996	1.011	818	1.159	932	1.105
Mid June	4104	1.058	868	1.137	1173	.952
Mid July	4255	1.062	898	.964	1047	1.122
Mid Aug.	4168	1.112	795	1.140	1071	.975
Mid Sept.	3443	1.001	689	1.040	954	1.027
Famine Begins						
Mid Oct.	3398	1.049	762	1.200	1033	1.146
Mid Nov.	2863	1.051	691	.887	1093	1.122
1945						
Mid Dec.	2152	1.088	686	1.104	1040	1.096
Mid Jan.	1813	1.098	608	1.218	1117	1.021
Mid Feb.	1688	1.104	611	.993	1063	1.028
Mid Mar.	2018	1.089	695	1.205	1060	1.044
Mid Apr.	2664	1.039	893	1.118	1086	1.152
Famine Ends						
Mid May	3900	1.074	995	.987	1099	1.138
Mid June	6889	1.060	1190	.995	1359	1.212
Mid July	7403	1.067	1105	1.072	1260	1.157
Mid Aug.	7730	1.097	1137	1.111	1367	1.076
Mid Sept.	7029	1.065	998	1.141	1211	1.127
Mid Oct.	6915	1.116	1035	1.099	1170	.940
Mid Nov.	6631	1.075	1012	1.124	1096	1.087
1946						
Mid Dec.	6158	1.076	954	1.131	1077	1.094
Mid Jan.	5811	1.030	923	1.090	1107	1.111
Mid Feb	5278	1.088	806	1.024	983	1.117
Mid Mar.	5680	1.045	830	1.013	1107	.994

In the famine cities the relationship between food rations and
fertility is strong and convincing below a threshold of caloric
rations of about 1500 calories. In the northern cities, too, a
decline in fertility is detectable. In the southern cities, there
is no such relationship. We believe that this is due to the fact
that in these cities, many of which were freed from occupation at
the time of the Hongerwinter, food supplies from the surrounding
countryside and the liberated armies were available over and above
the official ration.

    For each group of cities detailed comparisons were made,
month by month, of rations and births. We confirmed by study of
scattergrams and correlations that the relationship held up strongly
and consistently only when the ration fell below 1500 calories.
Thus, in the famine cities over the 11 months when the ration fell
below the threshold level, the correlation coefficient of calories
in the rations at conception with number of births was r = 0.92.
(The caloric standard is used for convenience. In practice, the
constituents of the diet, protein, fats and carbohydrates varied
together, and their individual effects were not separable).

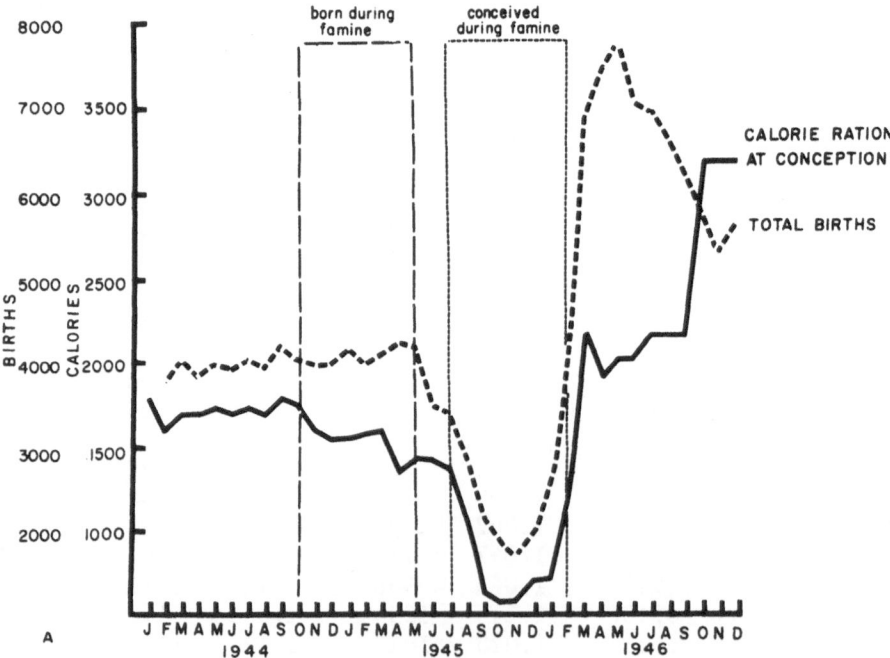

Figure 4A. Fertility and Caloric Ration. Famine Cities. Number
of births and official average daily caloric ration at estimated
time of conception for period June 1944 to December 1946, inclusive.

Decline in Births: Comparisons by Social Class

We found that infertility affected the social classes differently. Social class of births was most conveniently estimated from the occupation of fathers of the 18 year old men presenting to the military. This approximation was validated in its essentials from a sample of births registered during 1944-1946. Figure 5, based on the military data, shows that the decline in fertility in non-manual classes, though present, was less remarkable than that in the manual classes, in whom both the decline and the post-war rise was steeper. In the control cities, divergence between the classes was much less marked.

Decline in Births by Age and Parity

Some information is available on differential effects on fertility which the famine might have exerted on women of differing age and gravidity. Data relating to maternal age are available only on maternity hospital records. We found that among 2,521 women in famine cities whose babies were born in hospital, those

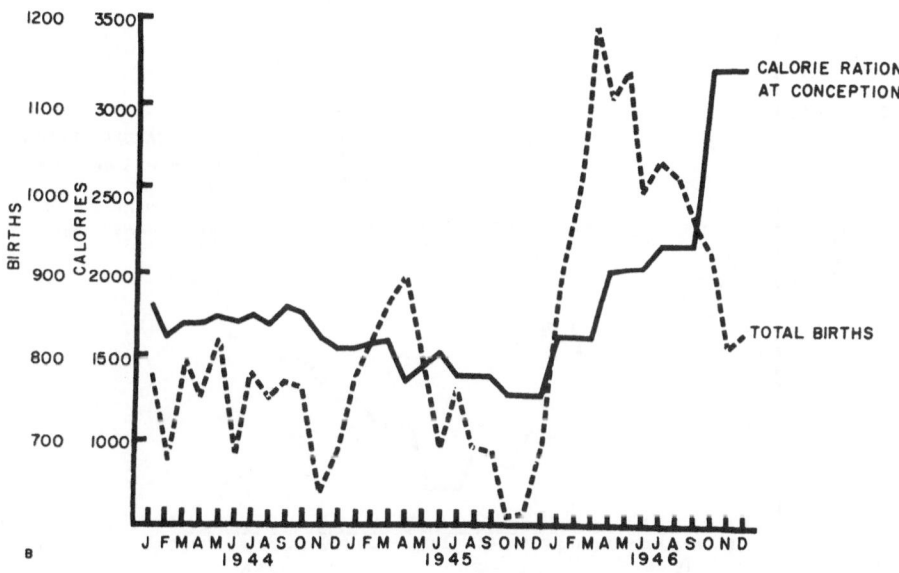

Figure 4B. Fertility and Caloric Ration. Northern Control Cities. Number of births and official average daily caloric ration at estimated time of conception for period June 1944 to December 1946, inclusive.

who conceived during the period of greatest hunger (numbering 528)
were somewhat atypical in that they were slightly younger. Their
average age was 27.5 years compared with an average age for the
rest of the period of 28.13 years (p<.025). No such differences
in maternal age were present in the maternity hospitals in control
areas.

   The birth rank of men in the Netherlands induction examination
is an index enabling us to compare the parity of childbearing
couples during the famine by time and place. We found a higher
than expected percentage of firstborn among those conceived at the
height of the famine, most marked in those with fathers in manual
occupations (Table 2). The effect was present only in the famine
cities. We infer that primiparae are able to continue fecundable
under conditions of starvation for longer periods than are multi-
parae. This inference is supported by the data from maternity
hospitals, which show an under-representation of grandimultips
(five or more previous births) in conceptions at the period of
greatest hunger, 9.7% where the expected is 12.9% (p<.05).

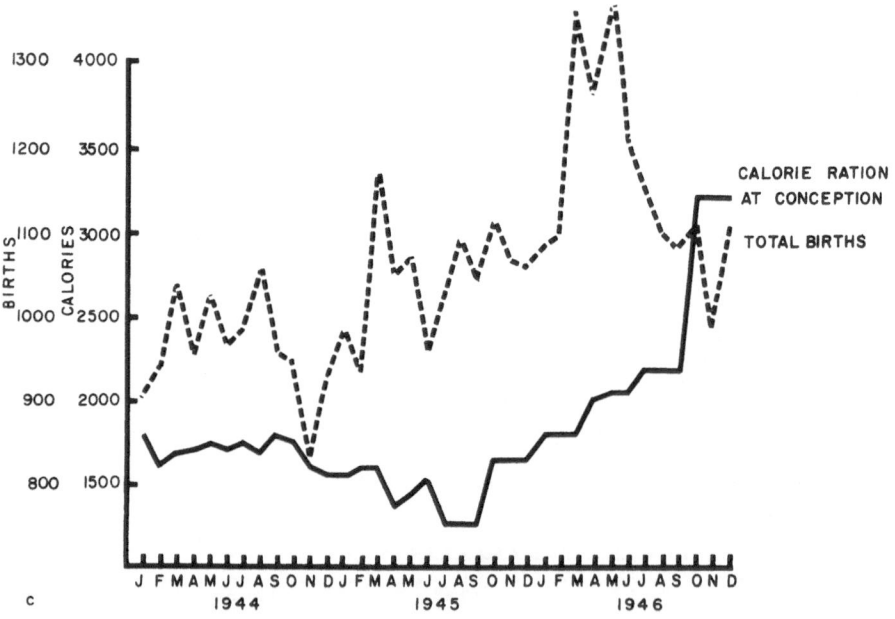

Figure 4C. Fertility and Caloric Ration. Southern Control Cities.
Number of births and official average daily caloric ration at
estimated time of conception for period June 1944 to December 1946,
inclusive.

The apparent effect of parity may be evidence for an advantage
of youthful childbearing rather than for a disadvantage of grandi-
multiparity. Both age and parity are recorded on maternity hospital
records, but the numbers are too small to provide a sensitive test,
and the hospital population is less representative than the induction series. We found that if maternal age is held constant, then
for older women there are slightly fewer women of high parity among
famine cohorts, 30% compared to 40% among those over 35 years, a
result that does not reach the .05 level of significance in the
numbers available.

There is, therefore, some suggestion in our data that both
youthfulness and lower parity conferred some protection against
infertility of couples during the Dutch famine but we cannot decide
the relative importance of these two conditions.

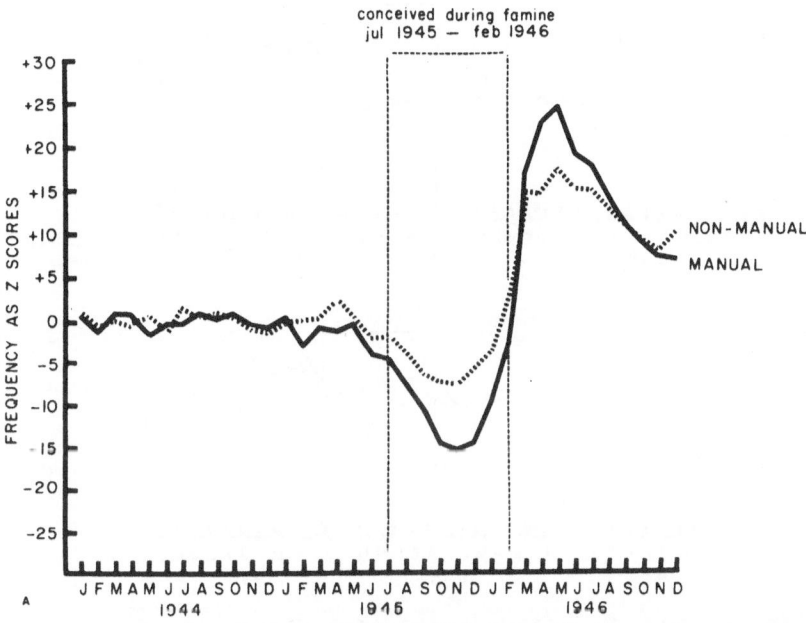

Figure 5A. Fertility and Social Class. Famine Cities. Frequency
of births, expressed as Z scores based on the number of male survivors at age 19 by social class (manual and non-manual according
to father's occupation) for the period January 1944 to December
1946, inclusive. Means and SD's for Z scores based on births from
January 1944 to December 1944.

Sex Ratio

In Table 1 we show boys and girls born alive each month over
a three year period in famine cities and control cities. We have
shown elsewhere the sex of those who died, by age at death (2).
The number of stillbirths is also shown there, so that stillbirth
rates can be considered in estimating perinatal mortality, but the
sex of the stillborn infants was not generally recorded. In the
last column of Table 1, the masculinity ratio (boys divided by
boys + girls) is given for all live births.

Our interpretation is that the masculinity ratio was not
modified, upwards or downwards, during the phase of a falling or
rising birth rate. Post-natally, there were more boys lost than
girls (2) and this was not true at all ages. The sex ratio of
those deaths did not change throughout the period of observation.

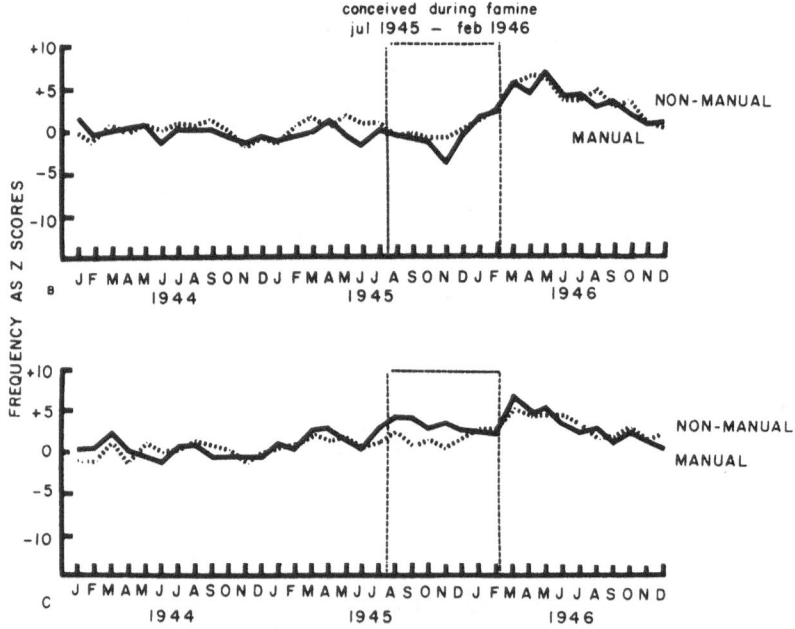

Figures 5B and 5C. Fertility and Social Class. B. Northern
Control Cities and C. Southern Control Cities. Frequency of
births, expressed as Z scores based on the number of male survivors at age 19 by social class (manual and non-manual according to
father's occupation) for the period January 1944 to December 1946,
inclusive. Means and SD's for Z scores based on births from
January 1944 to December 1944.

Table 2

Percent Distribution by Birth Order Among Netherlands Men Examined for Military Service, by Birth Cohorts and City, in the Famine Area (Amsterdam, Rotterdam, The Hague, Leiden, Utrecht, Haarlem), the Northern Control Area (Groningen, Enschede, Leeuwaarden, Helmond, Hengelo) and the Southern Control Area (Heerlen, Breda, Tilburg, Eindhoven, Maastricht)

Area	Birth Order	Birth Cohorts (See Figure 1)								
		A1	A2	B1	B2	C	D1	D2	E1	E2
Famine	1	41.1	39.8	36.7	34.8	35.3	35.2	38.2	33.8	36.1
	2-4	50.2	52.4	55.0	56.6	56.8	55.9	53.8	59.4	56.8
	5 +	8.7	7.9	8.3	8.6	7.9	8.9	8.0	6.8	7.1
North Control	1	38.1	37.7	38.8	32.7	33.8	34.6	34.9	33.5	35.5
	2-4	52.4	53.3	52.7	58.6	57.5	56.1	56.1	58.0	55.9
	5 +	9.5	8.9	8.6	8.7	8.7	9.4	9.0	8.5	8.6
South Control	1	32.0	29.6	28.4	27.8	30.8	28.4	25.3	28.0	29.1
	2-4	52.5	51.9	56.0	55.9	51.8	54.3	58.3	57.1	54.8
	5 +	15.5	18.5	15.6	16.3	17.5	17.3	16.5	14.9	16.1

The masculinity ratio among survivors of the cohorts that suffered the heavy infant mortality rate, however, would have been lower at older ages because the sex ratio among deaths is higher than that among births.

Rates of Twinning

Bulmer (18) studied the rates of twinning in selected European countries during the years 1940 to 1945. He was able to estimate rates of dizygotic twins and monozygotic twins from the frequency of pairs of like-sex and unlike-sex twins. In accord with his hypothesis, he found a marked decline in the dizygotic twinning rate (but not in the monozygotic rate) for maternities in the Netherlands in the period 1944-45. The findings are reproduced in Figure 6.

DISCUSSION

In attempting to understand the likely mechanism of famine infertility, we considered several possibilities. Following Davis and Blake (19), we deal with the "intermediate variables" (intercourse, conception, and gestation) in turn.

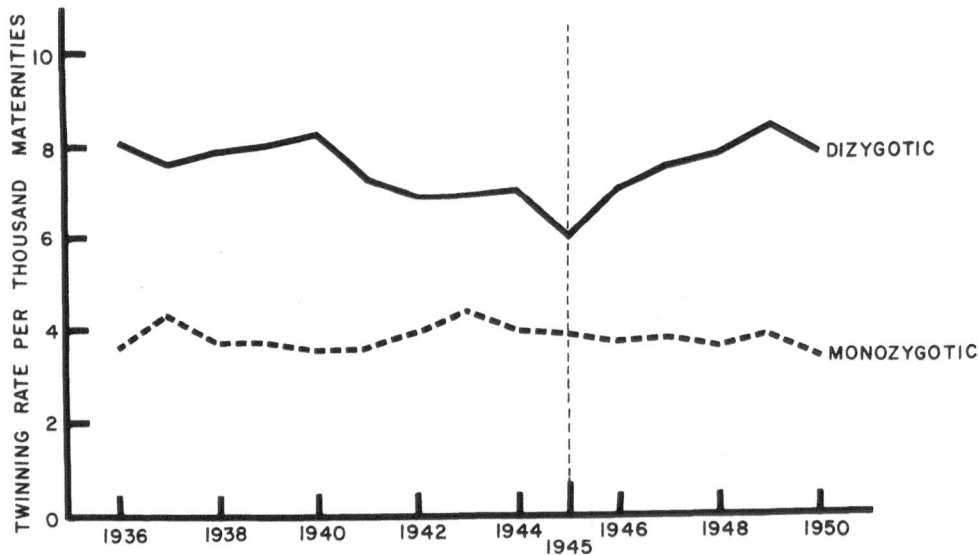

Figure 6. The twinning rate in the Netherlands during the second World War, standardized for maternal age (Bulmer, 1970).

First, with regard to intercourse, involuntary abstinence and
a decline in coital frequency were likely to have played some part.
Contemporary reports emphasize the lassitude of the starving population and diminished libido. In reports of prisoner of war camps
and under conditions of experimental starvation, a decline in male
libido has been documented (20). The hunger drive becomes so
powerful as to dominate thoughts and activities of the starving.

Second, with regard to conception variables, fecundability or
ovular cycles in women, or oligospermia in men must be considered.
We do know from the reports of gynecologists in practice at the
time, that amenorrhea was extremely widespread (21,10). Famine-
related amenorrhea has often been observed. It was also reported
in Greece where Valaoras (8) estimates it to have been present in
70% of women; in Leningrad (9); in Belsen (22); in prisoner of war
camps in the Far East (23); in a refugee camp in Egypt (24); and
on many occasions during World War I, summarized by Hytten and
Leitch (25); and by Keys et al. (20). We have no explicit statistical evidence on this point for the Hongerwinter, but there is
little doubt that amenorrhea was commonly experienced.

Third, with regard to gestation variables, we have considered
the possibility that births declined because of an excess of
spontaneous abortion (a failure of the conceptus to implant, or to
go to term). Although there is experimental evidence in rats linking early nutritional deprivation with a failure to implant (26),
human evidence of a relationship between starvation and early fetal
loss is in our view still anecdotal. Thus, Gopalan and Naidu (27)
refer to a pregnancy wastage rate of 30% observed by Sundar Rao.
It is not clear if what is meant by this statement is a probability
of fetal death, or of a fetal death ratio* (28). If it is a probability of fetal death based on a longitudinal study as appears
more likely, then 30% does not differ from estimates in other
populations not deemed to be starving. For example, from French
and Bierman (29) we estimate that 24% of pregnancies identified at
four weeks gestation will end in fetal death by the 40+ weeks
gestation. From Hertig et al. (30) we estimate that at least 30%
of fertilizations will abort at some stage.

If, on the other hand, 30% is a fetal death ratio, then the
Gopalan and Naidu estimate is somewhat higher than others. However, in this case we cannot judge whether it is truly raised

---

* The probability of fetal death is an estimate of the risk of
abortion. The gestational age at first observation is taken into
consideration through life table analysis. Fetal death ratios
relate the total number of abortions to the total number of pregnancies observed; the gestational age at which pregnancy is
identified is not taken into consideration.

without knowing the gestational distribution of the pregnancy wastage. If, for instance, a large proportion of pregnancies ended in the 4-8 week gestation period, then the fetal death ratio would be higher than most reports. Even then, the basis for diagnosing pregnancy is a problem, particularly if the diagnosis depends on the history of a delayed or missed period, for disturbed cycles are common with starvation. This type of indirect report is there- fore inadequate evidence to establish that there is an increased rate of early fetal loss in malnourished populations.

Similarly, Ifekwunigwe (31) says of the Biafran experience: "When pregnancy took place, the incidence of miscarriages was also markedly raised." Valaoras (8) in writing of the Greek famine mentions: "the numerous miscarriages and abortions observed during that time;" a similar impression of a rise in miscarriages and abortions was formed by many observers in Holland.

We gave considerable attention to a possible role of early fetal loss in causing the decline in births following the Honger- winter. The actual information on abortions available to us was also anecdotal, and induced and spontaneous abortions were in- distinguishable in the records. Instead, we turned to an indirect test. On the hypothesis that early fetal loss contributed in large part to the decline in births, we argued that the relief of the famine and the restoration of food from May 7, 1946 onwards should have enabled women who were at that time in the phase of pregnancy between conception and implantation to carry their preg- nancies successfully to term. In such a case, the restoration of fertility, marked by a rise in births, would have been evident before the whole of the normal mean gestation period had expired (i.e., before the end of January 1946). If the decline in fertility were related to spontaneous abortions after implantation, recovery of fertility should have occurred even sooner. On the alternative hypothesis, that a decline either in intercourse or in fecundity or both was responsible for famine infertility, then the restoration of fertility would not be detected before the elapse of the normal mean gestation period. In this case, the data favor the second alternative: the rise in births began about 290 to 300 days after the relief of the famine suggesting that the rise stemmed from an increase in conceptions after liberation.

To explain the differences in fertility between the social classes during the famine, we considered three interpretations:

1. Voluntary control of fertility.

2. Physiological resistance to infecundity (the intermediate variables based on pre-famine constitution.

3. Access to food.

We cannot distinguish between these three interpretations with certainty.* The first seems unlikely, the third most likely.

1. The social controls (sexual taboos, age at marriage, con-traception, abortion) that differentiated the fertility of the classes before and after the famine might have been altered during the famine, so that the upper classes relaxed their control of fertility, or the lower classes increased theirs.

This explanation is rendered unlikely because it requires a reversal of the usual pattern of fertility control among the social classes. Studies of family planning and sex behavior show that among the generation involved, higher social classes normally exercised stricter and more conscious controls on reproduction than the lower classes. In line with this behavior, many studies of social class values have described an upper and middle class ori-entation towards deferring gratification for the sake of future reward, and a lower class orientation, in the absence of such anti-cipation, towards accepting the gratifications of the present (32). Yet, during the famine, in a time of great uncertainty when con-trols on fertility might be expected to have been all the more strict among the majority of the higher classes, there was a relatively greater decline in lower class births.

2. At the onset of the famine, the higher social classes may have been in better health and, in particular, better nourished, than the lower classes. This advantage might have sustained rela-tive fecundity in the upper classes in the face of the famine. However, if physiological resistance were crucial, we would expect that the onset of a decline in fertility would be delayed among the higher social classes, and that persisting famine would in time exhaust the bodily resources of all, including the higher social classes, causing the rates of fertility of all classes eventually to converge. Yet the onset of infertility was simultaneous in all social classes as we have seen, and convergence of fertility rates did not occur. The low ration levels of the worst famine period continued for at least four months. During these months, the fertility rates of each social class persisted at a low level, but the gap between them widened.

3. Those who obtained more food would have been protected

---

* Another explanation, that men of different classes were absent in different proportions, seems unlikely from our limited historic-al knowledge, although there are no explicit data on this informa-tion.

against the severe effects of starvation. During the famine the
higher social classes with their resources in money, property, and
influence, may have obtained more food than the lower social classes. This explanation has most to commend it. The lower classes
were worst hit by the famine in many respects. During the famine,
the lower classes suffered a disproportionate increase in deaths,
and clinical signs of malnutrition seen in adults as well as children were most common in the poorer sections of the cities (17).
This third explanation of the social class differences in fertility
during the famine emphasizes the influence of current nutritional
state on fecundity.

To interpret the observation that fertility seemed to be less
depressed in younger women and/or in primiparae, it is reasonable
to assume that during famine less fecund women would be affected
first, and that those births that did occur would be concentrated
at the most fecund ages and parities. Changes in distribution of
births by age and parity could also point to changes in fertility
brought about by the mating behavior of couples, since age and
parity undoubtedly affect this behavior; perhaps libido persisted
more strongly in the young than in the middle aged, relative to
their usual drives.

The influence of possible delays in the onset of menarche, or
in the occurrence of ovular cycles (as suggested by Frisch (33)
could not be studied; certainly weight loss was widely reported in
all age-sex groups (17). The tendency for younger women and primiparae to continue fecund, however, might be read as evidence
counter to the view that the decline in births was due to such
factors.

Lactation was the rule in Holland during the war. We therefore reviewed reports on a relation between malnutrition and lactation, in prolonging infecundability. The evidence still seems to
us insecure (34,35,36,37). Reports relating the age of the lactating mother to infecundability seem more consistent (34,38). We
tentatively suggest here the possibility that age and starvation
could be synergistic in this respect.

With regard to the sex ratio, we could not infer that the
famine had effected a change either in primary sex ratio (occurring
at conception) nor in secondary sex ratio (occurring during early
fetal life, with abortions). There is certainly evidence for a
change in tertiary sex ratio, associated with the extraordinarily
high infant losses.

The reduction in the rate of dizygotic twinning (standardized
by maternal age) is of considerable interest. Bulmer (18) offers
two tenable explanations: a decline in male fertility (the number

and motility of sperm), or a decreased tendency of the ovary to produce two ovulations in one cycle. As dizygotic twinning is related to maternal rather than to paternal age and to parity, and since we have suggested above that infertility selectively affected women in the older age groups and those of higher parities, the evidence on twinning is coherent with the view that the famine served to depress ovulation, especially in older women of higher parity.

To explain the unprecedented rise in births after liberation and its distribution by social class, we have argued that women who conceived during the famine were more fecundable. Immediately after the famine such women (being already pregnant) would have been insusceptible and thus under-represented among fresh conceptions. The period of high birth rates would therefore be in some ways the mirror image of the period of low birth rates. The social class pattern provides some support for this notion.

CONCLUSIONS

Several propositions follow from the demonstration that starvation had a direct and current effect on fertility, and probably on its prerequisite, fecundability. Two are:

1. Infertility and infecundity caused by starvation are rapidly reversible. A steep rise in conceptions immediately after the liberation marked the restoration of susceptibility to fertilization. The main contribution to the rise in conceptions was made by couples, both of whom were resident in Holland throughout the famine period. The rise preceded in time a more gradual rise that followed the return home of soldiers, prisoners, deportees and refugees. The immediate recovery of fertility in the population suggests that there was immediate physiological recovery of sexual activity, normal ovulation, and fecundity in general.

One of the chief lessons to be learned from the famine is the great resilience of human populations exposed to the harshest environmental forces. Early in May 1945, the people were so weakened that the very survival of many was in doubt. The liberated armies were supported by emergency nutrition teams and brought plentiful supplies of food. Within one month of liberation from the Nazi occupation, many were restored to the normal activities of everyday life and to the business of rebuilding their families and their shattered cities.

2. The after-effect of a phase of infertility, followed by a phase of hyperfertility, will reflect variation between groups differently affected at different times. The variations have

consequences for the distributions of manifestations that may be used to detect effects of prenatal exposure to famine on the outcome of pregnancy. Thus, one consequence of the relative fertility of the higher social classes during the famine was an altered social class composition of cohorts conceived during the infertile months. The altered class composition of the famine cohorts contrasted particularly with the cohorts conceived immediately after the famine in the rebound from famine infertility. The different "mix" of social classes in successive cohorts can confound analyses of any outcome measures in which social class differentials exist. For instance, the altered mix was important in studying the effect of the famine on mental performance (2,39).

References

1. Aykroyd, W. In: Blix, G., Hofvander, Y. and Vahlquist, B., Famine Symposium with Nutrition and Relief Operations in Times of Disaster. Published for the Swedish Nutritional Foundation, Uppsala, Almquist and Wiksell, 1971.

2. Stein, Z., Susser, M., Saenger, G., and Marolla, F. Famine and Human Development: The Dutch Hunger Winter of 1944-1945. New York: Oxford University Press, 1975.

3. Stein, Z. and Susser, M. Fertility, Fecundity, Famine: Food Relations in the Dutch Famine 1944-45 Have a Causal Relation to Fertility and Probably to Fecundity. Hum. Biol. 47: 131-154, 1975.

4. Keys, A. B., Brozek, J., Henschel, A., Mickelson, O. and Taylor, H. L. The Biology of Human Starvation. Minneapolis: University of Minneapolis Press, 1950.

5. Aykroyd, W. The Conquest of Famine. New York: Readers Digest Press, distributed by E. P. Dutton, 1975.

6. Edwards, R. D. and Williams, T. D. The Great Famine. Dublin: Brown-Nolan, 1956.

7. Woodham-Smith, C. The Great Hunger: Ireland 1845-9. London: Hamilton, 1962.

8. Valaoras, V. G. Some Effects on Famine on the Population of Greece. Mil. Mem. Fund Quart. 24: 215-234, 1946.

9. Antonov, A. N. Children Born During Siege of Leningrad in 1942. J. Pediat. 30: 250-259, 1947.

10. Smith, C. A. The Effect of Wartime Starvation in Holland upon Pregnancy and its Product. Am. J. Obstet. Gynec. 53: 599-608, 1947.

11. Ryan, C. A Bridge Too Far. New York: Simon and Schuster, 1974.

12. Banning, C. Food Shortage and Public Health, First Half of 1945. Ann. Am. Acad. Pol. Soc. Sc. 245: 93-100, 1946.

13. Breunis, J. The Food Supply. Ann. Am. Acad. Pol. Soc. Sc. 245: 87-92, 1946.

14. Dols, M.J.L. and van Arcken, D.J.A.M. Food Supply and Nutrition in the Netherlands During and Immediately After World War II. Mil. Mem. Fund Quart. 24: 319-355, 1946.

15. Stare, F. J. Nutritional Conditioners in Holland. Nutr. Rev. 3: 225-227, 1945.

16. Burger, G.C.E., Sandstead, H. R. and Drummond, J. C. Starvation in Western Holland: 1945. Lancet ii: 282-283, 1945.

17. Burger, G.C.E., Drummond, J. C. and Sandstead, H. R. (eds.) Malnutrition and Starvation in the Netherlands: September 1944-July 1945. The Hague: General State Printing Office, 1948.

18. Bulmer, M. G. Twinning Rate in Europe During the War. Brit. Med. J. i: 29-30, 1959.

19. Davis, K. and Blake, J. Social Structure and Fertility: An Analytic Framework. Economic Development and Cultural Change 4: 211-235, 1956.

20. Keys, A. B. et al., op.cit.

21. Boerema, I. (ed.) Medische Ervaringen in Nederland Tijdens De Bezetting, 1940-1945. Groningen, J. B. Wolers, 1947.

22. Mollison, P. L. Observations of Cases of Starvation at Belsen. Brit. Med. J. i: 4-8, 1946.

23. Sydenham, A. Amenorrhorea at Stanley Camp, Hong Kong, During Internment. Brit. Med. J. ii: 159, 1946.

24. Grieve, W. P. Amenorrhorea During Internment. Brit. Med. J. ii: 243-244, 1946.

25. Hytten, F. E., and Leiten, I. The Physiology of Human Pregnancy. Oxford: Blackwell Scientific Publications, 1971.

26. Zamenhof, S., van Marthens, E., and Margolis, F. L. DNA (Ceu Number) and Protein in Neonatal Brain: Alteration by Maternal Dietary Protein Restriction. Science 160: 322-323, 1968.

27. Gopalan, C. and Naidu, A. M. Nutrition and Fertility. Lancet ii: 1077-1079, 1972.

28. Kline, J. Ph.D. Dissertation, Columbia University School of Public Health. Unpublished.

29. French, F. E. and Bierman, J. M. Probabilities of Fetal Mortality. Public Health Reports 77: 835-847, 1962.

30. Hertig, A. T., Rock, J., Adams, E. C., and Menkin, M. C. Thirty-four Fertilized Human Ova, Good, Bad, and Indifferent, Recovered from 210 Women of Known Fertility: A Study of Biologic Wastage in Early Human Pregnancy. Pediatrics 23: 202-211, 1959.

31. Ifekunigwe, A. In: Blix, G., Hofvander, Y., and Vahlquist, B. Famine Symposium Dealing with Nutrition and Relief Operations in Times of Disaster. Published for the Swedish National Foundation. Uppsala: Almquist-Wiksell, 1971.

32. Susser, M. W. and Watson, W. Sociology in Medicine. 2nd Ed. New York: Oxford University Press, 1971.

33. Frisch, R. E. Demographic Implications of the Biological Determinants of Female Fecundity. Paper presented to the Annual Meeting of The Population Association of America, April 1974. Reprinted in Harvard Center for Population Studies Research Papers Series, Paper Number 6, 1974.

34. Thomson, A. M., Hytten, F. E. and Black, A. E. Lactation and Reproduction. Bull. World Health Org. 52: 337-349, 1975.

35. Jain, A. K., et al. Demographic Aspects of Lactation and Post-Partum Amenorrhorea. Demography 7: 225-271, 1970.

36. Saxton, G. A. and Sevanadda, D. M. Human Birth Interval in East Africa. J. Repro. Fertil., Suppl. 6: 83-88, 1969.

37. Potter, R. G., et al. Applications of Field Studies to Research on the Physiology of Human Reproduction: Lactation and its Effects upon Birth Intervals in Eleven Punjab Villages, India. In: Sheps, M. C. and Ridley, J. C., ed. Public Health and Population Change. Pittsburgh: University of Pittsburgh, Pennsylvania, 377-399, 1965.

38. Perez, A. et al. Timing and Sequence of Resuming Ovulation and Menstruation After Childbirth. Population Studies 25: 491-503, 1975.

39. Stein, Z. S., Susser, M. W., Saenger, G., and Marolla, F. Intelligence Test Results of Individuals Exposed During Gestation to World War II Famine in the Netherlands. Science 198: 708-713, 1973.

EFFECT OF MATERNAL NUTRITION ON INFANT MORTALITY

Aaron Lechtig, Hernan Delgado, Reynaldo Martorell,
Douglas Richardson, Charles Yarbrough, Robert E. Klein

Institute of Nutrition of Central America and Panama
(INCAP), Guatemala City, Guatemala

INTRODUCTION

High infant mortality is a major health problem in many
countries of the world. In these countries the infant mortality
rate (IMR) remains a major determinant of life expectancy at birth
and the first year of life is the single most important risk
period that a person has to face. Maternal malnutrition has been
implicated as an important cause of the high IMR reported in many
developing nations. The objective of this paper is to review the
published data on the relationship between maternal nutrition and
infant mortality.

In order to examine this relationship we will first explore
the historical trends in the infant mortality rates of the developed countries. We shall then undertake cross sectional analyses
relating nutrient availability to IMR. Differences in infant
mortality associated with social class within countries will then
be studied and finally we shall review our field results in order
to document to what extent maternal nutrition is a determinant of
infant mortality.

SOCIOECONOMIC DEVELOPMENT AND INFANT MORTALITY

During the last four to five centuries infant mortality rates
in Europe fluctuated between 150-250/1000 live births (1-5).

147

reflecting the same situation seen in developing countries today
(6); however, infant mortality rates began to fall dramatically
in the late 19th century, first in Sweden and then in England,
France, Italy and the U.S.A. (1, 7-9). This appears to have been
a result of both improved sanitary practices and increased
standards of living and was relatively independent of improvements
in medical care (10,11). That economic factors had always played
a part is evident from the study by Peller (12) on mortality in
the ruling houses of Europe since 1500, which showed infant mortality comparable to modern standards as early as 1800-1899.

The same industrialized countries that decreased infant
mortality rates in the twentieth century, had a simultaneous
improvement in gross national product per capita. Admittedly,
gross national product per capita is a very crude indicator of the
nutritional condition of a population. Nonetheless, it is closely
associated with food availability per capita, and although the
shape and slope of this relationship varies from country to country,
it appears that there is a fairly consistent fall in IMR when per
capita income increases.

Figure 1, based on cross sectional data, shows that dietary
energy per capita per day, a measure of food availability and IMR,
are associated. Similar results have been shown previously with
the proportion of low birth weight (LBW) babies (13). The threshold appears to be around 2800 calories per capita, above which
IMR and the closely related LBW rates cease to decline significantly. Figure 1 reveals that for the same level of economic
development there is a wide range in IMR. This variability may be
partially due to variations in the efficiency of translating
economic growth into improved nutrition and health. For example,
in Sweden the drop in mortality occurred at a lower dietary energy
per capita than in the U.S.A.

In Figure 2, 123 countries have been divided into three
groups according to dietary energy per capita per day. It is clear
that no country with less than 2400 calories per day has "low" IMR
while most of the countries with more than 2800 calories have a
"low" IMR.

Figure 3 shows the infant mortality rates for the highest and
the lowest social classes in England during the last 100 years.
In general, offspring of wealthier parents died less frequently in
all periods (14). Death rates decreased proportionately the same
amount in both social classes (9). It can also be seen that the
IMR of social class I (professionals) in 1911 was not reached by
social class V (manual laborers) until 1941. Similar results
have been reported for France (15), the U.S.A. (16) and Finland
(17).

In summary, from three independent analyses: 1) examining the historical trends of IMR within developed countries; 2) comparing different values of dietary energy per capita per day with IMR in cross sectional analyses among countries; and 3) exploring differences in IMR across socioeconomic classes within specific countries; we can deduce a clear association between socioeconomic characteristics and infant mortality rate.

It should be pointed out that poor socio-economic conditions entail economic, cultural and biological deprivation. Lower class women are shorter (18,19), work more during pregnancy (17,20)and have generally poorer health (17, 21-23). They are also more likely to have a smaller pelvis and poorer diets during pregnancy (23, 34-44). Low SES mothers are also more likely to marry young, to be multiparous and to have illegitimate births (17,23). In addition, impoverished women are likely to show less than optimal care both for themselves during pregnancy and for their children. For instance, women of low social class are more likely to delay seeking antenatal care (45,46). Each of the above named factors has been shown to be associated with a high risk of infant loss (47,48). It would appear that the relationship between increased socioeconomic status and decreased IMR is mainly effected through the general improvement in health and nutritional status of the population due to a better standard of living. Our next task is to explore to what extent specific improvements in maternal nutrition may produce a decrease in IMR.

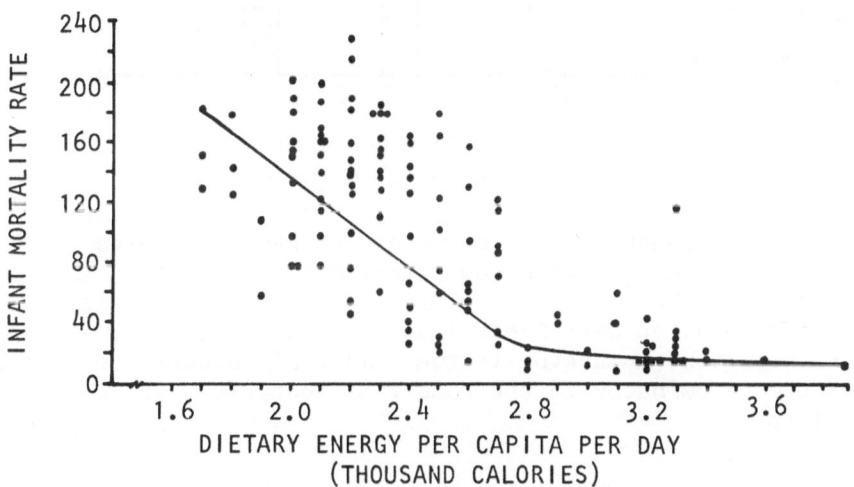

Figure 1. Relationship Between Dietary Energy per Capita and Infant Mortality Rate per 1000 Live Births. Computed from the World Population Data Sheet (Pop. Ref. Bureau Inc., 1975)

EFFECT OF MATERNAL NUTRITION ON INFANT SURVIVAL

Although there is no published data on investigations to assess specifically the relationship between maternal nutrition and infant mortality, the hypothesis of an effect of maternal nutrition on infant mortality rate seems reasonable and is supported by several studies. For instance, birth weight is consistantly associated with infant mortality (49,50). The majority of the racial mortality differential in the United States can be attributed to the higher proportion of low weight at birth of the black neonates (51,52), a difference that falls within the range of the effect of maternal nutrition on birthweight demonstrated through dietary surveys (53) or nutritional supplementation (54). Thus, maternal nutrition seems to be related to infant mortality through low birth weight*.

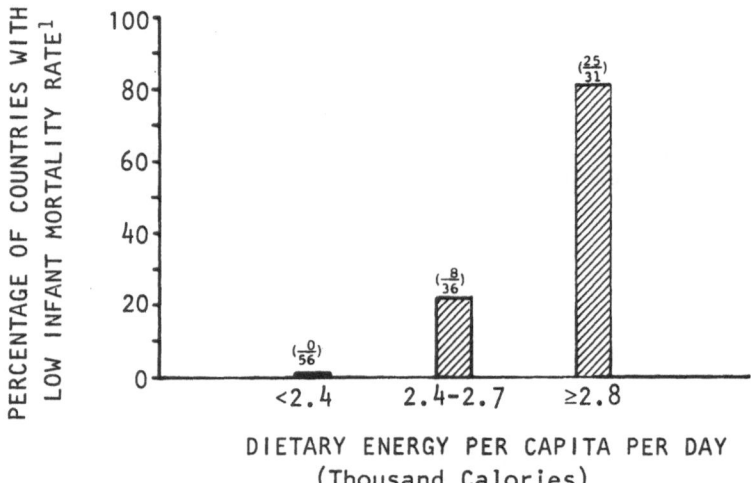

Figure 2. Relationship Between Dietary Energy per Capita and Percentage of Countries with Low Infant Mortality Rate. Low Infant Mortality Rate: <40/1000 Live Births. Computed from the World Population Data Sheet (Pop. Ref. Bureau, Inc., 1975). In parenthesis the numerator is the number of countries with low IMR and the denominator is the number of countries with available information.

----

*Low birth weight is defined as less than 2.5 kg.

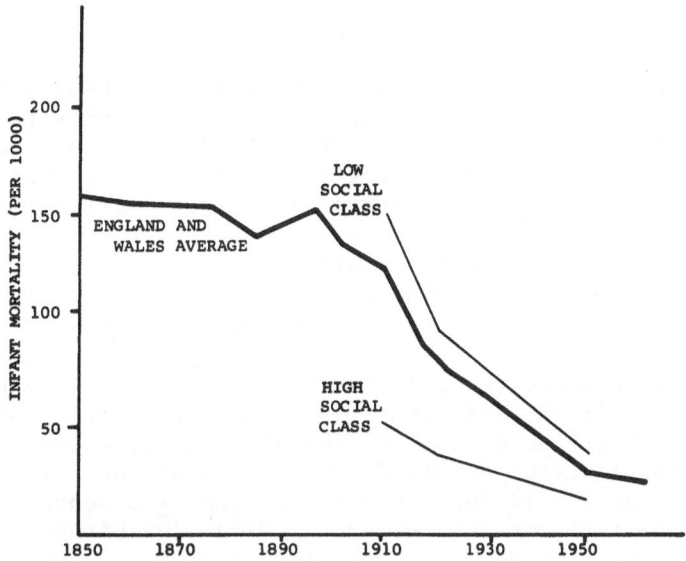

Figure 3. Trends in Infant Mortality by Social Class in England and Wales 1910-1950. Adapted from Morris and Heady 1955.

The next part of the hypothesis, that lower SES women have poorer diets during pregnancy has been demonstrated in developing nations where the social class gap is wide (19,53,55-59). In addition, placental size is smaller in low SES women, a factor that may contribute to fetal malnutrition (60-62). In other words, low socioeconomic status may lead to poor maternal nutrition, high prevalence of LBW babies and consequently high IMR. It has been argued that the accelerated drop in infant mortality rates which occurred during World War II could only be attributed to the wartime food distribution program which favored pregnant mothers (18). Further, maternal malnutrition during the mother's infancy and childhood could also produce an effect on infant mortality perpetuated through generations.

OBSERVATIONS IN GUATEMALA

We have explored the interrelationship between maternal nutrition and infant mortality in two different studies; the first one in a urban population of low social class from Guatemala City and the second one in four rural villages from eastern Guatemala.

Urban Study

In this study the design corresponded to a case-control retrospective study with the main purpose of identifying simple risk indicators of infant death. For this purpose we studied the records of 101 consecutive infant deaths from low social class during 1975 in a hospital of Guatemala City. These were compared with 199 children (control group) who survived the first year of life, were also of low social class and were being followed in the same hospital. From 42 variables examined 14 showed significant differences between the study and the control groups.

Table 1 presents the relative risk associated with these variables as well as their sensitivity and specificity as indicators of risk of infant death. Of the 14 risk indicators, 6 concern the nutritional status of either the infant or the mother. These are: weight for age ($\leq$ 80%), breast feeding ($\leq$ 6 months), weight for height ($\leq$ 90%), height for age ($\leq$ 87%), low birthweight ($\leq$ 2.5 Kg), and maternal arm perimeter ($\leq$ 24 cm). Two additional indicators probably affect infant survival by means of impaired maternal nutritional status. These are birth interval ($\leq$ 30 months) and maternal age ($\leq$ 19 years).

A risk scale was built on the basis of 7 of these indicators presented in Table 1, the possible score ranging between 0 and 7. The high risk population group, composed of those children with high score (from 5 to 7) in this scale, comprised 86 percent of the infant deaths and had a relative risk of dying during the first year of life 85 times higher than children with low score (from 0 to 4). Of the 7 components of this risk scale, 5 (weight for age, breast feeding, birth weight, birth interval and maternal age) concern the nutritional status of the baby, the mother or both. In conclusion, the results of the urban study bring support to the hypothesis that maternal nutrition is related to infant survival.

Rural Study

We have explored the interrelationship among these variables as part of a study in four villages of Guatemala (63). These are communities where chronic malnutrition and infectious diseases are highly prevalent, a situation unfortunately common to most of the rural populations of the third world. The economy is based on subsistence agriculture and corn and beans form basis of the local diet. Pregnant mothers, who average 149 cms. in height and 49 Kg in first trimester weight, have average daily dietary intakes of 1500 calories and 40 gms of protein. They deliver newborns weighing around 3 kg. and they breastfeed these children for a median of 17 months.

Until 1969, no "modern" medical services existed in these communities. Pregnancy and birth were supervised by midwives, home
remedies were used for minor illnesses, and serious medical
problems required transporting the patient to larger communities.

In 1969 INCAP provided a system of curative medical care in
these communities. Each village now has a clinic, staffed by an
auxiliary nurse, with weekly supervision by two physicians. Most
of the diagnosis and treatment is performed by a nurse who remains
in the community throughout the week. The doctors see patients on
a random basis as well as review the medical workups performed by
the nurses.

These clinics have cooperated fully with various national vac-
cination campaigns against measles, polio, diphteria, whooping
cough and tetanos. The out-patient problems today mainly encompass diarrheal, respiratory and dermatological conditions. The
infant mortality rates have been reduced from 160 per 1,000 in
1968 to about 50 per 1,000 in 1975.

The acceptance of our contemporary medical approach has been
very good. The villagers have expressed considerable confidence
in both the personnel and system of treatment. Midwives continue
to assist at childbirth in collaboration with the clinic. Thus,
the communities essentially have and use a system of medicine
which integrates the most favorable aspects of both traditional
and modern curative practices.

The study design and the principal examinations made in mothers
and preschool children are presented in Table 2. Two types of food
supplements are provided: atole* and fresco**. Two villages receive
atole while the other two receive fresco. Attendance at the supplementation center is voluntary and consequently a wide range of
supplement intake is observed. Table 3 presents the nutrient
content for both atole and fresco. It should be stressed that the
fresco contains no protein and that it provides only one third of
the calories contained in an equal volume of atole. In addition,
both preparations contain similar concentrations of the vitamins
and minerals which are possibly limiting in the diets of this
population.

As the home diet is more limiting in calories than in proteins (12), ingestion of supplemented calories was selected as the
criteria to assess supplement intake. We stress that while

---

* The name of a gruel, commonly made with corn.
** Spanish for a refreshing, cool drink.

Table 1

Urban Study - Risk Indicators of Infant Mortality

Indicator	Number of Cases		Relative[1] Risk
	Deaths	Control	
1. Hemorrhage during pregnancy[4]	101	199	23.2**
2. Weight for age $\leq 80\%$ [4]	101	197	21.1**
3. Breast feeding ≤ 6 months[4]	101	199	19.6**
4. Weight for height $\leq 90\%$	31	191	13.9**
5. Umbilical cord rolled in neck	101	199	12.6**
6. Height for age $\leq 87\%$	70	191	7.6**
7. Birth weight ≤ 2.5 kg.[4]	101	199	6.9**
8. Gestational age ≤ 37 weeks[4]	101	199	6.0**
9. Preceding Child dead	64	147	3.7*
10. Birth interval $\leq$ months[4]	64	147	3.0*
11. Arm perimeter ≤ 24 cm.	101	199	3.0*
12. Absence of perinatal medical care	101	199	2.9
13. Maternal age ≤ 19 years[4]	101	199	2.6*
14. Age of menarche ≤ 13 years	101	199	1.9*
Score of 5-7 in risk scale[5]	64	147	25.2**

* p < .05; ** p < .01
1. Computed increment of probability of death in high risk group
2. Percentage of deaths accurately predicted
3. Percentage of children alive accurately predicted
4. Components of risk scale
5. Score range: 0-7; high risk score: 5-7

calories are the main limiting nutrient in this population, other
populations may present very different nutritional situations.
Three additional independent variables were also included in the
present analysis: maternal height (an indicator of the nutritional
history of the mother during the age of growth); socioeconomic
score of the family; and birthweight (an indicator of fetal growth).
The socioeconomic score is a composite indicator reflecting the
physical conditions of the family house, the mother's clothing
and the reported extent of teaching various skills and tasks to
preschool children by family members. The principal outcome
variable was IMR in the cohort of children born from January 1,
1969 to February 28, 1975.

Table 2

Study Design for Four Villages*

Information+	When Collected
Obstetrical history	Once
Clinical examination[1]	Quarterly
Anthropometry[1]	Quarterly
Surveys[1]	
Diet	Quarterly
Morbidity	Fortnightly
Attendance at feeding center[1]	Daily
Amount of supplement ingested[1]	Daily
Socioeconomic status[1]	Annually
Birthweight	At delivery
Infant death	First year age

* Two villages received atole, a protein-calorie supplement, and two fesco, a calorie supplement.

+ Pregnancy was diagnosed by absence of menstruation; these surveys were made fortnightly.

[1] In mothers and preschool children.

Table 3

Nutrient Content per Cup*
(180 ml)

	Atole	Fresco
Total calories (Kcal)	163	59
Protein (g)	11	--
Fats (g)	.7	--
Carbohydrates (g)	27	15.3
Ascorbic acid (mg)	4.0	4.0
Calcium (g)	.4	--
Phosphorus (g)	.3	--
Thiamine (mg)	1.1	1.1
Riboflavin (mg)	1.5	1.5
Niacin (mg)	18.5	18.5
Vitamin A (mg)	1.2	1.2
Iron (mg)	5.4	5.0
Fluor (mg)	.2	.2

For the purpose of doing discrete variable analyses and due to the relatively small sample size, we will present analyses with dichotomous variables (categories "low" and "high). Table 4 presents the limits for partition of each variable in two categories. These limits were defined on basis of reported literature (i.e. low birthweight $\leq$ 2.5 Kg) or were based on results of prior analyses predicting birthweight.

Figure 4 explores the relationship between socioeconomic score (SES) maternal height, caloric supplementation during pregnancy and birthweight with the proportion of infant deaths in the four villages combined. In all four groups there is a lower proportion of infant deaths in the "high" category of each variable. However, the difference in the proportion of infant deaths in the "high" and "low" categories is statistically significant only with maternal height and birthweight.

Next, we studied to what extent each of these apparent associations with infant mortality held after controlling for the remaining three independent variables. Given the small sample size, we might not be able to measure the magnitude of the relationship between each of the variables presented in Figure 4 and proportion of infant deaths. In consequence, we explored mainly the consistency or replicability of the direction of these relationships across eight mutually independent comparisons.

Figure 5 shows the percentage of infant deaths for low and high categories of socioeconomic score within categories of birthweight, height and food supplementation. This analysis shows that once these last variables are controlled, there is no consistent association between socioeconomic score and infant death. This suggests that the original trend observed in Figure 4 may be due to the association between SES and the other three variables, maternal height, food supplementation, and birthweight.

Figure 6 presents a similar analysis comparing low and high categories of maternal height within categories of socioeconomic score, caloric supplementation during pregnancy and birthweight. It is evident that in all the eight comparisons the proportion of infant deaths is consistently lower in the groups with high maternal height than in those with low height. For instance, within the low birthweight category, the mothers with high height presented a lower proportion of infant deaths.

Women from poor populations are generally shorter in stature, mainly because of long-term malnutrition during the growth years (23,45,64,65). The inference is that in these populations height represents to some extent the nutritional history over the growth years, and that it is this which affects capacity of the offspring

Table 4

Limits Used to Form Dichotomous Variables

Variable	Category	
	Low	High
1- Supplemented calories during pregnancy	< 20,000	≥ 20,000
2- Maternal height (cm)	≤ 149	> 149
3- Socioeconomic Score	< mean + 1SD of four villages	> mean + 1SD of four villages
4- Birth weight	≤ 2.5 Kg.	> 2.5 Kg.

to survive. This gives rise to the idea of a generational mortality, determined during the mother's childhood.

The mechanisms through which short maternal stature are associated with poorer offspring survival remain obscure and may range from greater susceptibility of the fetus to infection to adequacy of the maternal nutrient supply to the placenta. In addition, smaller, stunted women are more likely to have contracted a pelvis, difficult labor and birth trauma (23). Whatever the mechanisms may be, it is evident that maternal height is, at least in these populations, a risk indicator of infant mortality.

Figure 7 shows a comparison between two categories of caloric supplementation during pregnancy within each category of socioeconomic score, maternal height and birthweight. This reveals that infant mortality was lower in the high supplemented group than in the low supplemented group in six of the eight independent comparisons. Of the remaining two comparisons in one there was no difference and in the other infant mortality behaved in the opposite direction.

In order to control for constant maternal factors, either measured or not measured, we explored the relationship between caloric supplementation during pregnancy and infant death within pairs of siblings of the same mother (see Figure 8). For this purpose the pairs of siblings were grouped according to the status of the preceding infant: alive or dead and then, substratified according to the status of the later infant (alive or dead). For each of these sub-groups we computed the proportion of mothers who decreased their caloric supplementation during the later pregnancy (vertical line of Figure 8). In the two independent comparisons presented in Figure 8 the proportion of mothers with decreased caloric supplementation during the latter pregnancy was higher in the groups in which the latter child died than in those in which the latter child survived.

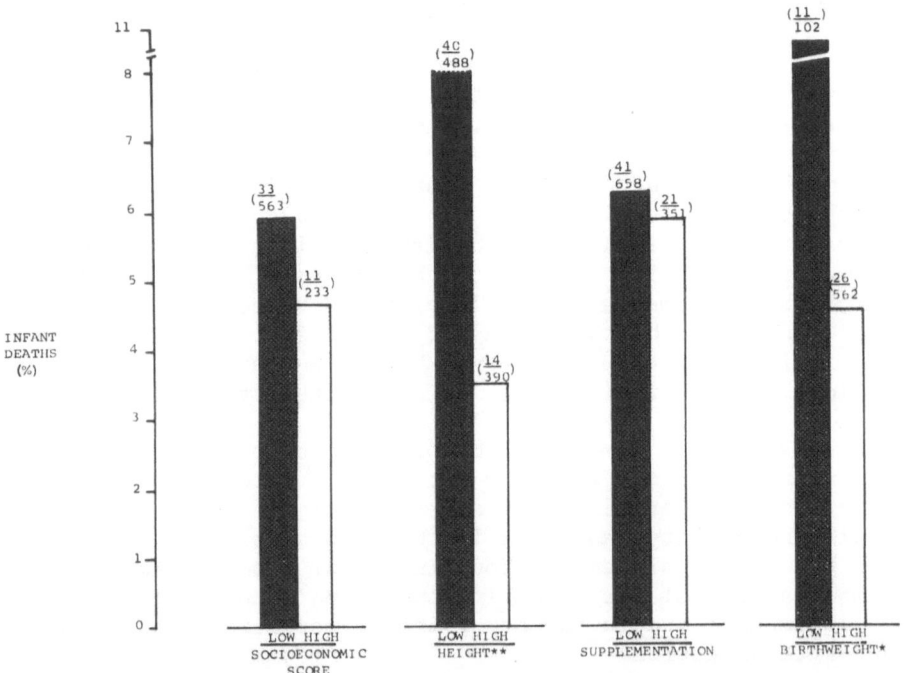

Figure 4. Percentage of Infant Deaths by Levels of Socioeconomic Score, Maternal Height, Food Supplementation During Pregnancy, and Birth Weight. In parenthesis the numerator is the number of infant deaths and the denominator is the total number of live births.

x^2 test: * p < .05
            ** p < .01

In consequence, in spite of the small sample size of the study groups, at present we believe that these results are compatible with the hypothesis that maternal nutrition is causally related to infant mortality. This conclusion arises from the following facts: 1) the results of Figure 6 suggested that maternal height, an indicator of nutritional history of the mother during ages of growth, is consistently associated with infant mortality, and 2) the results presented on Figures 7 and 8 suggest that caloric supplementation during pregnancy, an indication of maternal nutritional status during intrauterine life of the baby, is also associated with infant mortality in these populations.

The causal chain leading from maternal malnutrition to infant mortality may be composed by the following steps: 1) Maternal malnutrition may lead to smaller placental size and decreased

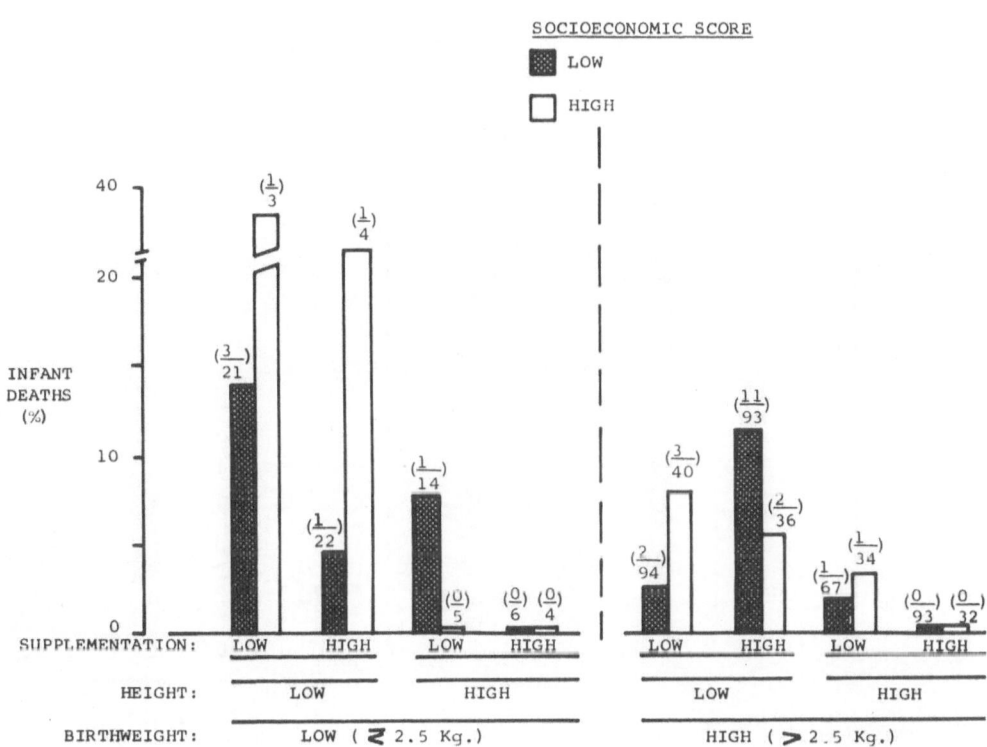

Figure 5. Relationship Between Socioeconomic Score and Infant Mortality After Controlling for Food Supplementation During Pregnancy, Maternal Height and Birthweight.

nutrient supply from the mother to the fetus. This would result
in developmental retardation during intrauterine life and therefore in decreased ability to survive during post natal life.
2) Maternal malnutrition may also produce sub-optimal lactation
performance which will contribute to the infant malnutrition,
growth retardation and, in consequence, may limit the infant's
potential to survive in its environment. Usually, this gradual
deterioration of the child's development may increase susceptibility to infections of the gastrointestinal and respiratory
tracts which in turn would worsen the health status of the baby
and end up as the "final" cause of death. There is available
evidence supporting the plausibility of several parts of this
hypothesis.

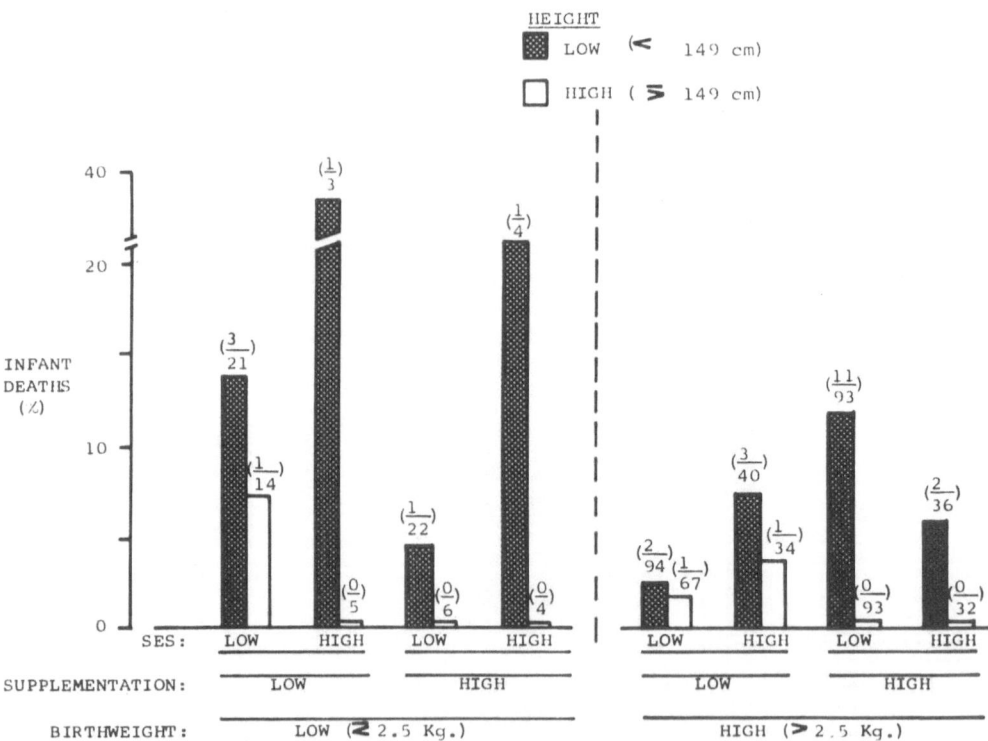

Figure 6. Relationship Between Maternal Height and Infant
Mortality After Controlling for Socioeconomic Score, Food
Supplementation During Pregnancy and Birthweight.

For instance, there is increasing information supporting the
hypothesis that maternal nutrition affects the materno-fetal
nutrient supply (60), and that fetal growth retardation is
accompanied by suboptimal immune response to some infectious
agents (69). It is becoming evident that the nutritional status
of lactating mothers may affect breast milk output (70-72) and
infant growth, at least during the first 3 to 6 months of age
(72,73). Finally, data on the literature (reviewed in 74) as
well as our own data (see Table 1), suggest that in poor populations the duration of breast feeding may be truly associated with
the probability of survival.

The finding (see Figure 7) that the association between

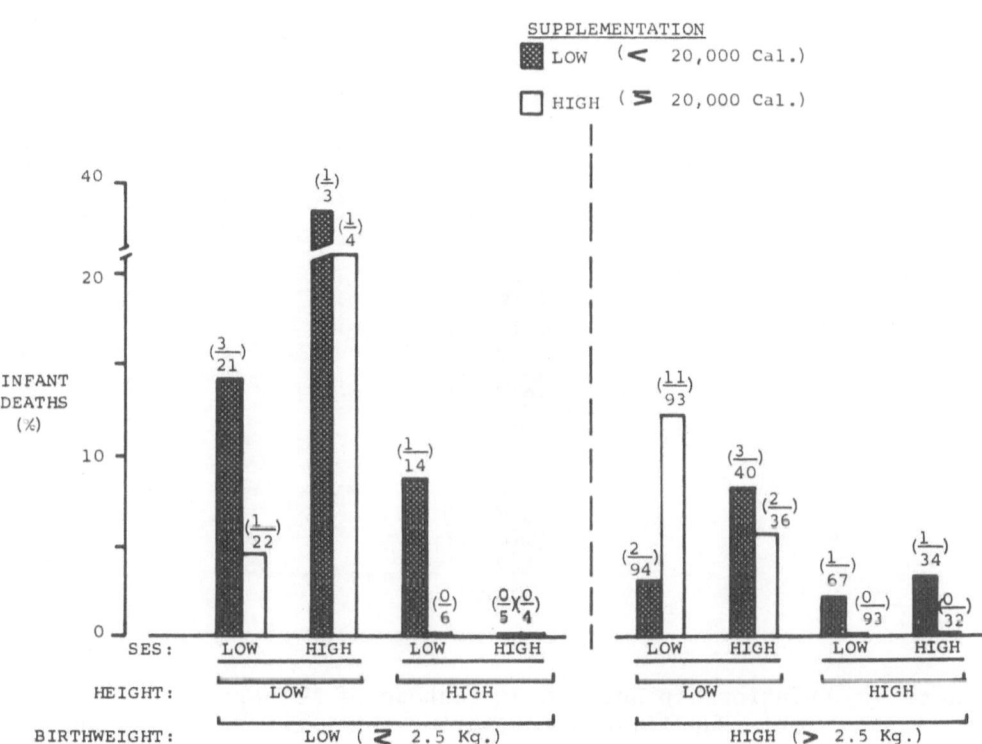

Figure 7. Relationship Between Food Supplementation During
Pregnancy and Infant Mortality After Controlling for Maternal
Height, Socioeconomic Score and Birthweight.

caloric supplementation and infant mortality does not disappear
after controlling for birthweight suggests that birthweight does
not contain all the prenatal information associated with infant
survival. An alternative explanation is that caloric supplementation during pregnancy not only affects birthweight but also post
natal maternal and infant nutritional status.

Finally, Figure 9 presents the relationship between two
categories of birthweight and proportion of infant deaths within
categories of socioeconomic score, caloric supplementation during
pregnancy and maternal height. It is clear that low birthweight
babies presented higher mortality rates in only four of the eight
comparisons presented in Figure 9. Of the remaining four, in two
there was no difference and in the other two the trend was to
higher mortality in the high birthweight group.

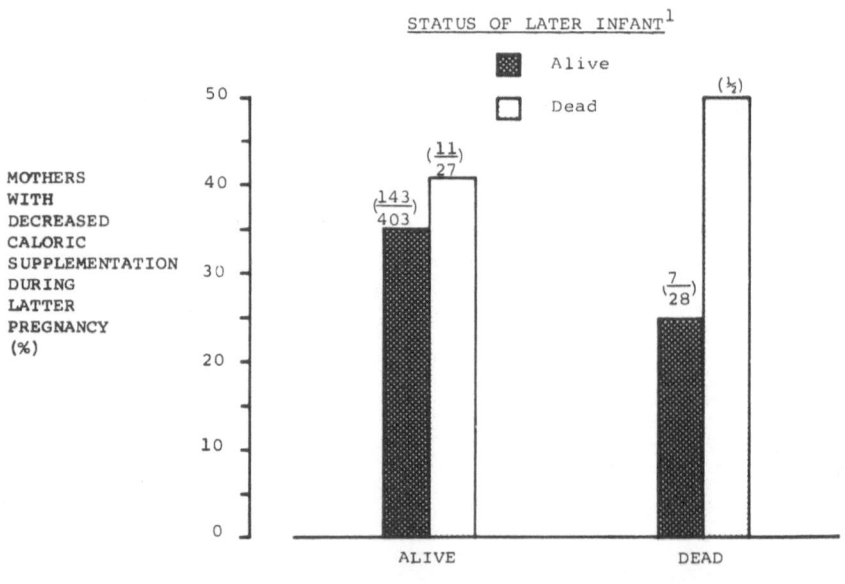

Figure 8. Relationship Between Percentage of Mothers with
Decreased Caloric Supplementation During the Later Pregnancy and
Death of the Later Infant During the First Year of Age.
In parenthesis the numerator is the number of mothers with
decreased caloric supplementation during the later pregnancy as
compared with the preceding pregnancy and the denominator is the
total number of pairs of siblings in the group.

Low birthweight (LBW) is considered the major predisposing factor of infant death in both developed and developing countries. Low birthweight infants who survive the first week remain at higher risk, being especially more susceptible to infection and severe malnutrition in developing countries. Even in developed countries where such factors play a lesser role, LBW survivors are 3-4 times more likely to die in the subsequent 11 months (49). It is recognized that the major factors influencing birth weight are of social, economic and biological origin, and that incidence of LBW may be a very sensitive indicator of social change (13,67, 68). The results presented in Figure 9 suggest that the association between birthweight and infant mortality may be explained, at least in part, by maternal characteristics such as height, socioeconomic score and food supplementation during pregnancy.

It should be noted in Figure 9 that the children with lower infant mortality were those delivered from mothers with high height and high supplement intake during pregnancy (deaths: 0;

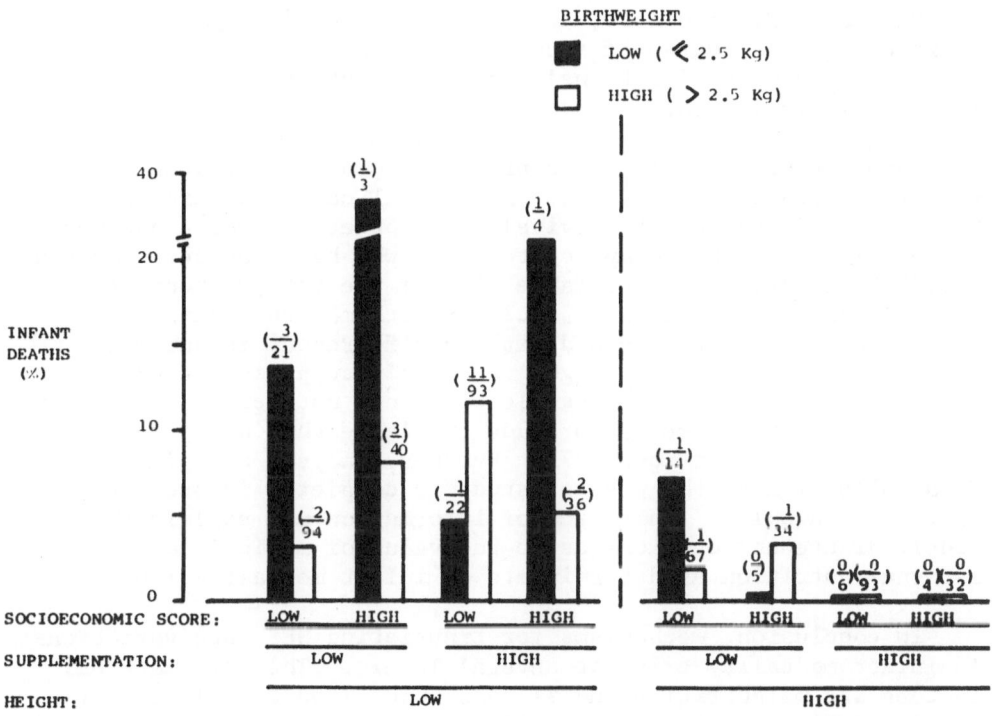

Figure 9. Relationship Between Birthweight and Infant Mortality After Controlling for Socioeconomic Score, Food Supplementation During Pregnancy and Maternal Height.

n = 135). In contrast, there were 9 deaths in the group of children delivered by mothers with low height and low supplement intake
(n = 158; t-test with arcsine transformation: t = 4.7; p < 0.001).

Conclusions

Our conclusion from these findings is that both short and
long term maternal nutrition status may be causally related to
infant mortality.

It should be pointed out that this conclusion does not mean
that other factors namely medical care and environmental sanitation are not important determinants of infant mortality in these
populations. Actually, it is probable that in these rural
populations in which medical care is available, infant mortality
is the end result of a complex interaction among several factors
including maternal nutrition. For instance, we have estimated
that in the four study villages the medical care system using
paramedical personnel and strict quality control systems is mainly
responsible for a decrement in IMR from 160/1000 in 1968 to about
85/1000 in 1969. The rest, from 85/1000 to 47/1000 may be
ascribed to the program of food supplementation or, in other words,
to the improvement of maternal and infant nutrition and to
improved medical care.

Some interactions are also probably occurring between both
programs, food supplementation and medical care. Several studies
have shown higher infant survival from mothers who have had more
antenatal visits when compared to those who have had less, or none
(16,25,26,27,32,74,75; see Table 1). If the mother's use of
medical care facilities is associated with maternal height or
supplement intake, this could explain differences in survival
associated with maternal height or caloric supplementation (75,
76). However, the present sample size does not permit us to solve
this problem and there is no study available that has placed an
answer to these questions (77). Further analyses are planned when
data collection of the present study is completed in order to
solve this problem. This lack of information may explain the
widely discrepant opinions as to the value of medical care and
maternal nutrition as determinants of infant mortality (20).

In conclusion, mechanisms for translating SES into variations
in infant mortality exist at several levels. The main maternal
factors are malnutrition and illness which lead to delivery of
poorly viable infants. These effects, aggravated by poor medical
care, lead to infant death.

These factors are heavily affected by access and utilization;

diet is affected by food availability, including food costs and individual purchasing capacity. The same holds for medical care, and home sanitary practices. Finally, each of these factors is influenced by socioeconomic status which affects income and attitudes and thus ability to afford medical care, adequate diet, and housing and sanitation. The relative contribution of each particular factor in a specific population and the variations among populations must be taken into account in program planning and study design. From this point we will turn our attention to the consideration of possible interventions.

RECOMMENDATIONS TO DECREASE INFANT MORTALITY

In the following paragraphs we will discuss the main aspects of action programs designed to decrease infant mortality in developing nations. We will mention the social, political and economic limitations to action; the need to implement immediate action programs and the main characteristics that these programs should have in poor populations.

Clearly, the nutrition and health problems in low income populations lie in the framework of the political, social and economical system. For example, poor communications, inadequate transportation, low availability of potable water, low purchasing power for basic foods are important nutritional determinants. Most intervention programs are dominated by political and financial considerations, and the scope of planning must necessarily work within (or against) these constraints since they affect the basic questions of what population is to be served, where, by by what method of intervention, and at what level of funding.

In some countries important improvements in socioeconomic conditions may not occur within the next one or two decades. Even in such cases action should not be delayed: the link between health services and political structure may be flexible enough to allow for an independent limited improvement of health. This is possible through integrated health care programs using paramedical personnel strongly emphasizing nutrition and preventive medicine and assigning first priority to high risk population groups.

Most efforts to reduce IMR are directed towards the mother during pregnancy. The data herein presented point out that in addition to these efforts, a long-term orientation is necessary for the malnourished girls of today may be the high risk mothers of tomorrow. In consequence, we believe that there is already sufficient knowledge in this field to justify planned action and evaluation. Based on both the literature reports and our own findings we believe it reasonable to assume that both short and

long-term maternal nutritional status are important determinants
of infant survival, growth and development. Waiting for firm
results and conclusions before acting will mean waiting for a
long time, sometimes longer than the life of the funding
government.

As implied above, actions to decrease IMR must be specifically
adapted to the needs of each population group. For instance, in
many developed countries IMR has begun a leveling trend as it
approaches a purely perinatal component. It seems that further
improvement in developed countries depends on advances in medical
science, whereas in the lesser developed countries it depends on
better nutrition and sanitation, and improved delivery of present
medical knowledge.

Projects to decrease infant mortality rates must be run by
local people, giving them confidence and a real awareness of their
usefulness in dealing with the prevailing conditions of their
societies. Although international coordinated effort is required;
this may be limited to promotion and technology. Local, national
personnel should establish their needs and programs and be in
charge of program implementation and evaluation.

SUMMARY

In summary, results of different analytic approaches indicate
a clear association between socioeconomic characteristics of the
mother and infant mortality rates. The reports available and our
own data support the hypothesis that short and long-term nutritional status of the mother are causally related to infant mortality
and are in part responsible for the association between socioeconomic status and infant mortality.

The actions to decrease infant mortality rates should be
specifically adapted to the needs of each population group, and
planners should take account of the socio-political constraints
that influence maternal nutritional status. As immediate actions
simplified health care programs with a strong nutritional component and using paramedical personnel may be very effective. In
the long-term, the most effective actions in developing countries
will be those oriented to a comprehensive attack of the causes of
underdevelopment. To be successful, this approach will require
positive socio-political changes focused on social objectives
and rational economic methods. The social changes are justified
not only because the ultimate goal of development is to improve
the quality of human existence but also because the quality of
human life is the key to development.

This research was supported by Contract No. N01-HD-5-0640 from the National Institute of Child Health and Human Development, National Institutes of Health, Bethesda, Maryland, and from Contract AID-TA-C/1224 from the Agency of International Development, Washington, D. C.

References

1. Cipolla, C. M. Four Centuries of Italian Demographic Development. In: Population in History: Essays in Historical Demography, 570-587. D. V. Glass and D.E.C. Eversley (eds.). London: Edward Arnold Publishers Ltd., 1965.

2. Aykryod, W. R. Nutrition and Mortality in Infancy and Early Childhood: Past and Present Relationships. Am. J. Clin. Nutr. 24: 480-487, 1971.

3. Deprez, P. The Demographic Development of Flanders in the 18th Century. In: Population in History: Essays in Historical Demography, 608-630. D. V. Glass and D.E.C. Eversley (eds.). London: Edward Arnold Publishers Ltd., 1965.

4. Gille, H. The Demographic History of the Northern European Countries in the Eighteenth Century. Pop. Studies 3: 3-65, 1949-50.

5. Henry, L. The Population of France in the 18th Century. In: Population in History: Essays in Historical Demography. D. V. Glass and D.E.C. Eversley (eds.), 445-448. London: Edward Arnold Publishers Ltd., 1965.

6. Verhoestraete, L. J. and Puffer, R. R. Challenge of Fetal Loss, Prematurity and Infant Mortality: A World View. J. Am. Med. Assoc. 167: 951-959, 1958.

7. Bourgeois-Pichat, J. The General Development of the Population of France since the Eighteenth Century. Population 6: 635-662, 1951 and Population 7: 319-329, 1952.

8. McCarthy, M. Infant, Fetal and Maternal Mortality USA 1963. Vital and Health Statistics, NCHS Series 20, No.3, 1966.

9. Morris, J. N. and Heady, J. A. Social and Biological Factors in Infant Mortality. V. Mortality in Relation to the Father's Occupation, 1911-1950. Lancet 1: 554-560, 1955.

10. McKewon, T. and Brown, R. G. Medical Evidence Related to
     English Population Changes in the Eighteenth Century.
     Population Studies 9: 119-141, 1955.

11. Hoffman, E. The Sources of the Italian Mortality Decline.
     California Institute of Technology Division of Humanities and
     Social Sciences, Working Paper No. 88, Pasadena, California,
     July 1975.

12. Peller, S. Mortality, Past and Future. Population Studies
     1: 405-456, 1948.

13. Lechtig, A., Margen, S., Farrell, T., Delgado, H., Yarbrough,
     C., Martorell, R., and Klein, R. E. Low Birth Weight Babies:
     World Wide Incidence, Economic Cost and Program Needs. Paper
     submitted for publication to World Health Organization,
     Special Supplement, 1976.

14. Morrison, J. N., Heady, J. A. and Morris, J. N. Social and
     Biological Factors in Infant Mortality. VIII. Mortality in
     the Post-neonatal Period. Arch. Dis. Childh. 34: 101-113,

15. Croze, M. La Mortalité Infantile en France Suivant Le Milieu
     Social. International Population Conference (Ottowa 1963),
     263-285. Liege: International Union for the Scientific Study
     of Population, 1964.

16. Kovar, M. G. Variations in Birth Weight - 1963 Legitimate
     Live Births. Vital and Health Statistics, NCHS Series 20,
     No. 8, 1966.

17. Rantakallio, P. Groups at Risk in Low Birth Weight Infants
     and Perinatal Mortality. Acta Paediat. Scand. 193: 1-93,
     Suppl. 1969.

18. Baird, D. Environmental and Obstetrical Factors in Prematurity,
     with Special Reference to Experience in Aberdeen. Bull. WHO
     26: 291-295, 1962.

19. Lechtig, A., Delgado, H., Lasky, R. E., Klein, R. E. Engle, P.
     L., Yarbrough, C., Habicht, J-P. Maternal Nutrition and Fetal
     Growth in Developing Societies: Socioeconomic factors. Am. J.
     Dis. Child. 129: 434-437, 1975.

20. Abramowicz, M. and Kass, E. H. Pathogenesis and Prognosis of
     Prematurity. New Engl. J. Med. 275: 878-885, 938-943, 1001-
     1006, 1053-1059, 1966.

21. Abernathy, J. R., Greenberg, B. G., Donnelly, J. F. Applica-

tion of Discriminant Functions in Perinatal Death and
Survival. Am. J. Obst. Gyn., 95: 860-867, 1966.

22. Anderson, U. M., Jenss, R., Mosher, W. E., Randall, C. L. and
Marra, E. High Risk Groups - Definition and Identification.
New Engl. J. Med., 273: 308-313, 1965.

23. Baird, D. Social Class and Foetal Mortality. Lancet 253:
531-535, 1947.

24. Bedger, J. E., Gelperin, A. and Jacobs, E. E. Socioeconomic
Characteristics in Relation to Maternal and Child Health.
Pub. Hlth. Rep. 81: 829-833, 1966.

25. Chase, H. C. and Nelson, F. G. Education of Mother, Medical
Care and Condition of the Infant. Am. J. Pub. Hlth.,
(Supplement) 63: 27-40, 1973.

26. Erhardt, C. L., Abramson, H., Pakter, J. and Nelson, F. An
Epidemiological Approach to Infant Mortality. Arch. Environ.
Hlth. 20: 743-757, 1970.

27. Erhardt, C. L. and Chase, H. C. Ethnic Group, Education of
Mother and Birth Weight. Am. J. Pub. Hlth. 63: 17-26, 1973.

28. Donabedian, A., Rosenfeld, L. S. and Souther, E. M. Infant
Mortality and Socioeconomic Status in a Metropolitan Community.
Pub. Hlth. Rep., 80: 1083-1094, 1965.

29. Greenberg, B. G. and Wells, H. B. Linear Discriminant Analysis in Perinatal Mortality. Am. J. Pub. Hlth. 53: 594-602,
1963.

30. Rider, R. V., Taback, M. and Knobloch, H. Associations
between Premature Birth and SES. Am. J. Pub. Hlth. 45: 1022-
1028, 1955.

31. Thompson, J. F. Some Observations on the Geographic Distribution of Premature Births and Perinatal Deaths in Indiana.
Am. J. Obst. Gyn. 101: 43-52, 1968.

32. Wiener, G. and Milton, T. The Demographic Correlates of Low
Birth Weight. Am. J. Epidemiol. 91: 260-272, 1970.

33. Willie, C., Rothney, W. Racial, Ethnic and Income Factors in
the Epidemiology of Neonatal Mortality. Am. Sociol. Rev.,
27: 522-526, 1962.

34. Chandrasekhar, S. Infant Mortality in India 1901-1935.

London: George Allen & Unwin Ltd., 1959.

35. Hedayat, S. H., Koohestani, P. A. and Kamali, P. Influences of Economic Status and Certain Maternal Factors on Birth-Weight. J. Trop. Ped. 17: 158-162, 1971.

36. Infante-Roldan, S., Puentes-Rojas, R., Rivera-Marfan, F., Gray-Gray, J., Maulen-Piña, J., Morales-Aedo, J., Zenteno-Travisany, M., Díaz-Zepeda, D., and Vargas-Jarmel, S. Epidemiología de la mortalidad infantil. Extudio comparativo con grupo control, area hospitalaria Vallenar, año 1967. Rev. Chilena Ped. 42: 281-292.

37. Jansen, A. A. Birthweight, Birthlength, Prematurity and Neonatal Mortality in New Guineans. Trop. Geogr. Med. 14: 341-349, 1962.

38. Jain, V. C. Some Social Components of Infant Mortality in India. Indian J. Ped. 35: 109-112, 1968.

39. Moodie, A. D., Hansen, J.D.L., Jordaan, H.V.F., Malan, A. F. and Davy, D. Low Weight Cape Coloured Mothers and Their Infants. South Afr. Med. J. 44: 1400-1408, 1970.

40. Rahimtoola, R. J., Mir, S. and Baloch, S. Low Birthweight, the "small for dates" Syndrome and Perinatal Mortality in a Low Family Income Group. Acta Paed. Scand. 57: 534-536, 1968.

41. Richardson, B. D. Studies on South African Bantu and Caucasian Pre-school Children: Mortality Rates in Urban and Rural Areas. Trans. Roy. Soc. Trop. Med. Hyg. 64: 921-926, 1970.

42. Shah, P. M., Udani, P.M. and Shah, K. P. Analysis of the Vital Statistics from the Rural Community Palghar. I: Foetal Wastage and Maternal Mortality. Indian Ped. 6: 595-607, 1969.

43. Shah, P. M., and Udani, P. M. Analysis of the Vital Statistics from the Rural Community, Palghar. II: Perinatal, Neonatal and Infant Mortalities. Indian Ped. 6: 651-668, 1969.

44. Timmer, M. Prosperity and Birthweight in Javanese Infants. Trop. Geogr. Med. 13: 316-320, 1961.

45. Baird, D. and Thomson, A. M. The Survey Perinatal Deaths Reclassified by Special Clinicopathological Assessment. In: Butler and Alberman, op.cit., Chapters 2,11,13,14, 1969.

46. Kincaid, J. C. Social Pathology of Foetal and Infant Loss. Brit. Med. J. 1: 1057-1060, 1965.

47. Butler, N. R. and Bonham, D. G. Perinatal Mortality: The
    First Report of the 1958 British Perinatal Mortality Survey.
    London: E.& S. Livingston, Ltd., 1963.

48. Butler, N. R. and Alberman, E. D. (eds.): Perinatal Problems:
    The Second Report of the 1958 British Perinatal Mortality
    Survey. London: E. & S. Livingston, Ltd., 1969.

49. Chase, H. C. Infant Mortality and Weight at Birth: 1960
    United States Birth Cohort. Am. J. Pub. Hlth. 59: 1618-1628,
    1969.

50. Lechtig, A., Delgado, H., Martorell, R., Richardson, D.,
    Yarbrough, C. and Klein, R. E. Socioeconomic Factors,
    Maternal Nutrition and Infant Mortality in Developing Countries.
    Paper presented at the VII World Congress of Gynecology and
    Obstetrics, Mexico, D.F., October 17-24, 1976.

51. Bergner, L. and Susser, M. W. Low Birth Weight and Prenatal
    Nutrition: An Interpretative Review. Pediatrics 46: 946-966,
    1970.

52. Habicht, J-P., Lechtig, A., Yarbrough, C. and Klein, R. E.
    Maternal Nutrition, Birth Weight, and Infant Mortality. In:
    K. Elliott and J. Knight (eds.): Size at Birth (Ciba Founda-
    tion Symposium 27), Amsterdam: Associated Scientific
    Publishers.

53. Lechtig, A., Habicht, J-P., DeLeón, E., Guzmán, G., and
    Flores, M. Influencia de la nutrición sobre el crecimiento
    fetal en poblaciones rurales de Guatemala: Aspectos
    dietéticos. Arch. Latinoamer. Nutr., 22: 101-115, 1972.

54. Lechtig, A., Habicht, J-P., Delgado, H., Klein, R. E.,
    Yarbrough, C. and Martorell, R. Effect of Food Supplementa-
    tion during Pregnancy on Birth Weight. Pediatrics 56: 508-
    520, 1975.

55. Arroyave, G., Hicks, W. H., King, D. L., Guzmán, M. A.,
    Flores, M., and Scrimshaw, N. S. Comparación de algunos
    datos bioquímico-nutricionales obtenidos de mujeres embara-
    zadas procedentes de dos niveles socio-económicos de Guatemala.
    Rev. Col. Med. Guate. 11: 80-87, 1960.

56. Arroyave, G., De Moscoso, Y., and Lechtig, A. Vitamina A en
    sangre de embarazados y sus recién nacidos de dos grupos
    socioeconómicos. Arch. Latinoamer. Nutr. 25: 283-290, 1975.

57. Institute of Nutrition of Central América and Panamá and
    Nutrition Program, Center for Disease Control (USPHS).

Nutritional Evaluation of the Population of Central America and Panama, 1965-1967. DHEW Publication No. (HSM) 72-8120.

58. Sebrell, W. H., King, K. W., Webb, R. E., Daza, C. H.,
     Franco, R. A., Smith, S. C., Severinghaus, E. L., Pi-Sunyer,
     F. X., Underwood, B. A., Flores, M., Conner, M. C., Townsend,
     C. T., Pezzotti, J. M., and Castillo, B. Nutritional Status
     of Middle and Low Income Groups in the Dominican Republic.
     Arch. Latinoamer. Nutr. _22_ (Supplement 1-190) 1972.

59. Venkatachalam, P. S. Maternal Nutritional Status and Its
     Effects on the Newborn. _Bull WHO_ _26_: 193-201, 1962.

60. Lechtig, A., Yarbrough, C., Delgado, H., Martorell, R.,
     Klein, R. E., and Béhar, M. Effect of Moderate Maternal Mal-
     nutrition on the Placenta. _Am. J. Obst. Gyn_. _123_: 191-201,
     1975.

61. Naeye, P. L. and Blanc, W. Poverty and Race: Effects on
     Prenatal Nutrition. _Pediatric Res_. _4_: 473, 1970.

62. Naeye, R. L., Diener, M. M., Horcke, H. T. and Blanc, W. A.
     Relation of Poverty and Race to Birth Weight and Organ and
     Cell Structure in the Newborn. _Pediatric Res_. _5_: 17-22, 1971.

63. Klein, R. E., Habicht, J-P. and Yarbrough, C. Some Method-
     ological Problems in Field Studies of Nutrition and Intelli-
     gence. In: D. J. Kallen (ed.), _Nutrition, Development and_
     Social Behavior, 61-75. Washington, D.C.: U.S. Government
     Printing Office, DHEW Publication No. (NIH) 73-242, 1973.

64. Thomson, A. M. Technique and Perspective in Clinical and
     Dietary Studies of Human Pregnancy. _Proc. Nutr. Soc_. _16_:
     45-51, 1957.

65. Lechtig, A., Delgado, H., Lasky, R., Yarbrough, C., Klein,
     R. E., Habicht, J-P. and Béhar, M. Maternal Nutrition and
     Fetal Growth in Developing Countries. _Am. J. Dis. Child_. _129_:
     553-556, 1975.

66. Illsley, R. Social Class Selection and Differences in Rela-
     tion to Stillbirths and Infant Deaths. _Brit. Med. J_. _2_:
     1520-1524, 1955.

67. Gruenwald, P., Funakawa, H., Mitani, S., Nichimura, T. and
     Takeuchi, S. Influence of Environmental Factors on Foetal
     Growth in Man. _Lancet 1_: 1026-1028, 1967.

68. Gruenwald, P. Fetal Growth as an Indicator of Socioeconomic
     Change. _Pub. Hlth. Rep_. _83_: 867-872, 1968.

69. Chandra, R. K. Fetal Malnutrition and Postnatal Immuno-
     competence. Amer. J. Dis. Child. 129: 450-454, 1975.

70. Lechtig, A., Martorell, R., Yarbrough, C., Delgado, H., and
     Klein, R. E. Influence of Food Supplementation on the Urinary
     urea/creatinine (U/C) Ratio of the Child. Submitted to J.
     Trop. Ped., 1976.

71. INCAP/DDH, unpublished data, 1976.

72. Lechtig, A., Delgado, H., Martorell, R., Yarbrough, C. and
     Klein, R. E. Maternal-feto Nutrition. In: D. B. Jelliffe
     and E. F. P. Jellife (eds.), Nutrition and Growth, New York:
     Plenum Press, in press.

73. Lechtig, A., Martorell, R., Delgado, H., Yarbrough, C. and
     Klein, R. E. Nutrition and Growth: Pre and Post-natal. In:
     M. Winick (ed.), Nutrition and Development: Pre-and Post-
     Natal. New York: Plenum Press, 1976, in press.

74. Lechtig, A., Delgado, H., Lasky, R., Yarbrough, C., Martorell,
     R., and Klein, R. E. Influencia de la nutrición materna
     sobre el crecimiento y desarrollo del niño hasto los 15 meses
     de edad. Paper presented at the X Congreso Centroamericano
     de Gineco-Obstetricia, Symposium on "Factors ambientales que
     afectan la salud de la madre y del niño en Centro América y
     sus implicaciones para la formulación de un programa materno-
     infantil." Guatemala, Nov. 27 - Dec. 2, 1974.

75. Levy, B. S., Wilkinson, F. S., Marina, W. M. Reducing Neo-
     natal Mortality with Nurse-midwives. Am. J. Obst. Gyn. 109:
     50, 1971.

76. Nold, B., Stallones, R. A. and Raynolds, W. E. The Social
     Class Gradient of Perinatal Mortality in Dependents of Mili-
     tary Personnel. Am. J. Epidemiol. 83: 481-488, 1966.

77. Yankauer, A., Goss, K. G. and Romeo, S. M. An Evaluation of
     Prenatal Care and Its Relationship to Social Class and Social
     Disorganization. Am. J. Pub. Hlth. 43: 1003-1010, 1953.

78. Richards, I.D.G. and Lowe, C. E. Changes in the Stillbirth
     Rate in England and Wales. Lancet 1: 1169-1173, 1966.

79. Parmlee, A. H. Prematurity and Illegitimacy. Am. J. Obst.
     Gyn. 81: 81-94, 1961.

80. Lechtig, A., Delgado, H., Yarbrough, C., Habicht, J. P.,
     Martorell, R. and Klein, R. D. A Simple Assessment of the

Risk of Low Birthweight to Select Women for Nutritional
Intervention. Am. J. Obst. Gyn. 125: 25-34, 1976.

81.   INCAP/DDH Publication/Working Group on Rural Medical Care:
      Delivery of Primary Care by Medical Auxiliaries: Techniques
      of Use and Analysis of Benefits Achieved in Some Rural
      Villages in Guatemala, 24-37. Washington, D. C.: PAHO/WHO
      Scientific Publication No. 278, Medical Care Auxiliaries,
      1973.

NUTRITION AND BREAST-FEEDING

INTRODUCTORY STATEMENT

Jeanne Clare Ridley

Georgetown University

Washington, D. C.

The declines in breast-feeding now occurring in developing countries have been viewed increasingly with alarm by professionals in several fields. Since breast milk is considered the best source of nutrition for infants and, in developing countries, has the added advantage of being the most sanitary source of food for infants, health personnel and nutritionists have become greatly concerned. Demographers have also voiced concern since, in the absence of family planning techniques, lactation has played an important role in maintaining fertility at a lower level than it would be if breast-feeding were not practiced.

In the paper by Van Ginneken, the state of knowledge concerning the relationship between lactation and fertility is summarized. Although considerable data exist as to the duration of breast-feeding for a large number of populations, less information is available concerning the degree of variability in the return of menstruation between women and among populations. While the return of menstruation among lactating mothers is not an accurate indicator of ovulation, few studies have been carried out to indicate when ovulation does occur. Moreover, the fact that some women become pregnant while breast-feeding and not menstruating, indicates the need for a better understanding of the contraceptive effect of the prolongation of amenorrhea by breastfeeding. As Van Ginneken suggests, there appears to be a limit to the contraceptive effect of lactation. The longer lactation lasts the less breast-feeding contributes to the prolongation of amenorrhea. The implication for family planning programs in defining the optimal time lactation can be expected to have a contraceptive effect is obvious. The need for detection methods of ovulation that are relatively inexpensive and reliable would greatly aid such programs.

Several other aspects of lactation are also in need of explora-
tion as suggested by Van Ginneken. First, little is known regarding
the impact of shifts from full to partial breast-feeding on the
return of menstruation and ovulation. Must full breast-feeding
always be maintained for lactation to have a contraceptive effect?
Alternatively, is there a level of partial breast-feeding that must
be maintained for a contraceptive effect to be present? In addition,
studies of the impact of lactation on fertility have not adequately
indicated the role of other factors that may tend to obscure the
relationship.

Not surprisingly, Van Ginneken's paper raises more questions
regarding the possible impact of lactation on fertility than it
answers. The author emphasizes the need for more studies utilizing
a prospective design. While such studies overcome the memory bias
inherent in retrospective studies, prospective studies must be of
sufficient length to ensure that a truncation bias is not introduced.

The paper by Wray provides an excellent review of data collected in the late 19th and early 20th century from the now
developed countries which indicate that the adverse consequence of
taking babies off the breast early were recognized and well documented a century ago. Though less definitive data are available,
it seems clear that the developing world is now following the
developed world in the transition from breast to bottle feeding,
with the attendant increases in infant morbidity and mortality.

Little is known about the effect of the nutritional level of
the mother in shortening or lengthening the period of amenorrhea
associated with breast-feeding. Variations in the length of
amenorrhea accompanying lactation observed for different populations, however, suggest that the nutritional level of the mother
may not be unimportant. Wray reviews data which suggest that
breast milk production, particularly volume and perhaps duration,
may be related to not only current maternal nutritional status,
but also childhood nutritional history. Because the infant nursing patterns are likely to be related to milk production, it is
possible that this may be a link relating poor maternal nutritional
status to prolongation of lactational amenorrhea.

The general hypothesis presented in the earlier paper by
Frisch as to body weight and fecundity suggests that the contraceptive effect of lactation may be overstated when estimates are
based on data for malnourished mothers. Indeed, very few studies
in well nourished populations of the period of amenorrhea associated
with lactation have been carried out. Studies that would dis-
entangle the role of such factors as nutrition, age of the mother,

infant survival and such cultural practices as abstinence need to
be initiated. Such studies could have important implications for
populations in developing countries if levels of nutrition are
improving.

    The paper by Butz presents a model from which a large number
of hypotheses regarding the determinants of breast-feeding practices may be derived. He identifies a large number of questions
to which future research should be directed if the factors associated with social choices relating to breast-feeding practices are
to be identified and policies initiated to stem the declines in
breast-feeding occurring in the developing countries. For example,
a crucial question is "what populations are at risk of breastfeeding declines and subject to the deleterious effects on infants
and on birth spacing?" The model proposed by Butz indicates a
wide range of factors that need investigation before effective
policies can be initiated. Although the discussion of the model
is focused on its application to developing countries, the model
also provides a framework for studying the factors contributing to
the low incidence in breast-feeding in developed countries. It
thus has policy implications if breast-feeding in such countries
is to be encouraged for purposes of ensuring better health among
future generations.

THE IMPACT OF PROLONGED BREAST-FEEDING ON BIRTH INTERVALS AND

ON POSTPARTUM AMENORRHOEA

Jeroen K. Van Ginneken

International Planned Parenthood Federation

London, England

INTRODUCTION

Many mothers in low income countries, particularly in rural areas, nurse their children from 1 to 2 years. The main purpose of this practice is, of course, to provide newborn children with the nutrition necessary for their survival. Many mothers continue to nurse for a long time, often until or after the next pregnancy occurs, because they believe it to be beneficial for their children (1,2).

Sustained lactation requires an adequate interval between births. In various countries it is believed that lactation itself postpones the next pregnancy and that adequate spacing between births can be achieved by means of this practice (3,4,5). In other societies spacing between births is realized through lactation together with abstinence from sexual relations after birth. This is particularly prevalent in polygynous societies in Africa, but also - with large variations in duration of abstinence - in many Asian countries* (2,6,7,8,9,10).

From a physiological point of view lactation postpones the next pregnancy by inhibiting ovulation and by delaying resumption of the menstrual cycle. Suckling of the infant is important for

---

* Reinforcing the practice of postpartum abstinence is the belief that intercourse during lactation reduces the supply of milk or spoils the milk. Abstinence is thus often practiced to make sure that mothers can nurse their children for 1 to 2 years uninterrupted by another pregnancy.

suppression of the menstrual cycle, because suckling leads to the release of prolactin which not only plays an important role in milk production, but also inhibits the release of gonadotrophins which initiate resumption of the menstrual cycle (11,12,13).

This paper will examine the birth spacing effect of prolonged breastfeeding and findings will be summarized which are derived from sample surveys conducted during the last 10 to 20 years. In these surveys women were interviewed concerning their breastfeeding practices and its impact on subsequent pregnancies and on resumption of menstruation. Questions on these topics were asked in many of these surveys as part of fertility and family planning surveys and in several epidemiological surveys.

This paper consists of four sections. In the first we will describe the kind of information that can be obtained by means of surveys and identify problems that can arise in the interpretation of survey data. Information on incidence and duration of breastfeeding derived from recent surveys will be provided in the second section. The third section will summarize results of the impact of lactation on the length of pregnancy and birth intervals. The fourth section will describe findings on the relationship of lactation with postpartum amenorrhoea together with the role of full versus partial breastfeeding.

METHODOLOGICAL ISSUES

Components of Birth Intervals

In order to determine the kinds of information that can be obtained with sample surveys it is useful to consider Figure 1, showing the three parts of birth intervals, for lactating and non-lactating women (14,15,16). The birth of a child is followed by a period of postpartum amenorrhea which is usually longer for nursing than for non-nursing women. This interval is followed by resumption of menstruation and a number of menstrual cycles leading to the next conception. This is the menstruating interval which is followed by a period of gestation. The data of conception is usually estimated at two weeks after the first day of the last menses. A birth interval, therefore, is the period ranging from one birth to the next and is composed of a period of amenorrhea, a menstruating interval and gestation. An (inter-) pregnancy interval is the period ranging from a birth to the next conception.

A period of amenorrhea can lead directly into a period of gestation indicating that pregnancies can occur during the first menstrual cycle after birth before resumption of menstruation.

Resumption of menstruation is, therefore, a less accurate indicator of return of fecundity after childbirth than is first ovulation after birth. Ovulation cannot, however, be determined with the type of surveys being discussed here.

On the basis of these definitions we can describe in more detail the information which can be obtained by means of sample surveys about lactation and its impact on fertility. Information is collected about the various dependent variables such as the length of pregnancy intervals, birth intervals and periods of amenorrhea. These dependent variables are related to independent variables, in particular nursing or non-nursing status, duration of nursing, and full versus partial nursing.

Interpretation of Data in Sample Surveys

Three problems often occur when interpreting survey results. One problem is how to isolate the influence of the independent variable under study (e.g., lactation) from the influence of other factors that affect the dependent variable (e.g., pregnancy intervals). This is often difficult and the possible role of extraneous variables should be kept in mind when interpreting results.

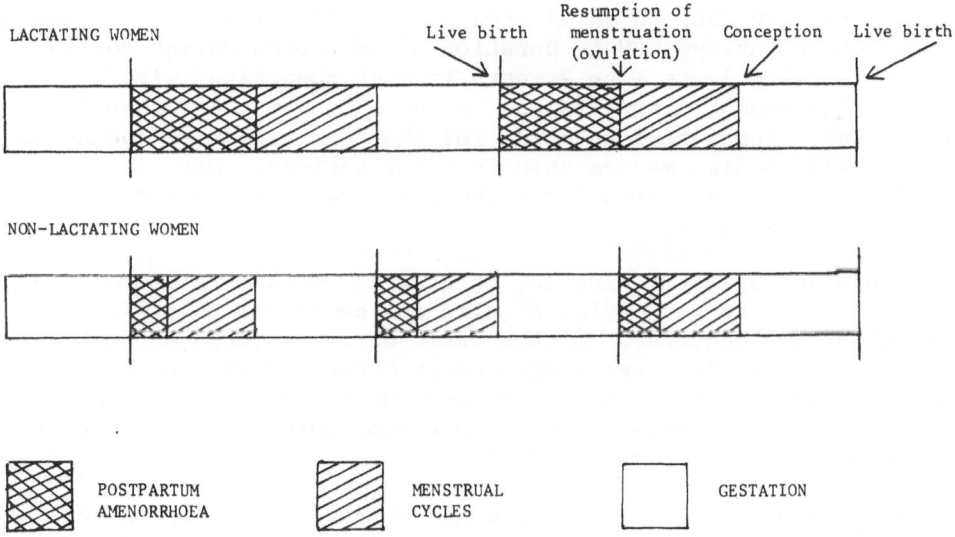

Figure 1. A Comparison of the Components of Birth Intervals of Lactating and Non-Lactating Women.

The second problem with surveys concerns the accuracy of the data obtained. This is particularly a problem with regard to retrospective surveys since respondents may not be able to give accurate answers about events which occurred one or two years earlier. For instance, with respect to the duration of breast-feeding, many more respondents are often recorded as having stopped nursing after 6, 12, 18, or 24 months.

The third problem is how to classify incomplete observations. An observation is incomplete when, for instance, women are still nursing at the cutoff date of a study. Data based on such incomplete observations can be included in the analysis by application of the life-table method (17,15). Generally, when incomplete observations are included, preference should be given to using medians instead of means when estimating variables such as duration of lactation or amenorrhea.

INCIDENCE AND DURATION OF LACTATION

Table 1 shows percentages of women who started breastfeeding after birth together with mean duration of breastfeeding (for those who practiced it). The studies represented in Table 1 were undertaken fairly recently (since 1967) and sample sizes were fairly large (at least 500 women or births). Table 1 indicates that lactation is nearly universal in rural areas of low income countries for which data are shown with the exception of Chile. The percentages of women who initiate nursing in urban areas are somewhat smaller than in rural areas, a result which is also found in many other surveys. Mean duration of lactation varies considerably. Nursing lasts 1 to 2 years in most countries, with a tendency for women in rural areas to nurse longer than those in urban areas. Women tend to nurse for shorter periods in countries in South and Middle America than in other regions. More quantitative information about incidence and duration of lactation is provided by Rosa (1).

Prolonged breastfeeding is, in general, much more common and practiced for a longer period of time in low income countries than in high income countries. On the basis of two surveys conducted in Paris, France, five years ago and in Great Britain ten years ago, for instance, it is estimated that only about half of the women began with nursing and that they continued for an average of 1 and 2 months respectively (18,19).

Many women begin with "on demand" nursing which ranges in most cases from 5 to 10 times per day. This decreases gradually to once or twice a day as the child grows older and solid food, with or without animal milk, is added to its diet. For more details on weaning practices in various countries, see Jelliffe

Table 1

Incidence and Duration of Lactation Derived from
Selected Surveys in a Number of Countries

Region and Country	Source	Residence (Urban/ Rural)	Percent Starting Lactation	Mean Duration of Lactation (for women whose children were weaned)
Africa				
Algeria	1	u/r	90-95	17.5
Nigeria	2	r	95-100	15
Senegal	1	r	95-100	24
Zaire	3	r	95-100	26
South and Middle America				
Chile	4	r	68	6
Colombia	1	u	79	5.5
Martinique	1	u/r	93	10
Venezuela, Colombia	1	u	84	7.5
Asia				
India,Calcutta	4	u	93	16.5
India, Tamil Nadu	4	r	-	22
Indonesia	5	r	99	25.5
Philippines	6	u	77	10
South Korea	1	u/r	96	24
Taiwan	1	u/r	93	16
Thailand	1	u	86	12
Turkey	1	u	95	13

Sources: 1. Original source cited in (5);   2.(7) (median);
         3. (21) (estimated from Figure 2, p. 439);
         4. Original source cited in (1);   5. (10);   6. (30).

(20). Fertility and family planning surveys have, in general,
provided little information about provision of supplementary nutrition at different intervals after birth and the time of its introduction. It is important to know for how long the infant was
dependent exclusively on breast milk and when and how often
artificial feeding was provided, because of implications for return
of fecundity.

A few surveys give information about supplemental feedings,
and they indicate that the average period of full lactation varies
a great deal. In the Nigerian survey represented in Table 1, the
median duration of full lactation was 11 months, while the median
period of full and partial lactation was 15 months (7). In the
survey in Zaire, on the other hand, it is estimated that supplementary feeding was generally introduced after 4 months, whereas
these women continued breastfeeding for more than two years (21).
In the Punjab (India) (4), full lactation was practiced for 6 out
of 21 months (medians), whereas in a survey in rural Bangladesh
(15) it was about 9 months out of 25 (also medians). In many low
income countries, in particular in urban areas, breastfeeding has
declined rapidly and has been replaced by bottle feeding (18,22).
This decrease in incidence and duration is related to a number of
"modernization" processes, such as widespread use of advertising
techniques to promote infant formulas, negative attitudes of medical personnel towards breastfeeding, employment outside the home,
and inadequate socialization in nursing techniques in nuclear
families (absence of relatives who have had experience with nursing) (18,22).

The influence of some of these modernization processes can be
inferred from survey data. Incidence and duration of breastfeeding are related to place of residence: it is more common and
practiced longer in rural than in urban areas. Many surveys have
also found a correlation with age at birth: among younger women it
is less common and practiced for a shorter time than among older
women. Another factor is education: women with higher levels of
education breastfeed less frequently and for a shorter time than
those with lower levels of education. Employment outside the
home is another factor of importance. Several surveys have found
that women who were employed and need to return to their jobs soon
after delivery nurse less frequently than those who are not working
(20,23).

LACTATION AND PREGNANCY AND BIRTH INTERVALS

Pregnancy Intervals of Nursing and Non-nursing Women

Figure 2 compares the average pregnancy intervals of nursing
mothers who had weaned their children with those of mothers who,
because of foetal deaths or stillbirths, had not nursed. In five
selected studies in populations who did not use contraception, or
only to a small extent, average pregnancy intervals were substantially longer for nursing than for non-nursing women. The difference
ranges from 13-15 months in Bangladesh, Nigeria and Senegal to 7
months in Taiwan. The duration of lactation averaged about two
years in the rural areas of Bangladesh, Nigeria, Senegal and Punjab

(India) in which these studies were undertaken, and about 16 months
in Taiwan. These survey results suggest that lactation lengthens
pregnancy intervals substantially.

    Figure 3, showing the cumulative percentages of nursing and
non-nursing women conceiving at various intervals after delivery
in two populations, illustrates in another way the substantial
effect of the practice of prolonged lactation on the rate of conception. Among nursing women, pregnancy rates remained low until
about one year after birth. After one year these rates increased

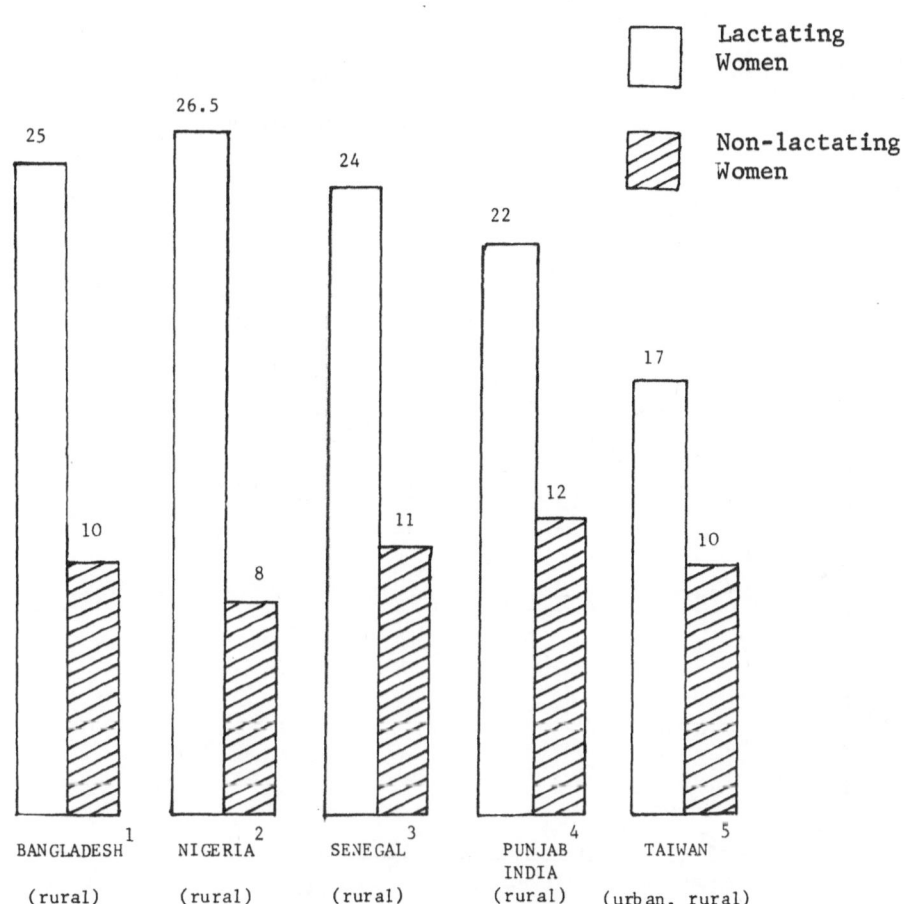

Figure 2. Average Length of Pregnancy Intervals (in months) of
           Lactating and Non-lactating Women
Sources: 1. (15) (estimate) (medians); 2. (31) (means);
          3. (32) (means); 4. (17) (medians); 5. (33) (means).

rapidly, suggesting that lactation protects against conception for a limited period of time.

One can estimate the relative effect of lactation on the overall birth interval by determining first how much longer birth intervals are for nursing than for non-nursing women. Next one can calculate to what extent this difference contributes to average birth intervals. In rural Bangladesh, for instance, birth intervals averaged about 36 months; lactation accounted for about 15 months, which means an effect of 15/36 or 42 percent. In many other low income countries, this impact on birth intervals is smaller than in rural Bangladesh. In Taiwan, for example, where

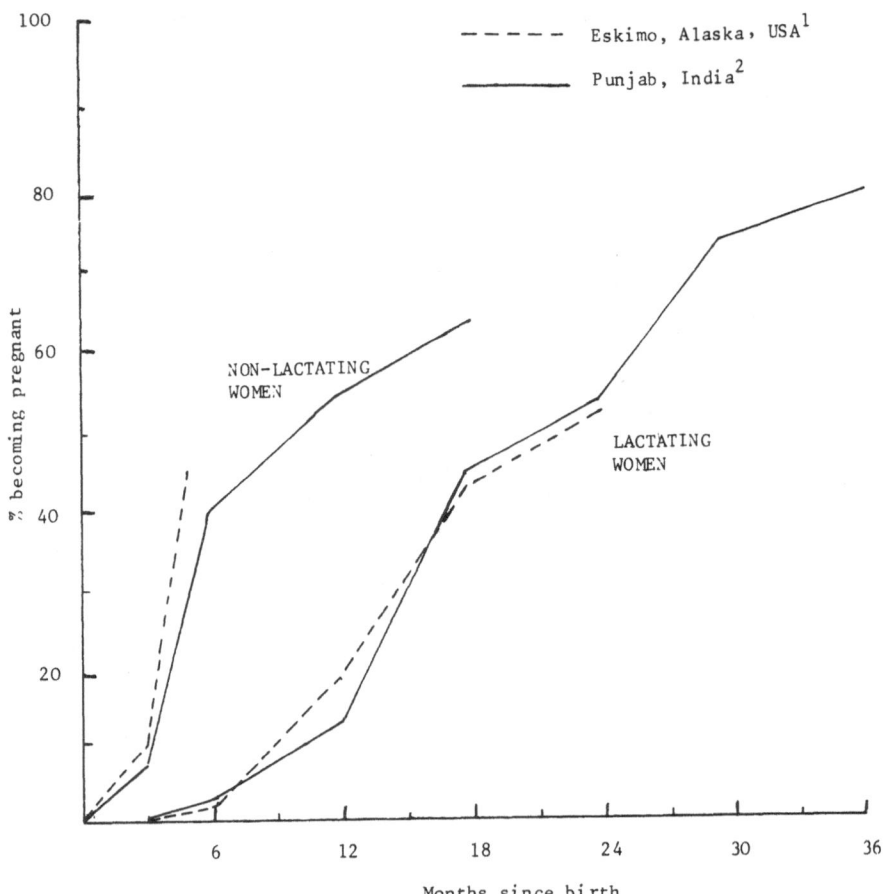

Figure 3. Cumulative Percentages of Lactating and Non-lactating Women Becoming Pregnant (by Months) Since Birth

Sources: 1. (27); 2. (17) (women 20-29).

birth intervals were about 30 months, the contribution of lactation was 7 months or 23 percent.

The data of Figures 2 and 3 should be interpreted with caution because several factors were not adequately controlled. One of these is malnutrition. Malnutrition may have an impact on amenorrhea independent from the effects of lactation (12,15). Other factors are the practice of abstinence from sexual relations after birth, or the frequency of sexual relations. In the Punjab (India) for example, postpartum abstinence lasted six months on average (17). It is also possible that the mothers who had experienced a foetal death or stillbirth wanted another child as soon as possible. Coital frequency may have been higher in that group of women than in the group of nursing women, thus influencing the pregnancy rates observed. Still another factor could be differences in the age composition of the study populations. Most studies have found that older women experience longer periods of amenorrhea than younger women; this relationship continues to exist after controlling for the duration of lactation (25).

Conception Before Resumption of Menstruation

It is important to know to what extent pregnancies occur before resumption of menstruation. Results of 4 studies using prospective designs are available on this subject. These studies in India, Bangladesh, Chile, and U.S.A. (Alaskan Eskimos) show percentages of women conceiving during amenorrhea of 7.0, 6.8, 7.0, and 2.6 percent respectively (4,15,26,27). These findings are consistent with results obtained by Perez et al., who demonstrated that the large majority of first menstrual cycles beginning more than two months after delivery were ovulatory (26).

Several other studies have reported on the incidence of pregnancies during amenorrhea, but these have not been used, either because retrospective designs were used, or because there were indications that some women had stopped nursing before becoming pregnant, or were using contraception.

A few studies have also measured pregnancy rates for nursing and non-nursing women after resumption of menstruation. These studies found no significant differences in the rate of conception after resumption of menstruation between nursing and non-nursing women (4,27). These studies suggest that the pregnancy preventing capacity of prolonged breastfeeding is probably to a large extent limited to the amenorrheic period.

LACTATION AND AMENORRHEA

Figure 4 presents data on average duration of lactation and of amenorrhea in nine selected surveys. The practice of nursing can have a substantial impact on the duration of amenorrhea; however, there is marked variability between different areas. The duration of lactation was a little more than 2 years on the average in rural areas of Zaire, Indonesia, and Bangladesh, with the duration of amenorrhea ranging from 19 to 22 months. In urban areas in Thailand, the Philippines and Colombia, on the other hand, duration of lactation ranged from 8 to 12 months, whereas periods of amenorrhea lasted from 4 to 6 months. The period of postpartum amenorrhea averaged about 2 to 3 months for non-nursing women (1). Thus, the impact of lactation alone on amenorrhea ranges from a maximum of about 18 months (in rural areas of Zaire, Indonesia and Bangladesh) to a minimum of about 2 months (in urban areas of Colombia).

The relationship of duration of amenorrhea to duration of lactation for groups of women in four different countries who nursed their children for different periods of time is shown in Figure 5. This reveals a linear relationship in all 4 studies between the two variables. The plateauing of the curves for Taiwan suggests that the longer lactation lasted, the less it added to the average duration of amenorrhea. The maximum duration of amenorrhea observed was about 15 months in the Taiwan study for women nursing between 30 and 36 months.

This Taiwan study also showed the influence of age on the relationship between lactation and amenorrhea. Periods of amenorrhea were in general shorter for women below 30 than for those who were 30 or older. Duration of amenorrhea levelled off for women below 30 at about 12 to 13 months for periods of lactation lasting 21 months or more (25).

Figure 6 shows cumulative percentages of nursing women resuming menstruation at various intervals after delivery. Comparison of the five groups of women who were nursing at the time of resumption of menses indicates that menstruation resumed faster for women in India, Taiwan and South Korea than for women in Bangladesh and Zaire. Comparison of these five groups of nursing women with the non-nursing group of women makes it clear that menstruation resumed much faster in the latter group than in the former groups. An important point to consider here is the variability of resumption of menses. Although the median duration of amenorrhea was about 12 months in India, Taiwan and South Korea, a considerable proportion of the nursing women experienced resumption of menstruation much earlier or much later than that average. The surveys in India, Taiwan and South Korea, for instance, show that among breast-feeding women 14 to 19 percent had resumed menstruation within 3

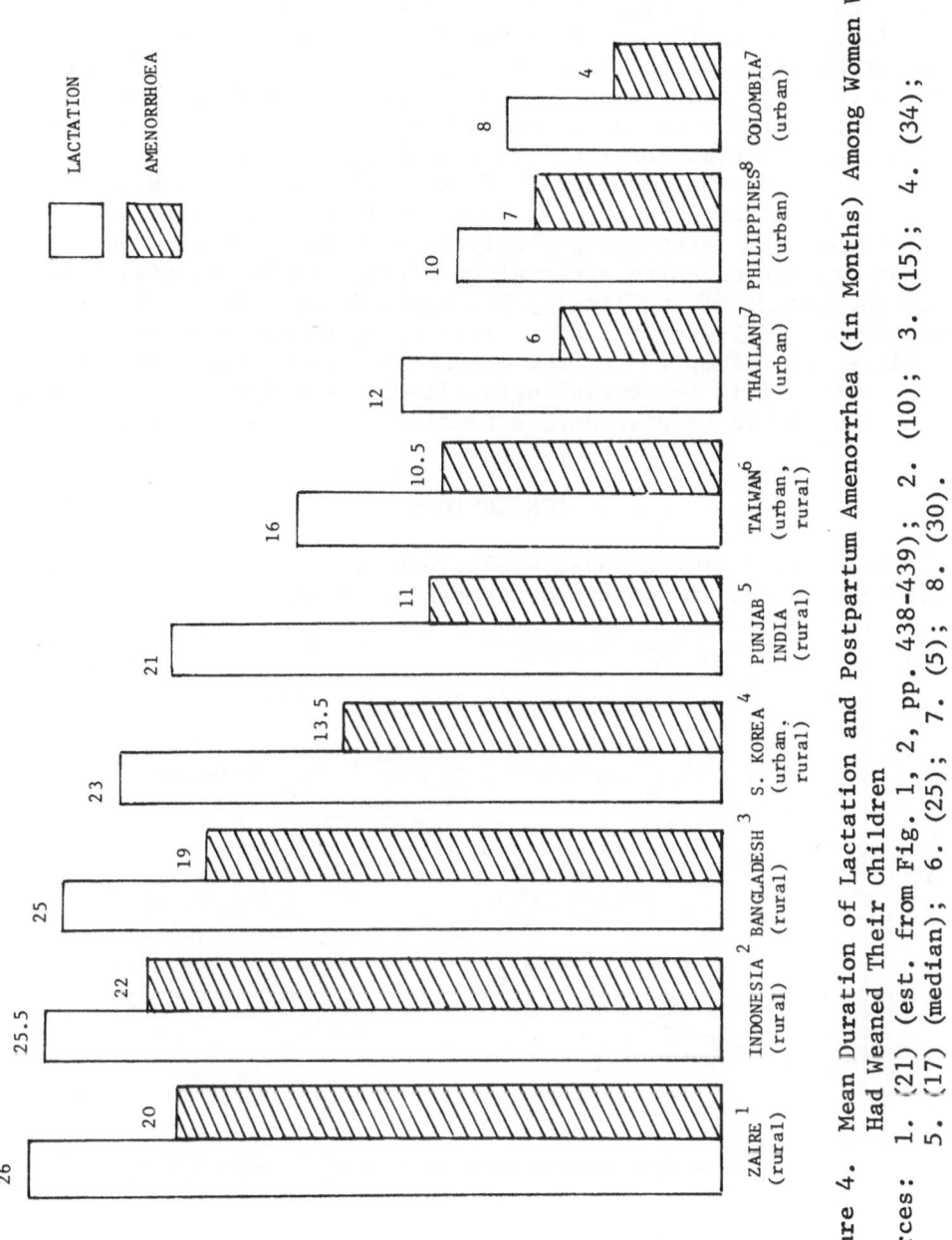

Figure 4. Mean Duration of Lactation and Postpartum Amenorrhea (in Months) Among Women Who Had Weaned Their Children

Sources: 1. (21) (est. from Fig. 1, 2, pp. 438-439); 2. (10); 3. (15); 4. (34); 5. (17) (median); 6. (25); 7. (5); 8. (30).

months after delivery.

Figures 5 and 6 indicated that lactation does not postpone amenorrhea indefinitely; the longer breastfeeding is practiced the more likely it is for menstruation to return and variability of resumption of menstruation is considerable. This is very likely due to the fact that women change from full to partial lactation at different intervals after birth. Perez, et al. and Chen, et al. found that menstruation (and ovulation) returned much sooner in women who gave supplementary foods to their infants than in women who were providing breast milk only (26,15). These changes from full to partial lactation probably explain why resumption of lactation can return quite early after birth. During partial lactation the amount of suckling by the child is much less intensive than during full breastfeeding, leading to hormonal changes which initiate the resumption of the menstrual cycle. The topic of changes from full to partial breastfeeding and its impact on return of menses should receive more attention in future surveys.

CONCLUSIONS

The effect of prolonged breastfeeding on birth and pregnancy intervals in low income countries can be substantial. In surveys

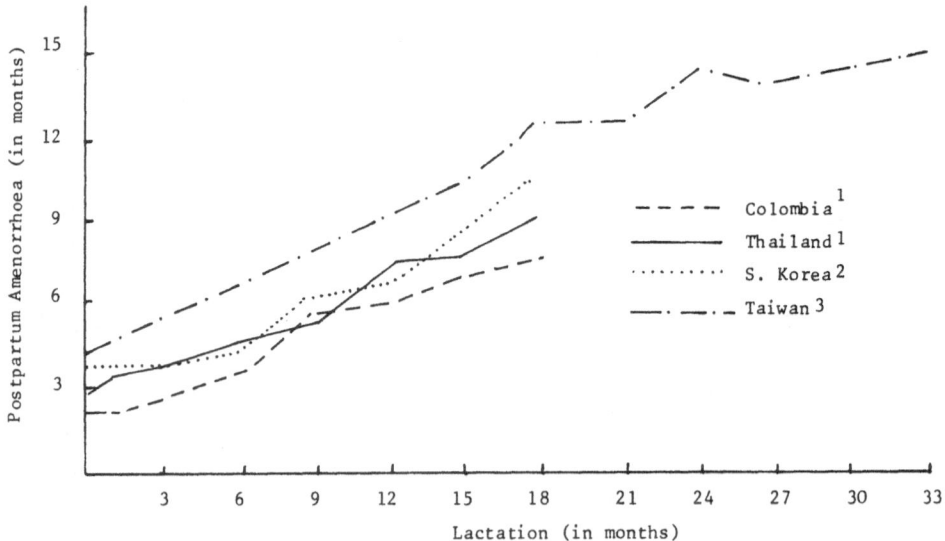

Figure 5.   The Relationship of Lactation with Postpartum Amenorrhea Among Women Who Had Weaned Their Children
Sources: 1. (5);   2. (35);   3. (25) (estimated from Fig. 2,p.262).

undertaken in the rural areas of some developing countries, it was found that lactational amenorrhea increased birth intervals by more than 15 months. An increase in birth intervals of 15 months accounts for about 40 percent of the average birth interval, implying a considerable impact on fertility. In most countries, the effect of breastfeeding is smaller. It is estimated that in most countries, lactation increases birth intervals from 5 to 20 percent.

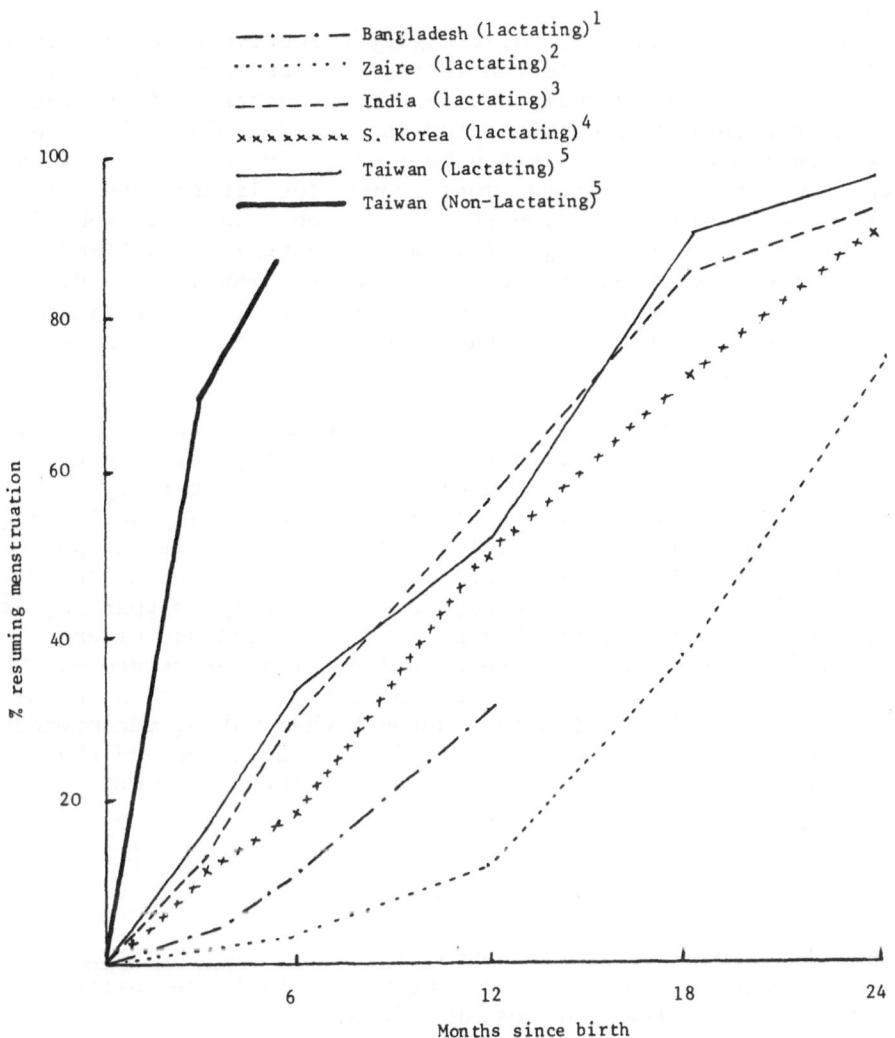

Figure 6.   Cumulative Percentages of Lactating and Non-lactating Women Resuming Menstruation (by Months) Since Birth
Sources: 1. (15);   2. (21) (estimated from Figures 1 and 2, pp. 438-439);   3. (17):   4. (34):   5. (25).

The incidence and duration of lactation in developing countries have decreased during the last two or three decades. In particular, in urban areas, it has been replaced to a considerable extent by bottle feeding. A consequence of this decrease in breastfeeding practices is that many more women are exposed to longer periods of risk of pregnancy. This means shorter birth intervals (which has probably happened in some countries) unless use of contraception increases at the same time.

Lactational amenorrhea, while highly effective as a fertility control measure at the population level, suffers from a lack of reliability at the individual level for two reasons. First, variability in resumption of menstruation is considerable. Although average duration of amenorrhea can be relatively long - for instance, one year - menstruation returns much sooner (or later) than this average for a considerable proportion of women. This is probably strongly related to the change from full to partial breastfeeding on return of ovulation and on resumption of the menstrual cycle. Second, from 3 to 7 percent of nursing women are likely to become pregnant during lactation amenorrhea since ovulation will precede the first menstruation in most cases.

Prolonged breastfeeding is thus by no means a perfect contraceptive method and women should - ideally speaking - initiate use of contraception at the beginning of the first ovulatory cycle after birth and not after return of first menses. Practical ovulation prediction methods do not exist, however, which leaves postpartum women who are interested in fertility control with the choice to initiate use of contraception immediately postpartum, at a certain point in time after birth, say 3 or 6 months, after changing from full to partial breastfeeding or after return of menstruation. Various cultural, health, nutritional and programmatic factors should be taken into account when making recommendations concerning use of contraception during lactation and the most appropriate time for its introduction. These have been discussed elsewhere (1,5,13,28,29).

References

1. Rosa, F. Breastfeeding in Family Planning. PAG Bulletin 5:5, 1975. Protein Calorie Advisory Group of the United Nations System (PAG), United Nations, New York.

2. Mandelbaum, D. G. Human Fertility in India. University of California Press, Berkeley, California, 1974.

3. Niehoff, A. and Meister, N. The Cultural Characteristics of Breastfeeding: A Survey. J. Trop. Paediatrics, 18: 16, 1972.

4. Wyon, J. B. and Gordon, J. E. The Khanna Study: Population Problems in the Rural Punjab. Cambridge, Harvard University Press, 1971.

5. Van Ginneken, J. Prolonged Breastfeeding as a Birth Spacing Method. Studies in Family Planning, 5: 201, 1974. Also in J. Env. Child Health 21: 59, 1975.

6. Okediji, F. O., Caldwell, J., Caldwell, P. and Ware, H. The Changing African Family Project: A Report with Special Reference to the Nigerian Segment. Studies in Family Planning, 7: 126, 1976.

7. Mott, F. L. Some Aspects of Health Care in Rural Nigeria. Studies in Family Planning 7: 109, 1976.

8. Nag, M. Factors Affecting Human Fertility in Non-industrial Societies: A Cross-cultural Study. Reprinted by Human Relations Area Files Press, Yale University Publications in Anthropology, No. 66, 1968.

9. Molnos, A. Cultural Source Materials for Population Planning in East Africa. Vol. 3, Beliefs and Practices, East African Publishing House, Nairobi, Kenya, 1973.

10. Singarimbun, M. and Manning, C. Breastfeeding, Amenorrhea and Abstinence in a Javanese Village: A Case Study in Mojolama. Studies in Family Planning 7: 175, 1976.

11. Tyson, J. E., Freedman, R. S., Perez, A., Zacur, H. A. and Zanartu, J. Significance of the Secretion of Human Prolactin and Gonadotropin for Puerpal Lactational Infertility. In CIBA Foundation Symposia 45, Breast-feeding and the Mother. Elsevier (Excerpta Medica), North Holland, Amsterdam, Netherlands, 1976.

12. Thomson, A., Hytten, F. E. and Black, A. E. Lactation and Reproduction. Bulletin World Health Organization 52: 337, 1975.

13. Buchanan, R. Breastfeeding - Aid to Infant Health and Fertility Control. Population Reports, Series J, 4, 1975.

14. Potter, R. G. Birth Intervals and Structure. Population Studies 17: 155, 1963.

15. Chen, L., Ahmed, S., Gesche, M., and Mosley, W. A Prospective Study of Birth Interval Dynamics in Rural Bangladesh. Population Studies 28: 277, 1974.

16. Leridon, H. Biostatistics of Human Reproduction. In:

Chandrasekaran, C. and Hermalin, A. (eds.) <u>Measuring the Effect of Family Planning Programmes on Fertility</u>. Ordina Editions, Belgium, 1975.

17. Potter, R. G., New, M., Wyon, J., and Gordon, J. Applications of Field Studies to Research on the Physiology of Human Reproduction. In: Sheps, M. and Ridley, J. (eds.), <u>Public Health and Population Change</u>. Pittsburgh: University of Pittsburgh Press, 1965.

18. Jelliffe, D. B. Community and Sociopolitical Considerations of Breastfeeding (and Discussion). In: CIBA Foundation Symposia 45, <u>Breast-feeding and the Mother</u>. Elsevier/Exerpta Medica/ North Holland, Amsterdam, Netherlands, 1976.

19. Langford, C. M. A Consideration of Some Retrospective Data on Breast Feeding in Great Britain (mimeographed). Population Investigating Committee, London School of Economics, 1976.

20. Jelliffe, D. B. <u>Infant Nutrition in the Subtropics and Tropics</u>, 2nd ed. World Health Organization Monograph No. 29, Geneva, 1968.

21. Vis, H., Bossuyt, M., Hennart, P. and Carael, M. The Health of Mother and Child in Rural Central Africa. <u>Studies in Family Planning</u> <u>6</u>: 437, 1975.

22. Berg, A. <u>The Nutrition Factor</u>. Brookings Institution, Washington, D. C., 1973.

23. Cleland, J. G. <u>A Study of Infant Care and Family Planning in the Suva Area</u>. Medical Department, Fiji, 1975.

24. Chowdhury, A., Khan, A., and Chen, L. The Effect of Child Mortality Experience on Subsequent Fertility in Pakistan and Bangladesh. <u>Population Studies</u> <u>30</u>: 2, 1976.

25. Jain, A., Hsu, T., Freedman, R. and Chang, M. Demographic Aspects of Lactation and Post-partum Amenorrhea. <u>Demography</u> <u>7</u>: 255, 1970.

26. Perez, A., Vela, P., Potter, R. and Masnick, G. S. Timing and Sequence of Resuming Ovulation and Menstruation after Childbirth. <u>Population Studies</u> <u>25</u>: 491, 1971.

27. Berman, M. L., Hanson, K. and Hellman, I. L. Effect of Breastfeeding on Postpartum Menstruation, Ovulation and Pregnancy in Alaskan Eskimos. <u>Amer. J. Obst. Gynec.</u> <u>114</u>: 524, 1972.

28. Morley, D. <u>Paediatric Priorities in the Developing World</u>.
    Butterworths, London, 1973.

29. Gray, R. H. Breastfeeding and Maternal and Child Health.
    <u>IPPF Medical Bulletin</u> <u>9</u>: 61, 1975.

30. Osteria, T. The Effects of Contraception upon Lactation.
    Analysis of Urban Data, 1973. Cited in Buchanan (13).

31. Martin, W., Morley, D. and Woodland, M. Intervals Between
    Births in a Nigerian Village. <u>J. Trop. Pediatrics</u> <u>10</u>: 82, 1964.

32. Cantrelle, P. and Leridon, H. Breastfeeding, Mortality in
    Childhood and Fertility in a Rural Zone of Senegal. <u>Population
    Studies</u> <u>28</u>: 505, 1971.

33. Jain, A. K. Pregnancy Outcome and the Time Required for the
    Next Conception. <u>Population Studies</u> <u>23</u>: 69, 1969.

34. Kang, K. W., Hong, J. W. and Cho, K. S. <u>A Study of the Inter-
    relationships Between Lactation and Postpartum Amenorrhea</u>.
    Seoul, Korean Institute for Family Planning, 1973.

35. Kwon, E., Kang, K., Hong, J., Park, C., Yun, B. and Whang, K.
    <u>A Study on the Interrelationships Between Postpartum Family
    Planning and Maternity Care</u>. College of Medicine, Seoul
    National University, Seoul, 1972.

MATERNAL NUTRITION, BREAST-FEEDING AND INFANT SURVIVAL

Joe D. Wray

Harvard School of Public Health

Boston, Massachusetts

INTRODUCTION

As important as breastfeeding may be to human survival - more so today in some places, of course, than in others - there is much that is not well understood, and much to be learned. A number of studies have been carried out to explore various aspects of the relation, but they vary widely in the problem addressed, in the variables examined - or omitted - in the methods used, in the population samples studied, and in the conditions under which they were conducted. Thus, if conclusions are to be reached, some of them will necessarily be tentative, if not downright speculative - and probably biased. In this presentation, I will address three questions:

1) Does maternal nutrition affect lactation?
2) Does lactation affect infant survival?
3) Do maternal nutrition and lactation affect fertility?

DOES MATERNAL NUTRITION AFFECT LACTATION?

An awareness of the importance of maternal nutrition in lactation must have been present in ancient times. Wickes, in his extensive review of the history of infant feeding (1), provides repeated references to the importance of health, and implicitly the nutritional status, as a critical criterion in the selection of wet-nurses. Such references go back to the time of Galen and appear in the Roman, Byzantine, and Arabic medical literature and can almost be said to dominate the Renaissance literature pertaining to child health.

In more recent times there has been a widespread notion that not only is the growing fetus nourished at the expense of the mother, but so indeed is the nursing infant. It is assumed that nutrients necessary for human milk production are mobilized from the mother's own tissues whether or not her diet is adequate. This seems to make "biologic sense." Given that the newborn is so dependent on the mother's capacity to produce milk, it should not be surprising that human mammals, like other mammals, have the capacity to produce the nutrients necessary for survival of their offspring.

If we examine the attempts to study the association between maternal nutrition and lactation, we find a modest number of useful studies. However, a failure to define, or to distinguish clearly between, maternal nutritional status and the nutritional adequacy of the mother's current diet is characteristic of the literature reviewed here, and is a source of potential confusion. Habicht et al. have asserted that the mother's nutrition during her own childhood and her pre-pregnancy nutritional status are factors which must be considered in evaluating the effects on birth weight of maternal dietary intake during pregnancy (2). Miller's study of Edinburgh mothers, in which he noted that women under 5 feet tall (only 10 percent of the sample) "were not as successful in breastfeeding their infants as the taller women" (3), suggests that childhood and pre-pregnancy nutrition may also affect lactation.

The problem is very relevant: in those populations where the potential effects of maternal diet on lactation are of most concern, the mothers have often been malnourished since childhood. Thus differences in quality and quantity of breast milk found in populations where dietary intakes are inadequate may be due to the mothers' current situation, their prior nutrition, or some combination. We could reasonably expect that the effects of acute nutritional deprivation would be less marked in women with adequate stores of body fat. Similarly, the effects of nutrition supplementation could vary with the inadequacy or adequacy of the mother's ordinary diet or with her basic nutritional status.

These study limitations must be kept in mind when we examine the different ways in which nutrition affects lactation. The areas I would like to focus on are: the effects of maternal nutrition on the quality of the milk, on the quantity produced each day, and on the duration of breastfeeding.

Quality of Breast Milk

Studies of the composition of breast milk are relatively straighforward. Methods for quantitative analysis of the important

nutrients are well known and can be carried out in many parts of
the world; samples of milk, sufficient for such analyses, are easy
enough to obtain. It is not surprising, therefore, that there are
far more studies of the composition of breast milk than there are
of any other aspect of lactation. Though many constituents of
human milk have been examined in such studies, this review concentrates mainly on proteins, fats and carbohydrates. There are a
number of studies by now which do show that there are significant
alterations in the composition of breast milk produced by women
who are themselves at the lower end of the nutritional scale.
Interestingly enough, fat, normally the source of over half the
calories in human milk, seems to be the component that varies
most, while protein and lactose levels are usually maintained at
more consistent levels. Studies of women in various tribal groups
in New Guinea (4) and women in India (5,6,7) and Pakistan (8),
where daily caloric intakes of lactating women are reported to be
1000-1500 calories per day below the recommended allowances, sometimes show quite low levels of fat in breast milk. In New Guinea
tribes, Bailey found several in which the mother's milk contained
less than 3 grams/100 cc (4). In South India, Gopalan reported
fat levels at about 3.34 grams/100 cc (5), and Karmarkar found
similar levels around Baroda (6).

Hanafy and colleagues in Egypt have reported the only available direct comparison of milk production in well nourished and
malnourished women (9). Nutritional status of the women, who were
from "a moderate to poor economic standard," was determined on the
basis of arm circumference, weight for height, serum albumin and
urea/creatinine nitrogen ratios. Caloric intake of the women was
not reported, but all of the 17 malnourished women reported diets
low in protein, while 5 of the 24 considered well nourished gave
such histories. Protein, lactose and fat content were found to
be lower in the milk of malnourished women, but only the protein
levels were significantly different. Total calories per 100 ml,
however, were also statistically significantly less in that group.

Quantity of Breast Milk

Measurement of the volume of breast milk produced each day is
much more difficult than simply measuring the composition of a
sample of breast milk. There are two alternatives: (1) weigh the
baby carefully (and his/her diapers) before and after each and
every feeding, around the clock, or (2) mechanically empty a full
breast and then multiply the amount obtained by some factor to
estimate the daily quantity. Both of these approaches are fraught
with a great variety of possible errors. Most studies are based
on weighing the babies and the difficulties are obvious. The
simple technical problems of weighing are complicated by the fact

that when a mother is brought into a hospital for the purpose of
determining milk output, the quantity she produces increases daily
for at least a week, with as much as a two-fold increase in output
(10). There are, of course, psychological and emotional factors
which probably affect this output. Older studies have shown that
output, at least as reflected by growth of the infant, is greater
on a demand schedule than it is on a fixed schedule; demand-fed
babies gain faster than clock-fed babies (11,12). Thus, if the
feeds are arranged at, say 4-hourly intervals, for the necessary
convenience of the staff, output is likely to be lower than it
might be if the baby were breastfed ad lib. Finally, Egli et al.
have shown that output also varies with frequency of feeds. They
found, for example, that when the number of feedings per day were
reduced from 6 to 5, output fell (13).

For these and other reasons, the number of reliable studies
of the quantity of breast milk produced are few. A scrutiny of
the literature, however, suggests that there may well be significant variation with maternal nutrition. It appears from studies in
Africa (10,14) that where the caloric intake of the mother is
adequate, the volume of milk produced is on the order of 700 to
800 cc/day, a level approximately equal to that of mothers in
Europe or North America (15). Where caloric intake is 2000 calories per day, or less, as observed in Mexico (16) and India (5,6)
or New Guinea (4), the volume tends to range from around 400 to
600 cc/day. In Egypt (9) the volume produced by malnourished
mothers (in a small sample) actually exceeded that of well nourished mothers in the 3rd and 4th months. Throughout the remainder
of the first year, however, their production fell far behind that
of the well nourished mothers. Studies by Chavez et al. in Mexico
(16) and by Gopalan in India (5) showed that when the diets of
these women is supplemented, the volume of milk produced increases
moderately, but there is little or no change in the composition of
the milk. What is especially interesting in Gopalan's study is
that he found that among hospitalized women on a daily diet providing 2900 calories, milk production increased about 100 cc per
day when protein intake was increased from 61 gm to 99 gm per day.
In Africa, where the mothers were receiving 3000 calories per day
and producing 700 or 800 cc/day, Edozian was able to provoke
increases on the order of 200 cc/day by increasing the daily
protein intake from 25 grams to 100 grams with diets that were
carefully isocaloric (14). It is obvious that much more information is needed in order to clarify and quantify the relative
effects of calorie versus protein deficiencies on human milk production, but clearly improvement of the maternal diet can increase
milk output.

Duration of Breastfeeding

Determining the relation between maternal nutrition and the duration of breastfeeding is immensely complicated by the fact that what determines the length of time a mother chooses to breast feed her infant depends on a variety of external factors, not the least uncommon of which is her next pregnancy. Whether or not she must return to work, the availability of other alternatives in feeding, advertising pressure, medical advice, and many other factors may also be involved. Add to those complications the necessity to follow, carefully, a sizable group of women over a period of many months, and it is by no means surprising that there are almost no studies which speak reliably to this issue.

In point of fact, I have been able to find only one such study, which was carried out at INCAP in Guatemala a few years ago (17,18). There, in conjunction with a longitudinal study of the effects of malnutrition on mental development in children, a population of mothers was followed over a period encompassing both pregnancy and lactation. In the population under study, it is the custom to breast feed as long as possible; the women are neither under pressure to return to work, nor is there any advertising or other pressure to persuade them to change to bottle feeding. Thus, each mother tends to nurse her infant until her milk production ceases.

Women were grouped according to the duration of lactation and mean values of the weight gains and losses were plotted for each group; results are shown in Figure 1. The mothers who were able to breast feed their babies only 9 months or less gained relatively less weight during their pregnancy, lost more weight in the postpartum period, and remained below pre-pregnancy weight levels until their milk "dried up." Those mothers who were able to breast feed for 21 months or more gained substantially more weight during their pregnancy, their postpartum weight loss was much less, and their body weights generally stayed well above pre-pregnancy levels throughout the period of lactation. Women who breast fed for periods intermediate between 9 months and 21 months gained proportionally more weight during pregnancy and lost less during lactation. These findings strongly suggest that maternal nutrition may be associated with duration of lactation in those situations where no other factors intervene.

The INCAP study is unique. There is other evidence which may be relevant, however. There are a number of places where, though breastfeeding is the cultural norm, the duration of lactation varies widely. In South India, Rao, et al. (7) found that "In spite of the general desire on the part of the mothers to continue suckling, nearly 40 percent had to wean their babies fully by the end of one year..." As shown in Table 1, in 29 percent of these

Table 1

Womens' Reasons for Discontinuing Breastfeeding
in the First Year of Life, as Reported in
Three Countries: India, Jamaica, Colombia *

Reasons	Percent Reporting		
	India	Jamaica	Colombia
Milk stopped	29.1	43	34.8
New pregnancy	46.8	-	21.1
Maternal illness or death	19.6	9	7.4
Working	-	13	4.2
Advertising	-	14	-
Miscellaneous	4.5	10	4.5

* Sources: References 19,20,21.

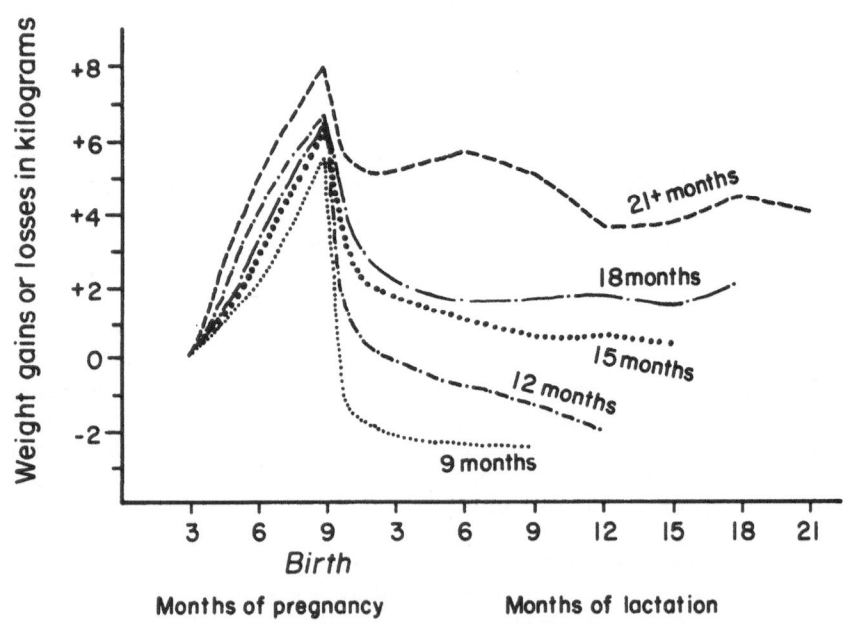

Figure 1. Weight gains and losses of mothers during pregnancy and
          lactation, by duration of lactation, Guatemala, around
          1970.
Source: Redrawn from Habicht and Behar (17) and Delgado (17a).

cases, milk production had stopped. No quantitative data concerning nutritional status or dietary intake in these women is provided, but we know from other studies (5,19) that the caloric intake among women in that part of India may be well below 2000 per day. Are the mothers whose milk "dried up" those at the lower end of the scale? Cessation of lactation is frequently reported where mothers are likely to be undernourished - some of them severely so. Examples of these are included in Table 1 - all from populations where other factors also are surely operating (20,21). These findings are consistent with those of Habicht and his colleagues at INCAP.

Conclusions

This brief review suggests some of the pieces of what I think is a fascinating puzzle. The evidence reviewed seems to suggest that the _quality_ of breast milk is affected only when the diet of the mothers is grossly inadequate. The _quantity_ of milk produced seems to decrease with less severe dietary inadequacy. Finally, the evidence available suggests that the effects of maternal nutrition on duration of lactation produce wide variation. In Figure 2 I have tried to summarize these possibilities graphically to sketch the whole puzzle. The quality of breast milk seems to be fairly consistent through a wide range of maternal dietary intake and suffers only at the lower end of the maternal nutritional scale where changes in composition (a decrease in fat content) produce at least a 10 percent fall in caloric content. The quantity of milk produced, as well as the duration of lactation, seem to be more sensitive to maternal intake and vary more widely. When maternal caloric intake is extremely low, daily volume appears to decrease by 40 to 50 percent; the Guatemalan findings suggest that duration of lactation decreases by as much as 60 percent. Thus, a maternal diet that is adequate for producing milk of normal quality may not support maximum output.

This phenomenon, if true, is biologically consistent with what we see in malnourished infants and young children. It is well known that over an extremely wide range of dietary intake the infant or child is able to maintain the composition of body tissues and the levels of serum constituents within quite normal limits. Many of us have seen infants with severe marasmus, who nevertheless had normal serum protein levels. The malnourished infant clearly adapts to dietary deprivation by maintaining biochemical integrity at the expense of growth, preferring, if you will, quality to quantity. Translated into breast milk production, the human mammary gland seems to adapt to dietary deprivation by maintaining compositional quality at the expense of quantity and duration.

Are these differences significant? If breast milk contains
only 3.5 grams of fat per 100 cc rather than the 4.5 grams that
might be expected in the milk of a well nourished mother, the difference might seem small when considered on a short term perspective. One less gram of fat per 100 cc means 10 calories less per
100 cc. If consumption averages 500 cc per day, there will be a
decrease of over 18,000 calories per year. Eighteen thousand
calories per year would have a protein sparing effect of approximately 4.5 kilos of protein needed for growth; this may not sound
like much, but it is the equivalent of 12 grams per day - a
significant amount for a growing infant.

Looked at another way, a mother producing 500 cc/day of 65-
calorie milk rather than the 800 cc of 75-calorie milk that a well
nourished woman can produce, will, in effect, produce 50 percent
fewer calories and equivalent deficits of other nutrients. Such a
mother can meet the nutritional needs of her growing infant for a
much shorter period of time than the well nourished mother. It is
likely that it is the average daily volume of breast milk that

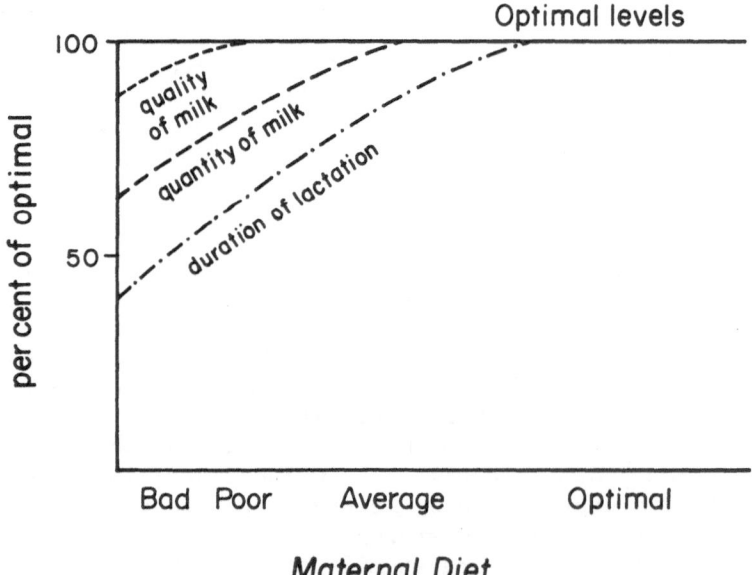

Figure 2. Postulated relation between maternal diet, quality and
           quantity of milk production, and duration of lactation.

determines the timing of growth faltering which inevitably occurs
in exclusively breast fed infants. We know that breast fed infants
grow according to European norms for the first six months of life
in many cultures (and among the elite in most); we also know that
in other cultures such growth persists for only three or four
months and then begins to fall behind. With data from careful
studies of different breast-feeding cultures, we might well be
able to predict the daily caloric intakes of the average mother
simply by knowing the age at which the growth of the average
infant begins to falter.

We have had to revise our concepts concerning the effects of
maternal nutrition on birth weights opposed to those of racial
factors; it may be time to reconsider our concepts about such
effects on lactation. My review of the literature suggests a sort
of taken-for-granted assumption that differences in breast milk
volume have a genetic or racial basis. The evidence reviewed
here, however, strongly suggests to me that where we find populations with a low average daily volume of milk, or poor quality,
we should look for poor maternal diets before assuming that racial
factors are responsible.

Thomson and Black recently prepared an extensive review of the
nutritional aspects of human lactation for the WHO (15) and concluded that breast milk volume and composition "are little influenced by the nature and amount of the maternal diet within a
remarkably wide range of intakes...", a conclusion that Thomson and
other colleagues had reached some years earlier (22). The evidence
reviewed here suggests to me that there are threshold levels of
maternal dietary intake which breast milk quality, quantity, and
probably duration, are affected. This is a potentially serious
issue: there are millions of women who fall below such levels. We
need to know much more than we do about the extent to which milk
production can be improved by better maternal nutrition, especially
in chronically malnourished women. The nutritional value of "more
and better" breast milk to millions of infants in poor countries
surely justifies further study.

We also cannot ignore the economic importance of breastfeeding.
Berg (23) calculated that hundreds of millions of dollars are saved
nationally when babies are breast fed rather than bottle fed.
More specifically, Habicht et al. (18) showed that in Guatemala
the cost of adequate bottle feeding is ten times greater than that
of extra food required by a mother for lactation. Similarly,
Reutlinger and Selowsky of the World Bank showed that a poor
mother in Calcutta who works must spend half her earnings to provide an adequate substitute for breast milk (24). For the world's
"poorest billion," breast-feeding is the only economically feasible
option.

DOES LACTATION AFFECT INFANT SURVIVAL?

Ancient testimony to the importance of human milk for infant survival comes, again, from historical references to wet-nurses. When a mother could not nurse her infant, the only reliable alternative was the milk of another woman. The biblical story of Moses provides the best known early example (though it was, in fact, his own mother who was hired as a wet-nurse) (25). According to myths, of course, Romulus and Remus survived because of a generous she-wolf, but details concerning the use of animal milk as an alternative to human milk in ancient times are simply unknown. Feeding vessels for infants found in graves dating back to 2000 B.C. suggest early use of animal milk, but Wickes found no reference to such in his review of the ancient literature (1), and Jamal Harfouche suggests in her review (11) that the use of animal milk was limited.

Wet-nurses began to be hired as social conveniences for the elite, rather than desperately needed alternative providers of the biologic mothers' milk, as early as Greek and Roman times. The practice continued and was widespread in Europe until well into the 19th century, and advice regarding wet-nurses is found in United States textbooks as late as 1920 (26). By the 17th century, however, sending babies to wet-nurses who did not, in fact, nurse them was a well documented European form of infanticide (1) (although by Langer's accounts, simple abandonment in the streets or garbage dumps was as common in many places through the 18th century and into the 19th) (27,28). Thus, like every other practice known to humankind, breastfeeding can be abused.

Breast-versus Bottle-feeding in the Western World:
Historical View

Alternatives to the use of wet-nurses in feeding babies were certainly available in the 19th century, and perhaps as early as the 15th (29,30). These usually consisted either of animal milks or of cereal paps. It has been reported for example that during the siege of Paris in 1870-71, when food supplies were cut off, the general mortality rate doubled, but the infant mortality rate fell from 330 to 170 per thousand live births. The reason offered was that the women had no other food to give their babies and therefore had to nurse them (31). A similar fall in the infant mortality rate was seen "during the Lancastershire cotton famine when mothers were not at work in the mills" (32). The practice of providing a cereal pap was widely used in some parts of Europe, especially in Bavaria and bordering districts of Austria (29). Infant mortality rates between 300 and 400 per thousand live births in districts where breastfeeding had been abandoned, in contrast to rates well below 200 in neighboring districts where breastfeeding

was the usual practice, provoked widespread concern on the part of
German physicians and led to the systematic collection of a great
deal of data concerning the relation between infant feeding and
mortality. The results of some of these studies were published by
Groth and Hahn in 1910 (33). Their data were re-analyzed by
Greenwood and Brown in 1912 (34) and again by Knodel and van der
Walle (29). Their findings are summarized in graphic form in
Figure 3; it is clearly apparent that there is a marked negative
correlation between infant mortality rates and the proportion of
babies in a given district who were breast fed for at least six
months. Breast-feeding nearly doubled an infant's chances of
survival.

Evidence collected from the turn of the century onwards suggests that the odds in favor of postneonatal survival among the
breastfed babies were even better. Studies carried out in Paris
in 1900 (35), in Derby, England, from 1900 to 1903 (36), in
Amsterdam (37) and Liverpool (38) in 1904, and in Boston in 1911 (39)
all showed a substantial excess of mortality among artificially fed

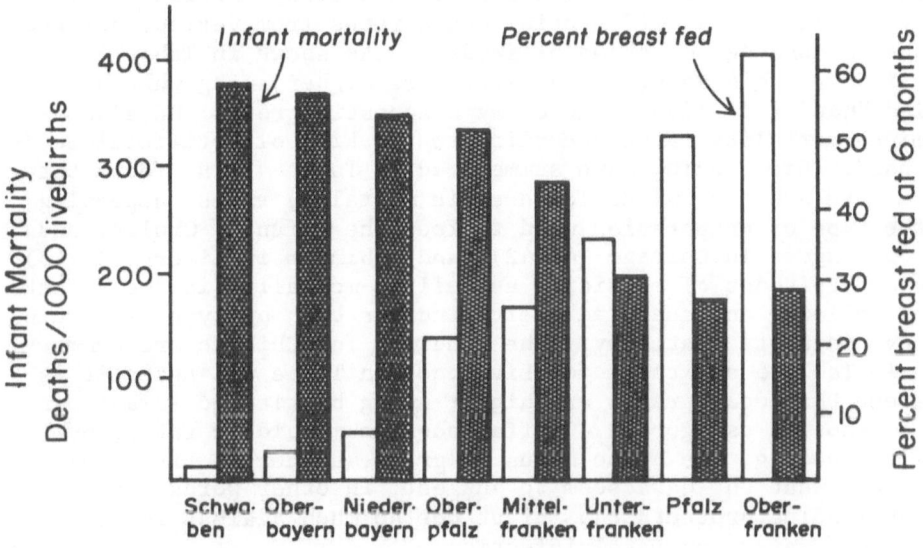

Figure 3. Association between breast-feeding practices and infant
           mortality rates in Bavaria, by district, late 19th
           century.
Source: Data from Knodel and van der Walle (29).

infants compared with those who were breast fed. Still later
studies were carried out in which the feeding of large numbers of
infants, and the mortality among them, were followed carefully during the first year of life: 22,422 infants in eight U.S. cities*,
carried out by the Children's Bureau, U.S. Department of Labor in
the early 1920s (40); 20,061 infants followed in Infant Welfare
Stations in Chicago from 1924 to 1929 (41,42), and in Liverpool
again from 1936 to 1942 (43). The differences in mortality found
in earlier studies persisted. Not until the late 1940s and early
1950s did they become insignificant in these affluent countries
(44,45,46). As late as 1946-47 in Great Britain, Douglas found
almost a two-fold difference (44). Mortality rates between the
ages of 8 weeks and 2 years in infants born in Great Britain during
March of 1946 and weighing between 6.5 and 9.5 pounds were 9.5 per
1000 in those breast fed more than 8 weeks and 17.1 per 1000 in
those breast fed 8 weeks or less.

The findings of these studies are summarized in Table 2.
Comparative mortality rates among partially breast fed infants are
also included when they were obtained. The survival-enhancing
value of breastfeeding is clearly apparent.

Several of the authors cited above did far more than simply
compare the mortality rates among breast fed and artificially fed
infants. Howarth (36) for example, in his study carried out in
Derby, investigated differential death rates from various disease
groups, according to method of feeding. As shown in Table 3,
modified from his data, death rates were higher among what he
called "hand-fed infants" in every diagnostic group. He also
examined mortality rates according to the kind of artificial feeding used. His findings are summarized in Table 4. He found that
there were substantial differences in mortality rates, depending
on the type of preparation used to feed the infant. Grulee, and
his colleagues in Chicago (41,42), and Robinson in Liverpool (43)
recorded episodes of morbidity as well as mortality in the infants
being followed and analyzed their findings both by type of feeding
and by diagnostic category. The findings for Chicago are summarized in Table 5 and those for Liverpool in Table 6. Again it is
apparent that death rates are higher among bottle fed infants in
all diagnostic categories. Differences in morbidity rates, by
type of feeding, are by no means so great, either in Liverpool or
Chicago. What the data seem to suggest, in other words, is that
breast-feeding protects the infant not so much against infection
as against severe or fatal infection.

---

* The cities were: Akron, Ohio; Baltimore, Maryland; Brockton,
Massachusetts; Johnstown, Pennsylvania; Manchester, New Hampshire;
New Bedford, Massachusetts; Saginaw, Michigan; and Waterbury,
Connecticut.

Table 2

Infant Feeding Practices and Infant Mortality Rates* by Type of Feeding
Various Western Cities or Countries, 1900-1950

Location (Reference)	Feeding practices in Total Population (Percent)			Mortality Rates (per 1000)			Ratio of Mortality Rates Bottle: Breast
	Breast	Partial	Bottle	Breast	Partial	Bottle	
Paris, 1900 (35)	-	-	-	140	-	310	2.2:1
Derby, 1900-03 (36)	63.3	17.3	19.5	69.8	98.7	197.5	2.9:1
Amsterdam, 1904 (37)	82	-	18	144	-	304	2.1:1
Liverpool, 1905 (38)	68.9	12.7	18.4	84.2	133.9	228.3	2.7:1
Boston, 1911 (39)							
1-5 months	73.4	-	22.6	15.34	-	145.5	9.5:1
6-11 months	66.2	-	33.8	15.0	-	77.7	5.7:1
Chicago, 1924-29 (41)	48.5	43.0	8.5	1.5	6.9	84.4	55.1:1
Liverpool, 1936-42 (43)	29.7	44.1	26.2	10.2	25.7	57.3	5.6:1
Great Britain, 1946-47 (44)	-	-	-	9.1	-	17.5	1.9:1

* Rates included in this table are not precisely comparable; most are post-neonatal and are
  intended simply to show the relative changes over time.

Table 3

Mortality Rates per Thousand Live Births by Diagnosis
Derby, England, 1900-1903*

Diseases	Mortality Rates per Thousand		
	"Breast-fed"	"Mixed"	"Hand-fed"
"Bronchitis and pneumonia"	14.4	12.6	26.5
"Diarrhoea and zymotic enteritis"	10.0	25.1	57.9
"Marasmus, atrophy and debility"	12.6	18.9	39.4
"Convulsions"	15.0	20.9	25.9
All other diseases	18.4	21.7	48.3
Total	69.8	98.7	197.5

* Source: Howarth (36). Adapted from Table 2.

In the Children's Bureau study of infant mortality by feeding
practice in 8 American cities (38) the type of feeding provided the
infant at each month during the first year of life was recorded.
Woodbury analyzed the data in a number of ways, and among other
things produced the findings that are shown in Figure 4.
Cumulative monthly death rates among infants exclusively breast fed
throughout the first year of life may be compared with the monthly
death rates among the infants in whom artificial feeding began during succeeding months of the first year. As Woodbury pointed out,
there is a cumulative effect of artificial feeding. For example,
death rates in the fifth month among infants artificially fed
from the first month are substantially higher than among infants
artificially fed from the third month. Also relevant is that
death rates among infants in whom exclusive artificial feeding did
not begin until late in the first year of life are not significantly
different from the death rates among infants who were breast fed
exclusively throughout the first year. In fact, the death rates
among infants weaned in the very latter part of the first year of
life are somewhat lower than those among breast fed infants.

I have summarized the findings of these studies in graphic
form, as shown in Figure 5, in order to show the trends in death
rates among breast- and bottle-fed babies in Western countries
over the past 100 years or so. Rates fell markedly in both groups
but, as the trends show clearly, breast fed babies had a distinct
advantage over bottle fed babies until rather recently, and this
advantage seems to have increased several-fold for a while during
the 1920s and '30s. Eventually, the bottle fed babies caught up.

Table 4

Number of Infants, Deaths, and Mortality Rates per Thousand
by Type of Feeding, Derby, England, 1900-1903*

Type of Feeding	Number Fed	Deaths	Rate/1000
Breast Milk	5278	368	69.8
"Hand-fed", total	1626	321	197.5
Diluted cow's milk only	895	158	177
Condensed milk only	149	38	255
"Bread, rusks, oatmeal, arrowroot, cornflour, sago, tapioca, and mixed foods"	159	40	252
"Patent foods"	482	85	202

* Source: Howarth (36). Adapted from Tables 1 and 3.

How can we account for the differences as well as for the
changes? The mortality differences are usually attributed to the
fact that breast milk is nutritionally ideal for the infant, provides some immunity, and is clean; artificial feedings, on the
other hand, are subject to contamination, sometimes grossly so,
and are often overly diluted. The fact, however, that mortality
fell so dramatically in breast fed infants, even though the fall
in artificially fed infants was greater in absolute terms, suggests that other factors must have been at work - the usually
recognized attributes of breast milk could not completely account
for the changes in mortality.

The mechanisms by which breastfeeding provides protection
against infection have been a matter of concern for decades. In
the early 1890s, Paul Ehrlich demonstrated with mice that mammary
secretion of antibodies was greater than trans-placental passage
(47). Such experiments could not be carried out in humans, of
course, and the issue remained in doubt for many years. As recently as 1958, an eminent European pediatrician reviewed the literature (48) and concluded that most of the immunity of the newborn
was obtained trans-placentally and not by breast milk.

By now, as noted in several recent reviews (49,50,51,52), it
is well known that a variety of immunoglobulins are secreted in
breast milk and are indeed able to protect the infant from a
variety of pathogenic viral and bacterial organisms. The studies
reviewed here, however, reflect an almost total concentration on

Table 5

Morbidity and Mortality Rates per 1000 Infants, Age 1 to 9 Months
and Fatality per 100 Cases, by Diagnosis and Type of Feeding
Chicago, U.S.A., 1924-1929*

Diagnosis	Breast Fed	Partially Breast Fed	Artifici- ally Fed	Ratios Breast:Bottle
Respiratory				
Morbidity	279.9	339.9	389.6	1:1.4
Mortality	.4	5.1	53.9	1:134.7
Case fatality	.15	1.5	13.8	1:92
Gastro-intestinal				
Morbidity	51.8	120.4	158.8	1:3.1
Mortality	.2	.7	8.2	1:41.0
Case fatality	.4	.6	5.2	1:13.0
"Unclassified"				
Morbidity	33.0	59.9	81.4	1:2.5
Mortality	.7	2.9	19.3	1:27.6
Case fatality	2.2	4.9	23.7	1:10.8
Infants at Risk	9,749	8,605	1,707	

*Source. Grulee et al. (41,42). Adapted from Tables 1 and 2.

the fact that breast fed infants are less subject to gastrointestinal diseases. Yet, it is clear that breastfeeding protects
infants from a variety of diseases. Although contaminated bottles
or feeds may indeed produce diarrheal diseases, the connection
between such contamination and respiratory infections, otitis
media, and other diseases is obscure.

How is it that death rates from a variety of infectious diseases were (and are still in developing countries) so much higher
in bottle fed than in breast fed infants while morbidity rates
were by no means so different? Breastfeeding, we noted, seems to
protect infants not so much from infection, but from dying. How
does this happen? If we attribute the decline in mortality among
breast fed infants in the West to some array of environmental
improvements, how do we account for the fact that mortality declines
in bottle fed infants eventually fell as far? Was that simply
environmental improvement also?

Table 6

Morbidity and Mortality Rates per 1000 Infants Age 1 to 7 Months
and Fatality per 100 Cases, by Diagnosis and Type of Feeding
Liverpool, England, 1936-1942*

Diagnosis	Breast Fed	Partially Breast Fed	Bottle Fed	Ratios Breast:Bottle
Respiratory infections				
Morbidity	102.9	167.9	170.9	1:1.7
Mortality	8.2	15.9	31.6	1:3.9
Case fatality	8.0	9.5	18.4	1:2.3
Gastro-enteritis				
Morbidity	6.1	38.8	78.4	1:12.9
Mortality	-	2.0	7.0	
Case fatality	-	5.3	8.9	
Other infections**				
Morbidity	110.1	254.6	320.7	1:2.9
Mortality	-	4.7	5.7	
Case fatality	-	1.9	1.8	
Infants at risk	971	1441	854	

** Includes: Otitis media, "infectious fevers", "unclassified
infections."

* Source: Robinson (43). Adapted from Table 2.

The answer to these questions, I believe, is that bottle feeds
were, and are still in places, often profoundly deficient in
nutrients. We know that such feeds are not only contaminated, but
highly diluted; somehow we ignore the latter. We tend to forget,
in short, the fact that bottle fed babies were and are often grossly
undernourished. If we consider the role of good nutrition in
general resistance to disease (53,54) and of the well demonstrated
association between malnutrition and diarrheal disease in preschool children in contemporary poor countries (55,56,57), then
nutrition, per se, must be accepted as a factor as powerful as all
the others in affecting mortality. Figure 6, for example, shows
the proportion of deaths from all causes and from three specific
causes in which malnutrition was found to be an associated cause
of death in 6 Latin American cities (58). I am prepared to assert
that in the West bottle fed infants caught up (or down) with
breast fed infants because, along with environmental improvements

and better food hygiene, the nutritional quality of the bottle
contents improved.

It is sobering to note that Dr. William Howarth, writing in
The Lancet in 1905, had reached basically the same conclusion:

"It is not easy to associate an increase of 12 per 1000,
or nearly 100 percent, in the mortality from bronchitis and
pneumonia with the manner of feeding...the probable reason is
to be found in the production of children suffering from what
might be termed 'lessened powers of resistence' or 'diminished vitality.' That these conditions are not the result
of marked differences in social position is shown...[by the
fact that, if anything] the hand-fed children are better
housed than the breast-fed and perhaps it is justified to
assume they are of at least equal social position. It is
more probable that these enfeebled constitutions are the

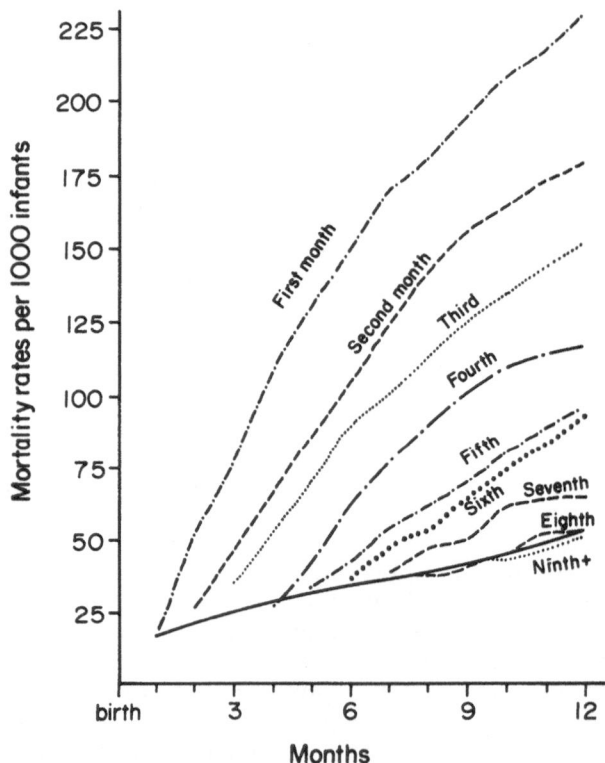

Figure 4. Cumulative infant mortality rates, by month in which
          artificial feeding was initiated, eight cities, U.S.A.,
          1920s.
Source: Data from Woodbury (40).

direct result of improper feeding, for when food constituents are not given to a child in their proper proportions,
or the substances...are unsuitable, it requires very little
imagination to suggest the evolution of a child who will
show...diminished resistence to attacks of the common
zymotic ailments" (36) (emphasis added).

Breast- versus bottle-feeding in the Third World:
Contemporary View

In many ways the so-called developing countries are following
the pattern set by the affluent countries of the West. Having seen
the changing patterns of mortality associated with infant feeding
practices in the West, what do we know about the current situation
in the so-called developing countries? Unfortunately, there are
by no means as many studies available, and none that are comparable
in scope or in sample size to some of those from the West. There

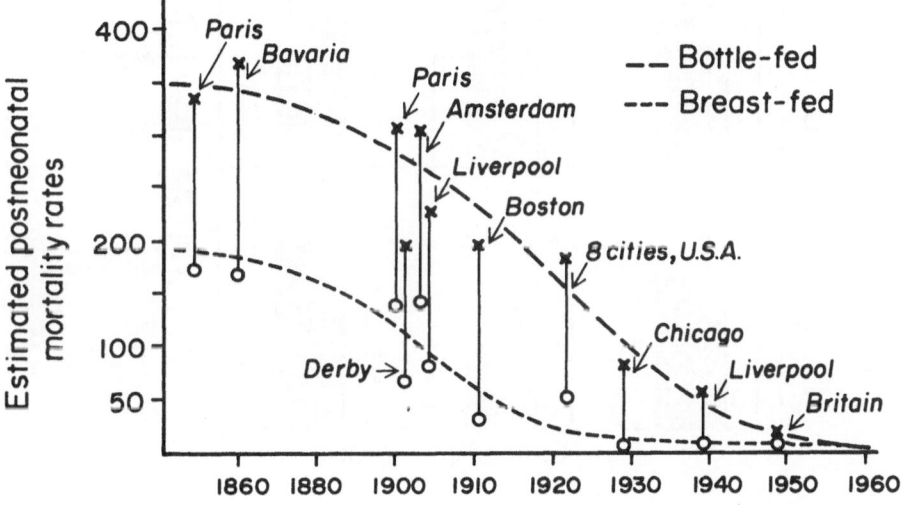

Figure 5. Trends in infant mortality rates, by type of feeding,
        in Europe and North America, 1860-1960.
Sources: References (29),(31),(35-44).

are a few, however, which provide some indication of the current situation.

      The limited data available show that the situation is similar to that which prevailed 50 to 100 years ago in the Western world. Almost 40 years ago, in fact, Cicely Williams pointed out that mortality rates of bottle fed infants were twice as high as those of breast fed infants in the coolie-laborers' families. Among the infants of shopkeepers rates were only moderately higher in bottle fed babies, and there were no differences in the infants of the upper classes (59). In the Khanna study, carried out in the Punjab from 1955 to 1959, Gordon, Wyon, and colleagues found that 19 of 20 infants artificially fed from birth died in the first year of life while the infant mortality rate among breast fed babies was 120 per thousand live births (55). In 1973, Plank and Milanesi reported much less marked, but nevertheless highly significant, differences in mortality in the first 9 months of life among

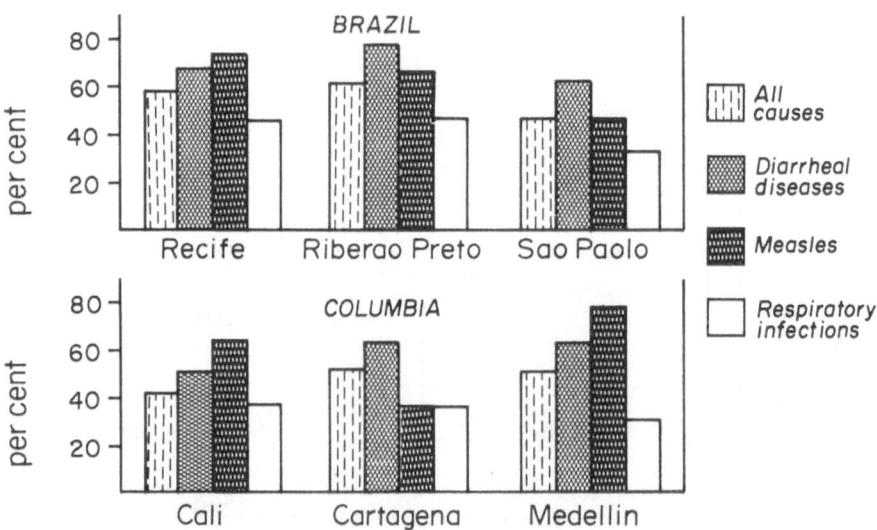

Figure 6.   Percentage of deaths in children under 5 years, with
            malnutrition as associated cause, various underlying
            causes, Latin American cities, 1970.
Source: Redrawn from Puffer and Serrano (58).

breast- and artificially fed infants in Chile (60), as shown in
Figure 7.

In the early 1970s, the PAHO study of infant and early childhood mortality in the Western hemisphere, reported by Puffer and
Serrano (58), showed that large proportions of the infants dying
of diarrheal diseases between the 6th and 11th month of life had
been artificially fed. Unfortunately, their report does not
include data concerning the breastfeeding practices among live
infants in their study populations, but such information is available for four populations from which they had mortality data.
Using the PAHO data showing the proportion breast fed six months or
longer among infants dying at 6-11 months of age, and the proportions in the total populations breast fed more than six months, it
is possible to calculate comparative mortality rates for four of
the PAHO study areas: rural El Salvador (61), Kingston, Jamaica
(20), Medellin, Colombia (21), and Sao Paolo, Brazil (62). The

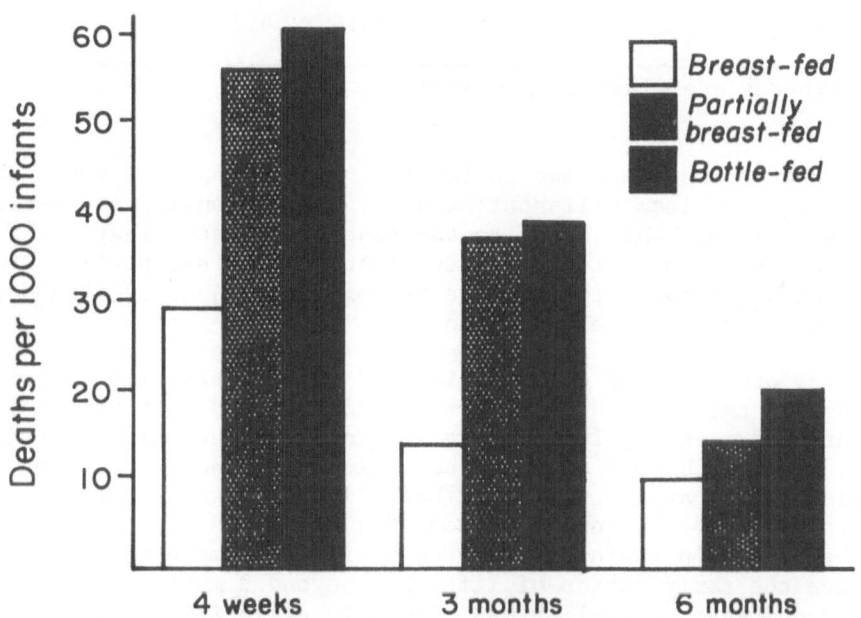

Figure 7. Mortality rates during the first year of life in breast-
          fed, partially breast-fed, and bottle-fed infants, among
          those surviving at 4 weeks, 3 and 6 months, rural Chile,
          1969-1970.
Source: Data from Plank and Milanesi (60).

Table 7

Percent of Infants Breast Fed Less Than 6 Months
or 6 Months and Longer in the Population,
and Among Infants Dying at 6-11 Months,
in 4 PAHO Study Areas, Around 1970,
and the Relative Risk of Dying
Among Short Breast Fed Infants

Study Area	Percent Breast Fed				Relative Risk of Death for Short Breast Feeding
	Total Infant Population		Infants Dying at 6-11 Months (		
	<6 mos.	≥6 mos.	<6 mos.	≥6 mos.	
El Salvador (61)	20	80	78.0	22.0	14.2:1
Kingston, Jamaica (20)	51	49	87.4	12.6	7.1:1
Medellin, Colombia (21)	61.8	31.2	91.3	8.8	6.4:1
Sao Paolo, Brazil (62)	77.2	22.8	95.9	4.1	6.8:1

* References are given in parentheses.

rates and ratios are shown in Table 7. These results, based on combining data from different studies, are obviously not precise, but they are probably close to the true differences that are found in such situations. Today in developing countries, bottle feeding produces a several-fold increase in mortality, just as it did in the West forty or more years ago.

One other aspect of mortality and feeding practices is worth noting: in the U.S. in the 1920s, Woodbury found that breast fed infants had markedly lower mortality rates in the early months of life, but that beyond seven or eight months infants receiving supplements or artificially fed had slightly lower rates, as we saw in Figure 4. Wyon and Gordon (63) found a similar situation in the Punjab in India: breast-fed babies were much more likely to survive the early months of life, but beyond 9 months and through the second year, mortality was higher in exclusively breast-fed infants than in those receiving supplements and the differences increased markedly with advancing age. Thus, in poor countries as elsewhere, breast-feeding is advantageous early, but is not sufficient as the only source of nutrients beyond the sixth month of life.

Further insights concerning the value of breastfeeding in poor countries are provided by studies in which the samples are too small to provide mortality rates, but which show lower rates of morbidity and better growth in breast fed infants. Such studies have been carried out, for example, among Alaskan (64) and Canadian (65) Eskimos, in the Caribbean (20,66), Colombia (56), Nigeria (67), and Thailand (68). In our studies in Thailand (68), we found that in rural villages, where mothers are well nourished and babies are routinely successfully breast fed, severe malnutrition in the first six months of life is rare; average heights and weights approximate North American norms throughout that period. In Bangkok slums, in contrast, where modernization has brought the bottle and many nothers must work outside their homes, severe malnutrition or marasmus was present in as many as one-sixth of the infants under 6 months of age, as shown in Figure 8.

Although the evidence shows clearly exclusive breastfeeding is insufficient beyond the sixth month, it is noteworthy that two of the studies (56,66) showed better growth of children when breast-feeding is prolonged <u>with</u> other foods.

Conclusions

The evidence that lactation affects survival in infants is far less equivocal than that relating maternal nutrition to lactation. More alarming is the fact that the evidence shows that the situation today in poor countries is very similar to that in Western countries 50 to 75 years ago. In poor countries now, as in Western countries then, the bottle feeding problem is mainly an urban one. The massive rural-urban migration that has occurred in poor countries during the past 25 years, and continues, bodes no good for babies.

DO MATERNAL NUTRITION AND LACTATION AFFECT FERTILITY?

From ancient times there were "old wives tales" to the effect that a nursing mother did not get pregnant. Such tales implied what has now been well substantiated. Lactation does indeed affect ovulation, and thus fertility. The question here is whether or not the effects of maternal nutrition on lactation have any effects, in turn, on ovulation.

The basic relationship between lactation and the duration of amenorrhea or the resumption of ovulation, is now well accepted and has been well reviewed (69,70-73). A growing literature, ranging from careful historical studies (29) on the one hand, to prospective clinical studies of the actual timing of ovulation (74) leave no doubt as to the basic phenomenon. These observations, of

course, have been borne out by a number of empirical studies in
which it has been observed that the duration of amenorrhea is
approximately 12 months longer in lactating women than it is in
non-lactating women.

The question here is whether or not maternal nutrition makes
a difference and the evidence is a bit confusing. Figure 9 from
Thomson and Hytten (70) shows the proportion of females who have
resumed menstruation by duration of lactation, as reported in
studies from several countries. Clearly, the pattern varies
greatly from place to place. In none of these studies was maternal
nutrition carefully examined, of course, but it might be assumed
that since lactating mothers in affluent countries are presumably
better nourished and, as shown in this figure, resume menstruation
more quickly while lactating, that better nutrition tends to
shorten the period of amenorrhea. This seems an unlikely explanation, however, for the differences in the same figure between
women in Calcutta and Taiwan. Given what we know about the general

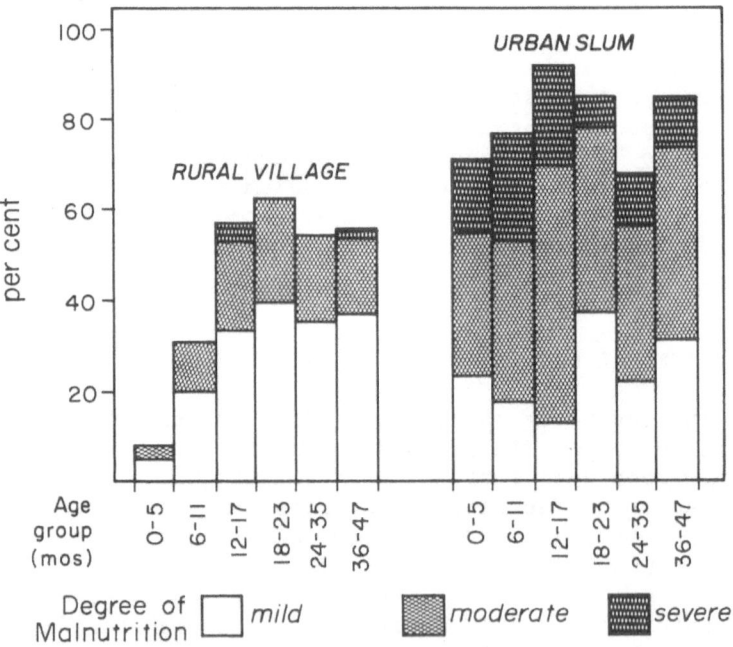

Figure 8. Prevalence of malnutrition among rural and urban
           children by age and severity, Thailand, 1872.
Source: Data from Khanjanasthi and Wray (68).

situation in Calcutta and Taiwan, it would seem reasonable to assume that the Taiwanese women were better nourished than those from Calcutta, although the Calcutta women might have been from the upper classes and well fed.

One study, that reported by Chavez and his colleagues, seems to support the idea that well nourished lactating mothers resume ovulation more quickly. Chavez _et al._ were interested primarily in the effects of maternal dietary supplementation on the growth of nursing infants and followed two small groups of women longitudinally, providing a generous supplement to one group of nursing mothers and not to the other. They observed in these two groups that the duration of amenorrhea in supplemented women was only approximately 7 months, while that in non-supplemented women was approximately 14 months. On the basis of this finding, they considered that improving nutrition in the Mexican women shortened the period of amenorrhea significantly.

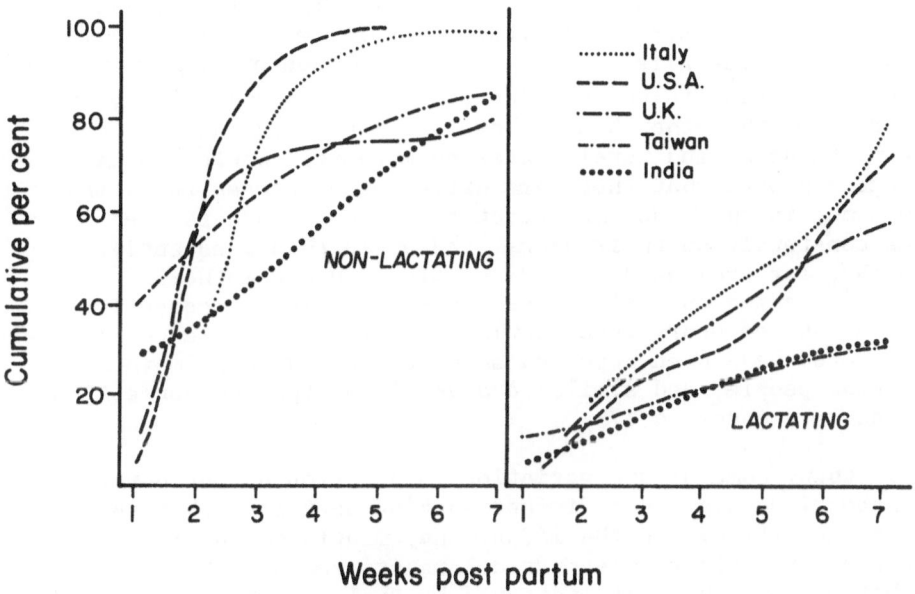

Figure 9.   Cumulative percentage of non-lactating and lactating women who were menstruating, by weeks post partum, various countries, 1960s and 1970s.

Source: Redrawn from Thomson and Hytten (70).

However, in the paper in which they reported that finding
(16) they did not mention the fact described in a report of other
aspects of the study (75), namely, that as soon as the growth of
the nursing infant of the supplemented mother faltered, they began
to supply the infants with generous supplements. Now we know that
under the best of circumstances, breast milk alone will sustain
normal growth only about 6 months at most. We also know, from a
careful work of Egli (13), for example, that if an infant is
supplemented and therefore sucks less vigorously or frequently,
milk production will decrease. This is indeed what seems to have
happened in the Mexican study. Their data show clearly that milk
production began to fall off in the supplemented mothers not long
after their infants began to receive supplementation. This suggests then that maternal nutrition is not the only variable that
could have affected the resumption of menstruation; perhaps it was
the nursing pattern of the infant.

This is the conclusion reached on clinical grounds alone by
Van Balen and Ntabomoura (76) who proposed that it may be the
vigor of the suckling, when what they called "natural lactation"
occurs, that inhibits ovulation. This is strongly suggested in
Figure 10, from the study of women in Rwanda by Bonte and her
colleagues (77), showing the conception rate among non-lactating
urban and rural females on the left, and among lactating urban and
rural females on the right. If there were significant differences
in the nutritional status of urban and rural women and nutritional
status differences affected the duration of amenorrhea, such effects
should be apparent in the non-lactating mothers and clearly there
are none. On the other hand, there are very clear differences
between the urban and rural lactating mothers. Bonte and her
colleagues report that there are differences between rural and
urban women in their nursing practices. Rural mothers keep their
babies constantly on their backs, and nurse them frequently, day
and night, for prolonged periods of time. Urban mothers do not
keep their babies on their backs, nurse them less frequently,
initiate supplementary feeds earlier. Similar differences in nursing patterns have been reported among urban and rural mothers of
the ! Kung people, and similar changes in postpartum conception
patterns were observed (78).

If then, some of the variation in duration of postpartum
amenorrhea is explained by infant sucking patterns, what about
maternal nutrition? In the INCAP study mentioned earlier the
women who were able to breastfeed longest seemed to be those who
were better nourished, as indicated by their weights. Bearing in
mind that this is a culture in which women have traditionally
tended to nurse their babies just as long as they had sufficient
milk, it does seem that nutrition affected the duration of lactation. Habicht reports that duration of amenorrhea in these women

was also prolonged (17). This was contradicted by other data from the same report, which showed that the duration of amenorrhea in lactating mothers receiving supplementation was slightly less than in unsupplemented mothers.

Conclusion

The evidence seems to suggest that improved maternal nutrition by its potential to prolong lactation <u>may</u> decrease fertility, although it is obvious that many other factors are operating to shorten lactation and to affect ovulation. There is at least a possibility that those women who wean their infants early because of cessation of lactation could nurse longer if they were better nourished and thereby delay pregnancy. There are surely many such women in the world, but obviously we need to know far more than we do about the many interactions involved.

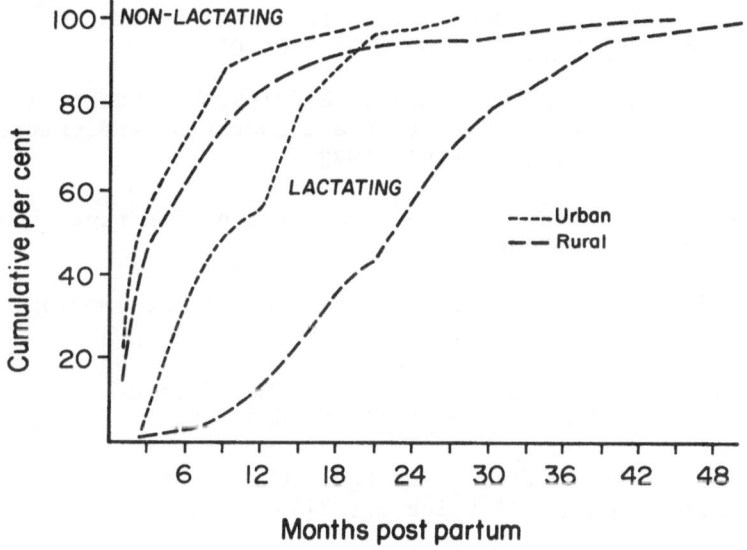

Figure 10.   Cumulative percentage of conceptions among non-
             lactating and lactating urban and rural women, by
             months post partum, Rwanda, 1970s.
Source: Data from Bonte <u>et al</u>. (72).

References

1. Wickes, I. G. A History of Infant Feeding (in 5 parts). Archives Diseases in Childhood, pp. 151-158, 232-240, 332-340, 416-422, 495-502, 1953.

2. Habicht, J-P., Yarbrough, C., Lechtig, A., Klein, R. Relationships of Birthweight, Maternal Nutrition and Infant Mortality. Nutrition Reports International 7: 1973.

3. Miller, R. A. Factors Influencing Lactation. Archives Diseases in Childhood 27: 187-208, 1951.

4. Bailey, K. V. Quantity and Composition of Breast Milk in Some New Guinean Populations. J. Trop. Ped., 1965.

5. Gopalan, C. Studies on Lactation in Poor Indian Communities. J. Trop. Ped., 87-97, 1958.

6. Karmarkar, M. G. Studies on Human Lactation. Indian Journal of Medical Research 47: 344-351, 1959.

7. Rao, K. Someswara. Protein Malnutrition in South India. Bulletin of the World Health Organization 20: 603-638, 1959.

8. Underwood, Barbara. Protein, Lipid and Fatty Acids of Human Milk from Pakistani Women During Prolonged Periods of Lactation. Am. J. Clin. Nut. 23: 400-407, 1970.

9. Hanafy, M. M., Morsey, M. R. A., Seddick, Y., Habit, Y. A. and el Lozy, M. Maternal Nutrition and Lactation Performance. J. Tropical Ped. 18: 187-191, 1972.

10. Sénecal, J. Alimentation de l'enfant dans les pays tropicaux et subtropicaux. Courrier 9: 1-22, 1959.

11. Harfouche, Jamal, K. The Importance of Breast-feeding. J. Trop. Ped. 16: 135-175, 1970.

12. Illingsworth, R. S. and Stone, D. G. H. Self-demand Feeding in a Maternity Unit. Lancet i: 683-687, 1952.

13. Egli, G. E. The Influence of the Number of Breast Feedings on Milk Production. Pediatrics 27: 314-317, 1961.

14. Edozian, J.C., Rahmin Khan, M. A. and Waslien, C. I. Human Protein Deficiency: Results of a Nigerian Village Study. J. Nutrition 106: 312-328, 1976.

15. Thomson, A. M. and Black, A. E. Nutritional Aspects of Human

Lactation. Bulletin of the World Health Organization 52: 163-176, 1975.

16. Chavez, A. and Martinez, C. Nutrition and Development in Infants of Poor Rural Areas. Nutrition Reports International 7: 1-8, 1973.

17. Habicht, J-P. and Behar, M. Nutricion, planificacion familia y salad en la madre y en el nino. Presented at the Seminar on Family Planning, San Salvador, 1974.

17a. Delgado, H. Personal communication, May 1977.

18. Habicht, J-P., Delgado, Y., Yarbrough, C. and Klein, R. E. Repercussions of lactation on nutritional status of mother and infant. In: Proceedings of the 9th International Congress of Nutrition, Mexico 1972, vol. 2, pp. 106-114. Basel: Karger, 1975.

19. Rajagopalan, S. Tamil Nadu Nutrition Project. Madras: Kalakshetia Publications Press, 1974.

20. Grantham-McGregor, Sally and Back, E. H. Breast Feeding in Kingston, Jamaica. Archives of Diseases in Childhood 45: 404-409, 1970.

21. Oberndorfer, Leni and Mejia, William. Statistical Analysis of the Duration of Breast Feeding (A Study of 200 Mothers of Antiquia Province, Colombia). J. Trop. Ped. 14: 27-42, 1968.

22. Hytten, F. E. and Thomson, A. M. Nutrition and the Lactating Woman. In: Milk: The Mammary Gland and its Secretion, S. K. Kon and A. T. Cowie (eds.), New York: Academic Press.

23. Berg, A. The Nutrition Factor: Its Role in National Development. Washington: The Brookings Institution, 1973.

24. Reutlinger, S. and Selowsky, M. Malnutrition and Poverty: Magnitude and Policy Options (World Bank Staff Occasional Papers, No. 23). Baltimore: The Johns Hopkins University Press, 1976.

25. Old Testament. Exodus 2: 7-9.

26. Morse, J. L. and Talbot, F. B. Diseases of Nutrition and Infant Feeding (2nd ed.). New York: The MacMillan Co., 1920.

27. Langer, W. L. Checks on Population Growth: 1750-1850. Scientific American 227: 93-100, 1972.

28. Langer, W. L. Infanticide: A Historical Survey. History of Childhood Quarterly: The Journal of Psychohistory 1: #3, 1974.

29. Knodel, J. and van de Walle, E. Breast-feeding, Fertility and Infant Mortality: An Analysis of some Early German Data. Population Studies 21: 109-131, 1967.

30. Knodel, J. Two and a Half Centuries of Demographic History in a Bavarian Village. Population Studies 24: 353-376, 1970.

31. Brehmer, Wochensehf f Saughingsfursorge, 1907. Cited in Morse and Talbot (26).

32. Devine: Hospital 41: 137, 1906-7. Cited in Davis (39).

33. Groth, A. and Hahn, M. Die sauglingsverhaltnisse in Bayern Munich, 1910. Cited in Greenwood and Brown (34).

34. Greenwood, M. and Brown, J. W. An Examination of Some Factors Influencing the Rate of Infant Mortality. Journal of Hygiene 12: 5-43, 1912.

35. Luling: These de Paris, 1900. Cited in Morse and Talbot (26).

36. Howarth, William J. The Influence of Feeding on the Mortality of Infants. The Lancet i: 210-213, 1905.

37. Jahresbericht der Gemeinde Amsterdam, 1904. Abteilung G. Cited by Knodel and van de Walle (29).

38. Armstrong, Hubert. A Note on the Comparative Mortality of Breastfed and Hand-reared Infants. British Journal Children's Diseases i: 115-116, 1904.

39. Davis, W. H. Statistical Comparison of the Mortality of Breastfed and bottle fed infants. American Journal of Diseases of Children 5: 234-247, 1913.

40. Woodbury, R. M. The Relation between Breast and Artificial Feeding and Infant Mortality. American Journal of Hygiene 2: 668-687, 1922.

41. Grulee, C. G., Sanford, H. and Herron, P. H. Breast and Artificial Feeding: Influence on Morbidity and Mortality of Twenty Thousand Infants. JAMA 103: 735-748, 1934.

42. Grulee, C. G., Sanford, H. and Herron, P. H. Breast and Artificially Fed Infants. JAMA 104: 1986-1989, 1935.

43. Robinson, M. Infant Morbidity and Mortality. A Study of 3266 Infants. Lancet i: 788-794, 1951.

44. Douglas, J.W.B. The Extent of Breast-feeding in Great Britain in 1946 with Special Reference to the Health and Survival of Children. J. Ob. Gyn. of British Empire 57: 335-361, 1950.

45. Westropp, C. Breast-feeding in the Oxford Child Health Survey. British Medical Journal 1: 138-40, 1953.

46. Mellander, D. and Vahlquist, B. Breast-feeding and Artificial Feeding. A Clinical, Serological and Biochemical Study in 402 Infants, with a Survey of the Literature. The Norrbotten Study. Acta Paediat 11: Suppl., 114-118, 1958.

47. Ehrlich, P. Ueber Immunitat Durch Vererhung und Baugung. Zeitshr. f Hyg. u Infectionskr. 12: 183-203, 1892.

48. Vahlquist, B. The Transfer of Antibodies from Mother to Offspring. In: Advances in Pediatrics, S. Z. Levine (ed.), Year Book Publishers Inc., Vol. X, 305, 1958.

49. Jelliffe, D. B. and Jelliffe, E.F.P. (eds.). The Uniqueness of Human Milk. Am. J. Clin. Nutr. 24: 968-1023, 1975.

50. Mata, L. J. and Wyatt, R. G. Host Resistance to Infection. Am. J. Clin. Nutr. 24: 976-986, 1971.

51. Béhar, Moises. The Role of Feeding and Nutrition in the Pathogeny and Prevention of Diarrhaeic Processes. Bulletin WHO 9: 1-9, 1975.

52. Gerrard, J. W. Breast-feeding: Second Thoughts. Pediatrics 54: 757-764, 1974.

53. Dubos, R., Savage, D. and Schaedler, R. Biological Freudianism: Lasting Effects of Early Environmental Influences. Pediatrics 38: 879-800, 1966.

54. Scrimshaw, N. S., Guzman, M., Flores, M. and Gordon, J. E. Nutrition and Infection Field Study in Guatemalan Villages, 1959-1964. V. Disease Incidence Among Pre-school Children Under Natural Village Conditions, with Improved Diet, and with Medical and Public Health Services. Arch. Environ. Health 16: 223-234, 1968.

55. Gordon, J. E., Chitkara, I. D. and Wyon, J. B. Weanling Diarrhaea. Am. J. Med. Sci. 245: 345-377, 1963.

56. Wray, J. D. and Aguirre, A. Protein-calorie Malnutrition in
    Candelaria, Colombia. I. Prevalence: Social and Demographic
    Factors. J. Trop. Pediat. 15: 76-98, 1969.

57. Pharaon, H. M., Darby, W. J., Shammout, H. A., Bridgforth, E. B.
    and Wilson, C. S. A Year-long Study of the Nutriture of
    Infants and Pre-school Children in Jordan. A Monograph issued
    in conjunction with J. Trop. Pediat. 11: 3-39, 1965.

58. Puffer, R. T. and Serrano, C. V. Patterns of Mortality in
    Childhood. Washington: Pan American Health Organization
    (Sc. Pub. 262), 1973.

59. Williams, Cicely. Milk and Murder. Address delivered to the
    Rotary Club of Singapore (mimeo.), 1939.

60. Plank, S. and Milanesi, Lucilla. Infant Feeding and Infant
    Mortality in Rural Chile. Bulletin WHO 48: 203-210, 1973.

61. Menchú, M. T. Lactancia y destete en el area rural de Centro
    America y Panamá. Archiv. Latinoamericanos de Nutrición 22:
    83-89, 1972.

62. Iunes, M., Sigulem, Dirce and Campino, A. C. Estado Nutricional
    de Criances de 6 a 60 Meses no Município de São Paolo. 11.
    Analise de Dadas, São Paolo: Escola Paulista de Medicina, 1975.

63. Wyon, J. B. and Gordon, J. E. The Khanna Study. Cambridge
    (Mass.): The Harvard University Press, 1971.

64. Maynard, J. E. and Hammes, L. M. Study of Growth, Morbidity
    and Mortality among Eskimo Infants of Western Alaska.
    Bulletin WHO 42: 613-622, 1970.

65. Shaefer, O. An Epidemiological Study of Infant Feeding Habits
    and Incidence of Recurrent and Chronic Middle Ear Disease in
    Canadian Eskimos. Canadian Journal of Public Health 62: 478-
    489, 1971.

66. Antrobus, A.C.K. Child Growth and Related Factors in a Rural
    Community in St. Vincent. Env. Child Health 17: 188-210, 1971.

67. Morley, D. et al. Growth and Nutrition in a Nigerian Village.
    Trans. Roy. Soc. Trop. Med. and Hyg. 62: 164-195, 1968.

68. Khanjanasthiti, Pensri and Wray, J. D. Early Protein-Calorie
    Malnutrition in Bangkok Slums, 1970-1971. J. Med. Assoc.
    Thailand 57: 468-476, 1974.

69. Buchanan, R. Breast-feeding. Aid to Infant Health and Fertility Control. Population Reports (Series J): 49-67, 1975.

70. Thomson, A. and Hytten, F. E. Lactation and Reproduction. Bulletin WHO 52: 337-349, 1975.

71. Van Ginniken, J. K. Prolonged Breast-feeding as a Birth Spacing Method. Studies in Family Planning 5: 201-206, 1974.

72. Rosa, F. Breast-feeding in Family Planning. PAG Bulletin 5: 5-10, 1975.

73. Gray, R. Breast-feeding and Maternal and Child Health. IPPF Medical Bulletin 9: 1-3, 1975.

74. Perez, A., Vela, P., Masnick, G. S. and Potter, R. G. First Ovulation after Childbirth: The Effect of Breast-feeding. Am. J. Ob. Gyn. 114: 1041-1047, 1972.

75. Chavez, C., Martinez, C., Bourges, H., Coronado, M., Lopez, M., Basta, S. Child Nutrition Problems During Lactation in Poor Rural Areas. In: Proceedings of the 9th International Conference on Nutrition, Mexico, 1972. Basel: Karger, 1975.

76. Van Balen, H. and Ntabomoura, V. Methods of Birth Spacing, Maternal Lactation and Post-partum Abstinence in Relation to Traditional African Cultures. Environmental Child Health 22: 50-52, 1976.

77. Bonte, M., Akingeneye, E., Gashakamba, M., Mbarutsa, E. and Nolens, M. Influence of the Socio-economic Level on the Conception Rate during Lactation. Int. J. Fert. 19: 97-102, 1974.

78. Kolata, G. B. !Kung Hunter-gatherers: Feminism, Diet, and Birth Control. Science 185: 932-934, 1974.

ECONOMIC ASPECTS OF BREAST-FEEDING

William Butz

The Rand Corporation

Santa Monica, California

INTRODUCTION

For thousands of years, the popularity of breast-feeding among women of different cultures has fluctuated widely (1,2,3,4). The longest known trend in this history has occurred in Western Europe and North America during the last century, when increasing proportions of women have failed to nurse their infants at all. The mean length of both full and partial breast-feeding of those who nursed has also steadily declined during this period (5,6,7,8,9,10). More recently, a pervasive decline in breast-feeding activity is also underway in urban areas of many less developed countries, with similar tendencies suggested in some rural areas as well (11,12, 13,14).

Concern about this most recent phenomenon is acute among many public health researchers and officials because of accumulating evidence that inadequate and contaminated food consumption is contributing to the death, disease, or poor physical development of many non-nursing infants in poor areas (15,16,17,18,19,20,21,22). Concern is also growing in light of strong clinical and field evidence that something about the lactation process inhibits the return of a woman's postpartum ovulations (23,24,25,26,27,28,29, 30). Hence, reduced lactation activity may induce shorter pregnancy intervals causing detrimental effects on child and maternal health and leading to faster population growth and larger families. Some have expressed concern, in addition, about an unnecessary strain on family and national resources when mothers substitute other infant foods for their own milk (31,32,33,34).

Scientific evidence concerning these <u>results</u> of declining breastfeeding activity, incomplete as many feel it to be, is considerably stronger than evidence concerning the <u>causes</u>. Most lacking are empirically supported prescriptions of: 1) what can be done to slow or stop the emerging breastfeeding trends, and 2) how to lessen their undesirable biomedical and demographic effects.

The important aspects of the first question, in my opinion, are:

- What are the characteristics of populations most at risk of declining breastfeeding activity?

- What factors are responsible for the declines?

- What factors might be altered by public policy to prevent or arrest the declines (these need not be the same factors that are directly responsible).

For each alternative set of policies (if there are alternatives) that might be pursued,

- What is the aggregate effect on breastfeeding activity that can be expected to result?

- What is the cost of the policy?

- What are the policy's significant side effects?

Concerning the second question - how to lessen undesirable effects of declining breastfeeding - one would like to know:

- What populations are at risk of breastfeeding declines and subject to deleterious effects on infants and birth spacing?

- For these populations, how can policy increase the supply of effective substitutes for breastfeeding in its functions as contraceptive and contributor to infant survival and development?

This paper offers a general framework for thinking systematically about these questions. Breastfeeding is not a costless activity for many women: it requires time and nutrients, both of which are often available only at a cost. Under unusual conditions, it can detract from the mother's health as well. The fact that this costly activity is ever undertaken suggests that it also produces benefits that people value. The important ones are presumably survival and improved development of the child, and delay of the subsequent pregnancy.

In looking for determinants of variations in breastfeeding behavior (intensity and duration), one might usefully look, then, at variations in the costs of breastfeeding, in the value to parents of the results of breastfeeding, and in the cost and availability of substitute methods of attaining those results. Such a search would hopefully lead to biological, institutional, and economic factors that influence these costs and returns and account empirically for some of the observed variations in breastfeeding behavior. These factors would be targets for public policy action.

In the next section I develop a simple economic model describing interactions among some potentially important factors and derive from it a number of refutable predictions concerning breastfeeding behavior. [The verbal explication of the model is tedious; I hope the range and interest of its predictions repay the reader's effort.] Concentrating on those predictions linking breastfeeding to economic factors, I then review relevant empirical evidence from several studies. Finally, I offer a concluding recommendation for policy and research.

A CONCEPTUAL MODEL OF BREASTFEEDING BEHAVIOR*

In trying to explain and predict how a particular scarce resource is allocated among competing uses, economists generally find it helpful to investigate determinants of the supply of that resource and of the demand for it that arises out of each competing use. This effort, when it is productive, results in predictions concerning the effects of changes in particular factors that influence either the supply or the demand. In the present case, the scarce resources of interest are a woman's time and her stock of nutrients. Among the competing uses of these resources may be sleep, work in the home, work in the fields, work in the labor market, social activities, and breastfeeding. Each competing use has a value to the woman or her family. Some values, like wages for market work, are relatively easily measured. Others, like the value of sleep or social activity, are conceptually and empirically very difficult to evaluate. At our level of abstraction, however, all alternative uses share the important characteristics of being undertaken or produced only by the expenditure of a woman's time and calories, and of having value to her or to her family.

---

* This model is developed algebraically and more tightly in a forthcoming paper that investigates empirical determinants of length of breastfeeding in a Guatemalan population (35).

We can think of the amount of breastfeeding as the number of feedings per day, the number of minutes of nursing per day, the total number of days the child nurses, or any combination of these. A woman's (or her family's) demand schedule for breastfeeding tells the amount of breastfeeding she or they will choose, for whatever reasons, at each cost of a unit of breastfeeding. I assume that they demand more at lower costs, so that the demand curve, D, in Figure 1 is negatively sloping. For the moment, let us assume that this demand can only be satisfied by the woman's own lactation (wet nursing does not occur). The higher the value of a unit of breastfeeding, the more she will choose to lactate; hence, her supply curve of breastfeeding, curve S in Figure 1, is upward sloping.

If the woman breastfeeds her child at all, the two curves intersect in the indicated quadrant, implying a positive amount of breastfeeding q_0 at a "price" p_0. P_0 and q_0 are equilibrium values to which the "price" and quantity of breastfeeding are predicted to return if disturbed. For example, if the woman finds herself breastfeeding q_1 minutes, times, days or whatever, the marginal cost, P_1, of this use of her resources exceeds the marginal value, P_2. The last unit of breastfeeding costs more than it is worth to her. By breastfeeding less, she reduces the cost of the last unit

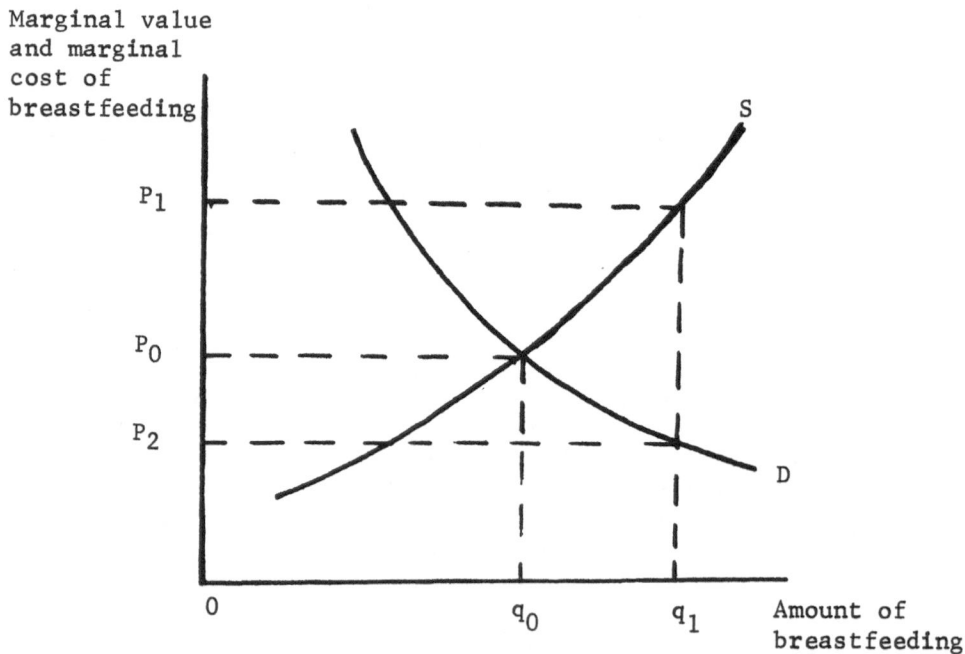

Figure 1.

and increases its value. Equilibrium is at q_0 where marginal cost
equals marginal value.

Our task in this section is to identify factors that influence
the positions of the supply and demand curves for breastfeeding
and to predict the breastfeeding consequences of particular changes
in these factors. On the supply side, the amount of breastfeeding
a woman produces depends in a systematic way on the amount of time
she devotes to the activity and on her nutrition. The form of
this technical production relationship influences the shape and
position of her supply curve of breastfeeding which, in turn,
depends on (1) the opportunity cost of her time spent breastfeeding, and (2) the marginal cost of nutrition required.* If relatively high paying jobs become available that cannot easily be done
while caring for an infant, then the opportunity cost of a unit of
her time spent breastfeeding rises, and the amount of breastfeeding
she is willing to offer declines at each value of an additional
unit of breastfeeding: S_1 shifts to S_2 in Figure 2. The same
shift would result from an increase in the amount of nutrients the
mother's system requires to produce an additional unit of milk or
from an increase in the cost of nutrients, since either raises the
marginal cost of nutrition for breastfeeding.

Whatever the cause, the backward shift in S induces the mother
to reduce breastfeeding to q_1, where the marginal cost and marginal
value of this activity are both higher than at q_0, but still equal.
There is a new equilibrium position.

---

* These are the relevant costs because mother's time and mother's
nutrition are the only two factors assumed important in the underlying production function that describes how breastfeeding is produced. A more complete model might include one or more maternal
morbidity variables as well.

This is an appropriate point to introduce the difference
between lactation and breastfeeding. The former is a biological
process produced, in our model, using maternal nutrition. The
second is a behavioral cum biological process produced using nutrition and the mother's time. This might suggest thinking of the
lactation process as the first stage in a separable production
relationship -- first comes production of milk, then comes production of infant feeding or health, using the milk. Instead, I
view the two components as part of the same production process
because of the fact that they are technically related, as discussed
below.

Shifts may also occur in the demand curve. Since I assume
that a woman or her family value her breastfeeding for its survival
and development effects in infants and/or for its contraceptive
effect, the demand function depends on the value to her or them of
the amount of these results that an additional unit of breastfeeding provides. Accordingly, more breastfeeding is desired at each
cost of an additional unit if (1) that unit produces more child
survival and development and/or more contraception, (2) the other
means of attaining child survival and development and/or contraception that exist are less effective compared to breastfeeding,
(3) those substitutes that. exist are more costly to obtain and use,
or (4) the value to the family of an additional "unit" of child
survival and development and/or contraception is higher. The first
two factors are characteristics of the biological relationships
determing child survival probabilities, physical and mental development patterns of children, and birth probabilities. These
factors - in economic terms, the marginal productivity of breastfeeding and the elasticities of substitution between breastfeeding
and other contributors - depend exclusively on biological relationships. As I discuss below, the form of these relationships changes
greatly with the age of the child and the amount of breastfeeding,
and perhaps slightly with the age and parity of the mother.

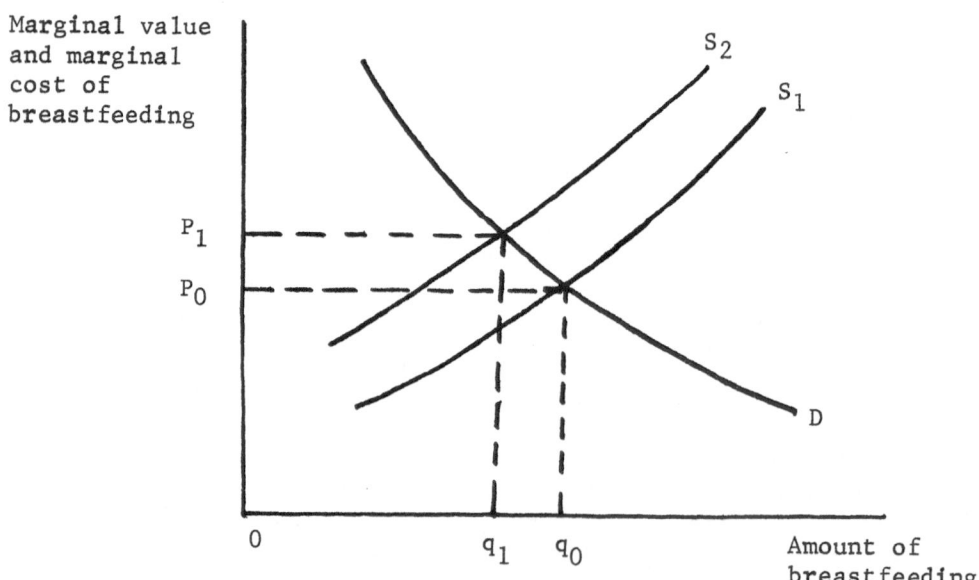

Figure 2.

The last two sets of factors that determine the position of the demand curve for breastfeeding are predominantly behavioral and economic. Given the relative productivities of breastfeeding and its substitutes (factors 1 and 2), the family chooses among them on the basis of their relative costs (factor 3). It minimizes the cost of producing a unit of child development or contraception at the point where the ratios of marginal product to marginal cost of each input (breastfeeding and others) in the production relationship are equal. The only remaining question, then, is the "amount" of child survival and development and the "amount" of contraception that are desired. These desires can be summarized in two marginal value schedules. One gives the marginal value to the family of an additional unit of child survival and development, for every amount of these goods. The other similarly relates marginal value of birth aversion to length of birth interval. In both relationships, I assume that the value of an additional unit declines with the number of units.

Figure 3 pictures the equilibrium positions of two families with the same supply curve but different demand curves (or it could be the same family at two times or two places). Demand curve D_2

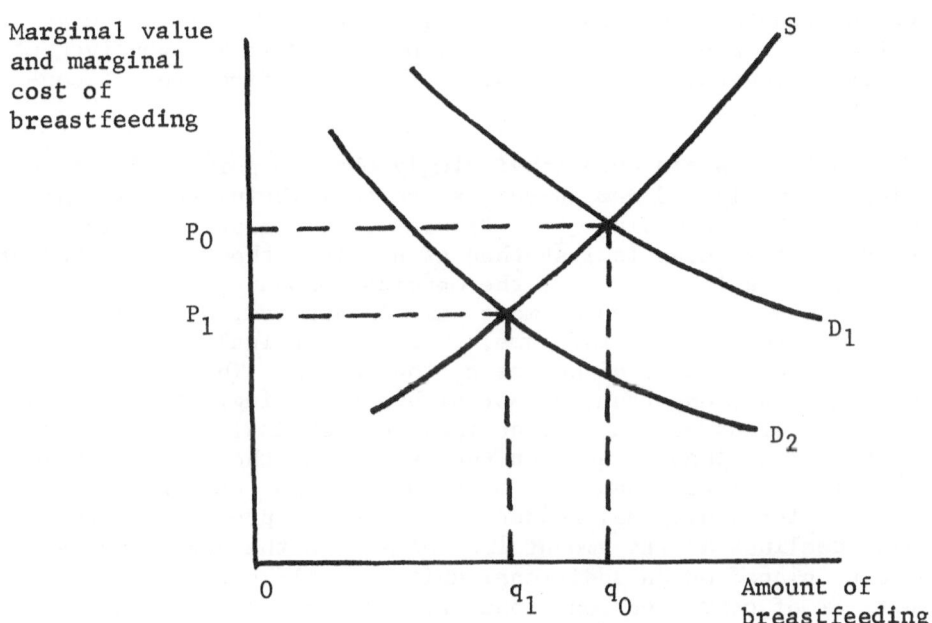

Figure 3.

may be lower because nutritious hygienic weaning foods are cheaper, because modern contraceptives are cheaper, because the family places less value on the survival and development of its children, or because it places less value on delaying the subsequent birth (wants births rapidly).* These reasons are behavioral and economic. On the biological side, to the extent that women(and children) differ significantly in the amount of child survival and development and the amount of contraception produced by an additional unit of breastfeeding, at given amounts of breastfeeding and age of child, curves D_1 and D_2 will differ accordingly. In any case, the family with the lower demand curve, D_2, has less breastfeeding (q_1) at a lower equilibrium "price" (p_1).**

We are now in a position to examine in more detail the changes in breastfeeding that are expected to result from changes in particular factors. In general, a shift in the supply (demand) curve, for whatever reason, causes a larger shift in breastfeeding amount when the demand (supply) curve is more elastic. Elasticity of the supply curve depends in this case only on how fast the opportunity cost of the mother's time and the price of nutrition

---

* Demand curve D_2 in Figure 3 might also be lower if prices are lower for weaning foods women wrongly think are as effective as breast milk in producing child development, or if inexpensive but ineffective contraceptives are believed to be effective. I consider these cases below.

** We can now explain more convincingly why the points of intersection of supply and demand curves are equilibrium points. At quantity of breastfeeding q_1 in Figure 1, the amount of time devoted to other uses is less than at q_0 since the total number of available hours is fixed. If the marginal productivity of time in these other uses declines as more time is applied, holding the amounts of other inputs the same, then the marginal product of time in these other uses is higher at q_1 than at q_0. This is the definition of a higher opportunity cost of breastfeeding. A similar but less simple argument can be made that the marginal cost of nutrition is higher at q_1 than at q_0. At the same time, the marginal value of q_1 units is lower than that of q_0 units. In the first place, we posit that for biological reasons the marginal product of breastfeeding declines as its amount increases. In the second place, the value placed on an additional unit of child survival and development, or of contraception produced, may decline as the number of units increases. Beginning at q_1, then, the mother's incentive is to lower the marginal cost and increase the marginal value. She does this by reducing her amount of breastfeeding until q_0 is reached.

rise as she uses more of them in breastfeeding. If there are close
substitutes for her time (older children, perhaps, or modern conveniences) in other household production activities or if there is
a labor market in which she can work as much as she wants at a
wage that is high relative to her household marginal productivity
schedule, her supply curve will tend to be elastic. It will also
tend to be elastic if the marginal nutrition cost of breastfeeding
does not rise much or at all as she breastfeeds more. This may
occur because she has adequate calorie stores with no alternative
use.

   Elasticity of the demand curve depends on the goodness of
available substitutes for breastfeeding, how their cost changes
with the amount of them used, and how quickly the marginal values
of pregnancy aversion and child survival and developmant fall as
the couple obtains more of them.

   Figure 4 represents two situations in which the demand for
breastfeeding has fallen by the same amount, D_1 to D_2, due, say,
to the introduction of commercial formula in local stores. From
the same initial position, q_o, the amount of breastfeeding in one

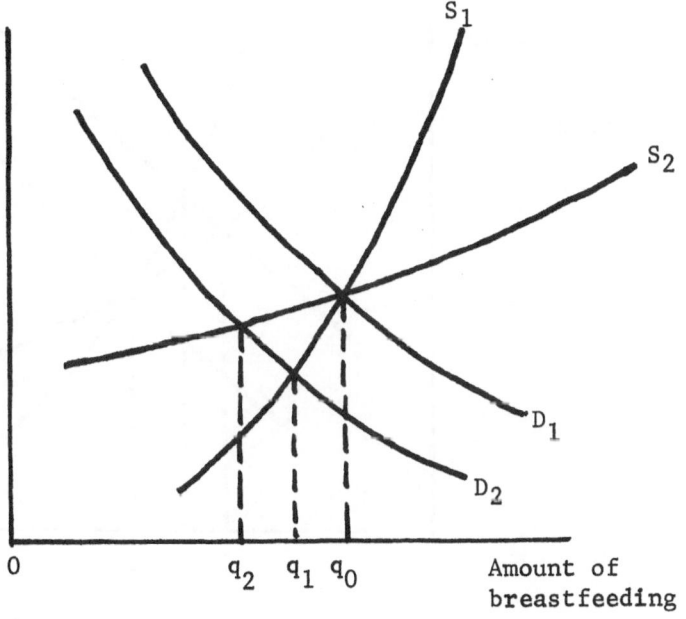

Figure 4.

community (S_1) falls relatively little (to q_1) since the supply
curve is inelastic. It takes a large fall in the breastfeeding
demand schedule to induce movement of mother's time and nutrition
to other purposes. The same contraction of the demand curve
induces women with elastic supply curve S_2 to reduce their breastfeeding considerably more (to q_2). These women more readily
take advantage of the cheapening of a nursing substitute or any
other factor that lowers their demand curve for breastfeeding.

With Figure 5, one may concoct his own examples of the difference made by the elasticity of the demand curve when the supply
curve shifts, say, because a factory opens that pays high wages to
female workers.

Consider now several other cases. In Figure 6, S represents
a woman who, for nutrition or health reasons, can breastfeed more
than q_1 units (per day, per child) only at rapidly increasing
medical risk. Large shifts in the demand curve will not affect
her breastfeeding much until demand falls consideraly. S could
also have such a shape due to a cultural norm restricting breastfeeding to some amount; the result is the same.

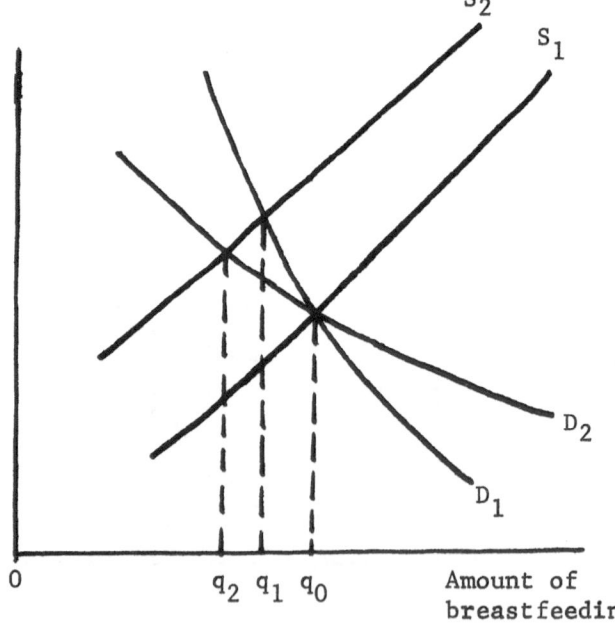

Figure 5.

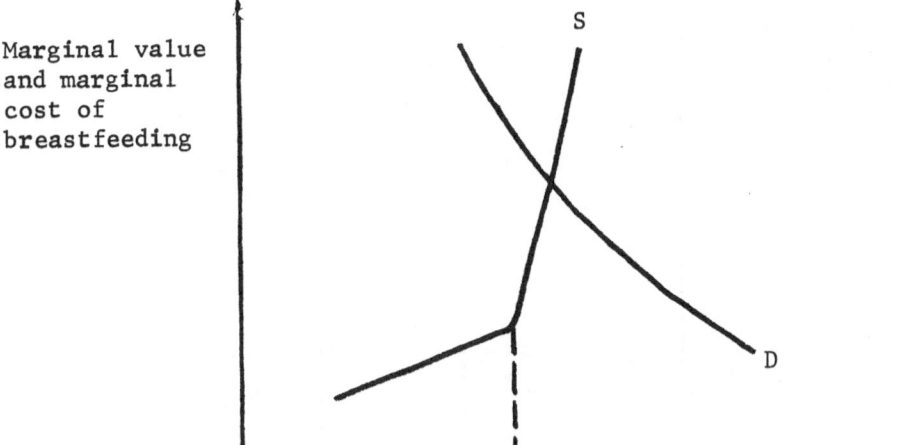

Figure 6.

Taking another example, in Figure 7 there is a market supply of breastfeeding, S_m, that is far enough down to be relevant. In the cases so far considered, this market supply curve (not pictured) is too high to intersect the demand curve to the right of its intersection with the woman's supply curve, S. In the case pictured, the market can supply all the services desired at a constant price, p . In equilibrium, the woman breastfeeds q_1 amount and hires a wetnurse to nurse her child q_0-q_1 amount. The wetnurse receives an amount equal to abq_1q_0 in compensation. A shift in the demand curve has its maximum effect in the area to the right of point b, since it can be easily accommodated in the market for wetnursing. On the other hand, left of point a, shifts in the supply curve have no effect on the amount of breastfeeding the child receives, though they do affect the mother's amount of lactation.

Hence, as is reasonable, where there is an active wetnursing market, variations in factors that underlie women's breastfeeding supply curves may affect their period of post-partum amenorrhea but not the survival or development of their children (if the wetnurse is a good substitute for the mother). Alternatively, shifts in factors that influence women's demand for breastfeeding may affect their infants' development and survival but not their fecundity.

The case in which the demand curve for breastfeeding is

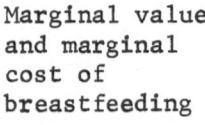
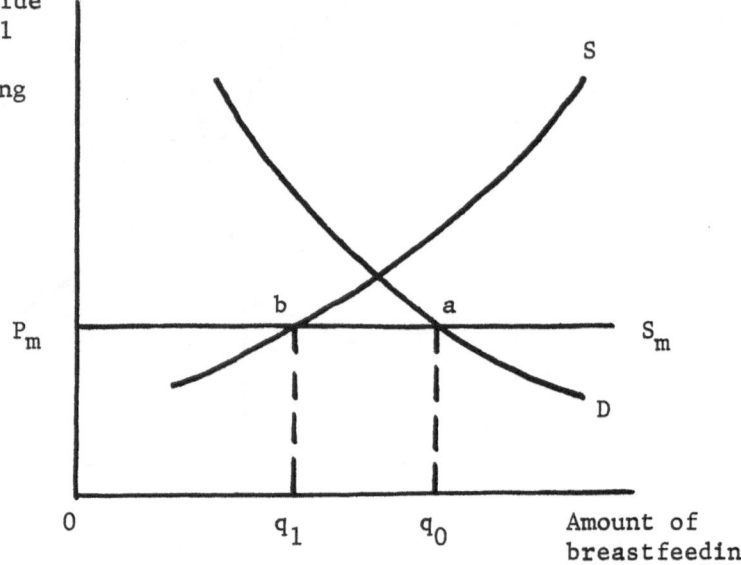

Figure 7.

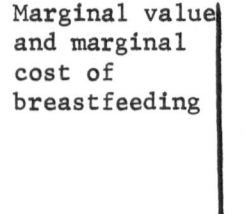
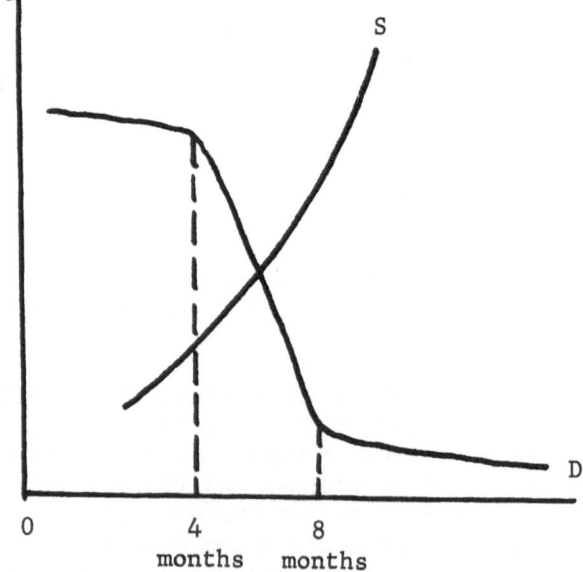

Figure 8.

dominated by the shape of its marginal value in producing child
survival and development is pictured in Figure 8. This marginal
value curve is characteristically high for the first four to six
months, declines rapidly to about eight months, and then continues
to fall slowly, according to current evidence (15,16,17,18,19,20,
21,22). In the inelastic portion of the curve, between four and
eight months, large changes in the determinants of the woman's
breastfeeding supply curve have little effect on her equilibrium
quantity.

A similar situation arises when the demand curve is dominated
by the shape of its marginal value in spacing pregnancies. Here a
particular woman's demand curve would be high and declining until
her first post-partum menstruation, when it falls to the horizontal
axis.* For a community of such women, the average demand curve
would decline rapidly to the axis in the range of months during
which most first menstruations occur, frequently 10 to 14 months
for full breastfeeding populations (23,24,25,26,27,28,29,30).
Large contractions in the supply of breastfeeding are predicted to
induce relatively small decreases in breastfeeding activity in this
range.

Some Implications of the Model

My emphasis on the distinction between demand and supply
factors in determining breastfeeding patterns masks another distinction - between behavioral and biological factors. I don't
believe the loss is a great one. Lactation is a biological function, but it can be influenced by a woman's food intake and health
status, both of which are known to respond systematically to changes
in income and relevant prices. Moreover, breastfeeding is a use
of time, whose allocation is influenced by other economic and
social factors. Correspondingly, the number of hours a person
works at a job is usually considered an economic variable to be
studied as part of an economic system, but it can be significantly
influenced by health and nutritional status, especially in poor
populations. These systems appear richly connected. People's
activities set in motion biological processes whose results influence, in turn, the relative costs and rewards of pursuing those
activities in the future.

_____

* Lactation and amenorrhea are not causally related in this simple
temporal way, but a woman cannot know that the sterility producing
effects of her breastfeeding have ended until her first menstruation, or pregnancy.

I am interested here in breastfeeding, child survival and development, and birth spacing. I have contended that, although breastfeeding affects the other two through biological processes, both it and its effectiveness can be systematically influenced behaviorally. The interesting question is whether these behavioral effects are quantitatively important. As a way of organizing the relevant empirical literature, it may be useful to state and briefly discuss some predictions that arise from the model outlined above.

First, to make two fundamental assumptions explicit, the propositions to follow suggest that people act _as if_ they allocate their available time, income and other resources in such a way that their utility or satisfaction, as they see it, is maximized. Underlying this, it is also assumed that people act _as if_ they are familiar with their relevant biological production functions: whether nursing depletes their energy for other tasks, and if so how much more they must eat to compensate; how much nursing adds to their infant's chance of survival and development at different ages; and how much nursing of different intensities and lengths increases their probability of infecundity by month post-partum.* The comparative equilibrium positions discussed in the previous section reflects criteria of optimal resource allocation derived from these assumptions.

I now turn to some implications of the model, all of which concern partial effects, holding other important factors constant.

1. An increase in the market demand for female labor tends to reduce breastfeeding if the jobs are less than fully compatible with maternal child care. The increase may come about because the family moves to an urban area for unrelated reasons, because new firms are established or old ones expanded near the community, or because the supply of "traditional" workers contracts (due perhaps to seasonal migration of men).

2. An increase in the supply of female labor to the market (resulting from factors unrelated to breastfeeding motivation) tends to reduce breastfeeding if many labor market jobs are less than fully compatible with breastfeeding. The increase may result from poor weather that ruins the crop and reduces women's marginal productivity in their fields. Or it may occur because jobs

---

* This set of as-if assumptions concerns knowledge of the amounts of outputs that result from various combinations of inputs into biological processes, not understanding of the underlying biological mechanisms.

normally held by men become less available or less well paying, inducing a positive labor market supply response by their wives.

3. An increase in the price of food staples consumed by adults tends to reduce breastfeeding in populations suffering mild to moderate or worse malnutrition. Bad weather or rapidly increasing prices of nitrogen fertilizer might be the cause.

4. An increase in the marginal value product schedule of a woman's time in home agriculture or cottage industry tends to reduce breastfeeding if these activities are less compatible with child care than alternative activitis engaged in. Favorable prices for crops or cottage industry products, or higher prices of substitutes for the woman's time in these activities could lead to this result by raising the equilibrium amount of time the woman spends in them.

These first four implications follow from hypothesized shifts in the woman's supply curve of breastfeeding. In each case, the reduction in breastfeeding tends to be more if the demand for breastfeeding is elastic. The next four implications concern this aspect.

5. Factors that reduce the supply curve of a woman's breastfeeding (as in the first four implications) tend to reduce her actual breastfeeding more if alternative weaning foods are hygienically available at a constant price.

6. The same factors tend to reduce breastfeeding more if modern contraceptives are available at a constant price.

7. The same factors tend to reduce breastfeeding more if the marginal value of birth aversion does not decline much as the length of the birth interval increases. This would occur if the couple has access to substitutes for the economic and/or non-economic benefits they receive from children and if the supplies of these substitutes - say social security provisions, hired labor, disability insurance, modern household appliances - are elastic.

8. The same factors tend to reduce breastfeeding more if the marginal value of a surviving and healthy child does not decline much as the probability that the infant will be strong increases. This would happen if the couple has access to substitutes of the type listed directly above.

9. Changes in these same factors may have little effect on breastfeeding for awhile and then begin to produce large declines if women customarily breastfeed four to eight months to insure survival of their infant, or ten to fourteen months (on the average)

until ovulation begins. In either case, the demand curve for
breastfeeding is likely quite inelastic in the indicated ranges.
The supply curve can contract considerably before having a noticeable effect. However, continuing contractions due to the factors
listed in the first four implications above can suddenly induce
large declines in breastfeeding.

10. Changes in these same factors tend to reduce a woman's
lactation without affecting how much her child is breastfed,
where an active market exists in the services of wetnurses.

These implications concern predicted effects of changes in
particular factors that influence women's supply of breastfeeding.
The next implications concern changes in demand-determining factors.

11. An increased supply of modern contraceptives from local
stores or family planning outlets tends to reduce breastfeeding.

12. An increased supply of infant weaning foods in local
stores or through public distribution channels tends to reduce
breastfeeding. In this and the previous case the increases in
effective supply could come about through better quality products,
lower prices, or more widespread distribution.

13. An increased supply of substitutes for breastfeeding, as
in implications 11 and 12, tends to reduce breastfeeding more if a
large family, relatively inexpensive modern household conveniences,
or laundromats, restaurants, barbershops and other specialized
suppliers of home production substitutes are available in elastic
supply for the mother to use in place of her own time.

14. An increased supply of substitutes for breastfeeding
tends to reduce breastfeeding more if an active female labor
market exists in which women can work as many hours as they want
at the same wage.

15. An increased supply of substitutes for breastfeeding
tends to reduce breastfeeding more among women who are well
nourished. (These women may breastfeed more than poorly nourished
women both before and after the change in the supply of substitutes,
but the amount of their decrease is predicted to be greater.)

16. An increased supply of substitutes for breastfeeding
tends to reduce the amount a child is breastfed without reducing
its mother's lactation, where an active market exists in the services of wetnurses. Child survival and development, but not birth
spacing, would be affected.

17. No unambiguous predictions arise concerning the effects

of changes in the value of children to parents, as might accompany
expansion of private or public insurance and old-age security
programs or effectively enforced school attendance laws (but see
implications 7 and 8). These changes do tend to reduce the
marginal economic value schedules of children to their parents,
but the resulting pressures on breastfeeding can work both ways.
As the total number of children desired falls, the marginal value
curve for breastfeeding as contraceptive shifts out. Simultaneous-
ly, however, the marginal value curve of breastfeeding as contributor to child survival and development shifts in. The net effect
on the demand curve for breastfeeding is ambiguous, a priori.

REVIEW OF EVIDENCE

It is a remarkable fact that not one of the above predictions
has received testing adequate for making even a preliminary judgment as to support or refutation. Most of the predictions have not
been tested at all. We are unfortunately in the position of looking around for empirical generalizations that seem consistent or
inconsistent with particular predictions.

One such generalization is that physiological and hereditary
factors are usually unimportant. The lactation process is well
protected from mild to moderate malnutrition and general morbidity
(36,37,38,39,40). Furthermore, it is economically improving populations that generally suffer more declines in breastfeeding (41).

Another useful generalization is that the Western European
and U. S. breastfeeding declines, as well as the recent trends in
less developed areas, took place first and most strongly among
urban dwellers and migrants. Looking over the predictions, one
sees many hypothesized causes of breastfeeding decline that are
known to characterize most urban environments: more women's job
opportunities that are not fully compatible with child care
(implications 1 and 14); cheaper weaning foods and modern contraceptives available at a constant price (implications 5, 6, 11, and
12); higher price of food staples consumed by adults (implication
3); lack of an active market for wetnursing (implications 10 and
16); more elastic supply of modern household appliances as well as
restaurants, laundromats and other suppliers of home production
substitutes (implications 7 and 13); more women who are well
nourished (implication 15); more elastic supply of medical, life,
and old age insurance from private sources or government plans
(implications 7 and 8). I cannot find any prediction from the
model that is inconsistent with usual patterns of economic and
institutional change during urbanization, though particular cities
can be cited as exceptions to various of the generalizations.
Accordingly, it is no surprise to find breastfeeding declines among

urbanizing populations, and it is safe to predict that recent and prospective urban migrants are among the high risk population.

Existing evidence is much less helpful in answering the other questions with which this paper began. The model developed here points to a number of specific factors that, though they may not be responsible, might be changed by public policy in order to off-set the deleterious effects. If one occurrence has contracted women's supply curves of breastfeeding, policies might be initiated to induce counteracting movements in other determinants of supply or to increase the demand for breastfeeding. Similarly, a contraction in demand might be reversed, or met with action to expand supply. Finally, it might be most cost-effective to give up on the declines and work to lessen their undesirable effects. Informed operational choices among the alternatives await empirical evidence indicating which linkages, implied by this or other models, are quantitatively important.

Venturing farther from convincing evidence than I would like, I can venture some guesses about what will emerge from careful empirical research.

● My guess is that the good or bad advice that hospital personnel give will prove unimportant except in the short run. I also suspect that commercial advertising of baby formula and other foods that end up getting contaminated before ingestion is not of enduring importance. Distribution of powdered milk that mothers water down excessively is in the same category. These factors are prominent in current public health discussions about reasons for the decline (42,43,44,45,46,47,48,49,50).

When the environment changes rapidly, as it does for new urban migrants in a less developed country, there is much learning to be done. It is natural that people make mistakes while learning, and bad advice extends the trial-and-error period. However, evidence suggests that traditional peasant farmers learn quickly about the profitability in their own fields of new agricultural technologies and react appropriately, in some cases against the incorrect advice of agricultural extension workers (51,52,53). Why not expect mothers to do as well in another matter of great importance to them?

I do not deny that the short run, the trial-and-error learning period, is a very costly time: many infants die and many birth intervals are shortened during it. Correct medical advice and responsible commercial advertising can probably help much. But the hypotheses presented here suggest that more fundamental factors are at work, and that breastfeeding declines will continue to spread even if these deficiencies are corrected. Mothers knew what they were doing in the traditional environment (54,55,56), and they will learn in the new.

● Little will probably be learned by asking women why they
don't nurse their children. It is easier to blame "lack of milk,"
"child's unwillingness," or "sickness" than to admit a growing
interest or economic incentive to spend time in other ways (57,58).
Such changing incentives can also interfere quite unconsciously
with the physiological "let-down reflex" that initiates lactation
(59,60) leaving women uncertain why their lactation has "failed."

● Estimates of the national cost of bottle feeding now
reported (31,32,33,34) will probably look far less impressive when
compared to estimates of the national cost of breastfeeding. The
total caloric cost is probably large in some malnourished populations (61,62,63,64,65), and the total time cost, which is nearly
always ignored in the calculations, is surely large in most urban
areas and many rural ones.

● Variations in breastfeeding by sex of child will probably
suggest better care of male infants in societies where parents are
independently known to favor boys. Available evidence points this
way (66,67).

● Variations in the opportunity cost of mother's time with
children will probably be found to account for significant amounts
of the variation in breastfeeding. The little existing evidence
shows negative simple and partial correlations between length of
breastfeeding and different measures of women's work activity,
wages, and schooling level (58,68,69,70,71,72,73). More sophisticated attempts to discover the direction of causality in these
correlations are in the offing (58,74). The implications in the
previous section point to a number of family and community factors
that can alter this opportunity cost. Knowledge of these factors'
empirical importance awaits research with household-level data on
persons' characteristics and activities, including breastfeeding.

A CONCLUDING RECOMMENDATION

The European and U.S. breastfeeding declines and the current
stampede from the practice in many less developed countries are
obviously the result of powerful and pervasive forces. Few pockets
of traditional behavior are left intact in their wake. People of
diverse religions, cultures, and social and economic systems have
been similarly (not identically) affected. This generality of the
phenomenon suggests that common ingredients of the socioeconomic
development process, itself, may be responsible. I suggest that
the key is the movement of increasing numbers of functions from
the home to specialized outside institutions during economic

development, and the increasing proliferation of market-produced goods that substitute for human time in household production. This process of specialization and the physical transfer of productive processes is at the center of - may be the essence of - economic development. It probably occurs in part because of long-term increases in the value of human time (75,76).

Whatever the reasons, declines in breastfeeding seem a natural part of this process. They do not appear different from mothers coming to use clothing stores, bakeries, medical clinics, schools, canned foods, gas stoves, and electrical appliances instead of the time of themselves and their families that were used in a previous generation to make clothes and bread, care for and teach children, and cook and keep house. Mothers similarly come to substitute market produced weaning foods and contraceptives for their own time spent breastfeeding, as specialization of labor and the economic cost of human time increase during economic development.

Viewed in this way, the most effective solution in many situations may be to work in league, rather than at cross purposes, with the economic development process. If public policy can rapidly increase the supply of effective contraceptives and the hygienic, effective use of weaning foods, mothers will have means to maintain and even increase their birth spacing and the survival and development of their infants.* Ironically, the model developed here suggests that these policies will speed the breastfeeding declines at the same time that they make them irrelevant. The only practical alternative is research to identify particular factors in families' surroundings - factors indicated by the model developed here and by others - that governments can alter to induce women to maintain their time and energy spent breastfeeding, even as their overall time allocation patterns change dramatically.** Action on both fronts is certainly warranted.

---

* This has apparently been the outcome in the U.S. and Western Europe where increasing supplies of hygienic infant foods and effective contraceptives have made breastfeeding nearly irrelevant to birth spacing and infant survival (77). It is interesting to note that infant mortality rates and fertility decreased during much of this period of declining breastfeeding without government participation in the markets for infant foods and contraceptives.

** Research strategies that rely on cross-tabulations of data, simple correlations, and even methods of partial correlation such as path analysis will not get far here. One can expect their estimates to be significantly biased, in light of the joint determination of many nutritional and economic variables in family behavior (78).

This paper was written under a grant from the Rockefeller
Foundation to the Rand Corporation. The views expressed here are
those of the author and not necessarily those of either organization.

References

1. McGeorge, M. Current Trends in Breast Feeding, New Zealand
    Medical Journal, 35-36, January 1960.

2. Shorter, E. Mothers and Infants, The Making of the Modern
    Family, 175-190, Basic Books, New York, 1975.

3. Newton, N. and M. Newton. Psychological Aspects of Lactation,
    The New England Journal of Medicine, 277, 1183, November 30,
    1967.

4. Knodel, J. and E. Van de Walle. Breast Feeding, Fertility and
    Infant Mortality: An Analysis of Some Early German Data,
    Population Studies, 21, 109-131, September 1967.

5. Mead, M. and N. Newton. Cultural Patterning of Perinatal
    Behavior, in S. A. Richardson and A. F. Guttmacher, eds.,
    Childbearing--Its Social and Psychological Aspects, 183-184,
    The Williams & Wilkins Compnay, 1967.

6. Ross, A. I., and G. Herdan. Breast-Feeding in Bristol,
    The Lancet, 630, March 17, 1951.

7. McGeorge, M. op.cit., 31-32.

8. Rouchy, R., M. Taureau and M. J. Valmyre. Current Trends in
    Maternal Breast-feeding, Bulletin de la Federation des
    Societes de Gynecologie et d'Obstetrique de Longue Francaise,
    471-473, 1961 (French).

9. Meyer, H. F. Breastfeeding in the United States: Extent and
    Possible Trend, Pediatrics, 22, 116-121, July 1958.

10. Harfouche, J. K. The Importance of Breast-Feeding. Journal
    of Tropical Pediatrics, 16, 154-155, September 1970.

11. McGeorge, M. op.cit., 33.

12. Wong, H. B., K. Paramathypathy and N. B. Tham. Breast-Feeding

Among Lower Income Mothers in Singapore, _Journal of the Singapore Paediatric Society_, 5, 89-93, October 1963.

13. Romaniuk, A. Modernization and Fertility. The Case of the James Bay Indians, _Canadian Review of Sociology and Anthropology_, 11, 355-356, 1974.

14. Buchanan, R. Breast-feeding--Aid to Infant Health and Fertility Control, _Population Reports_, J, 54-55, July 1975.

15. Berg, A., portions w/ R. J. Muscat. _The Nutrition Factor, Its Role in National Development_, 94-95, The Brookings Institution, Washington, D. C., 1973.

16. Wade, N. Bottle-Feeding: Adverse Effects of a Western Technology, _Science_, 184, 45, April 5, 1974.

17. Oomen, H.A.P.C. The Pauan Child as a Survivor. _J. of Tropical Ped._, 103, March 1961.

18. Potter, R. G., M. L. New, J. B. Wyon and J. E. Gordon. Lactation and Its Effects upon Birth Intervals in Eleven Punjab Villages, India, _J. Chronic Dis._, 18, 1131, 1965.

19. Jelliffe, D. B., and E.F.P. Jelliffe. Human Milk, Nutrition, and the World Resource Crises, _Science_, 188, 557, May 9, 1975.

20. Jelliffe, D. B. Culture, Social Change and Infant Feeding. _Am. J. Clinical Nutrition_, 10, 36-39, January 1962.

21. Mellander, O., B. Vahlquist, T. Mellbin and collaborators. _Breast Feeding and Artificial Feeding_, 48, 11-99, Almquist and Wiksells Bektryckeri AB, Uppsala, 1959.

22. Douglas, J.W.B. The Extent of Breast Feeding in Great Britain in 1946, with Special Reference to the Health and Survival of Children. _J. Obstet. and Gynecol._, 57, 349-359, 1950.

23. Berman, M. L., K. Hanson, and I. L. Hellman. Effect of Breast-feeding on Postpartum Menstruation, Ovulation, and Pregnancy in Alaskan Eskimos. _Am. J. Obstet. and Gynecol._, 114, 524-534, October 15, 1972.

24. Chen, L. C., S. Ahmed, M. Gesche and W. H. Mosley. A Prospective Study of Birth Interval Dynamics in Rural Bangladesh. _Population Studies_, 28, 277-297, July 1974.

25. Gonzalez, N. L. Solien de. Lactation and Pregnancy: A Hypothesis. _American Anthropologist_, 66, Part 1, 873-878, August 1964.

26. Potter, R. G., M. L. New, J. B. Wyon and J. E. Gordon. op.cit., 26.

27. Buchanan, R. op.cit., 56-58.

28. VanGinneken, J. K. Prolonged Breastfeeding as a Birth Spacing Method. Studies in Fam. Plan., 5, 201-203, 1974.

29. Knodel, J. Infant Mortality and Fertility in Three Bavarian Villages: An Analysis of Family Histories from the 19th Century. Population Studies, 23, 297-318, November 3, 1968.

30. Romaniuk, A. op.cit., 357.

31. Jelliffe, D. B., and E.F.P. Jelliffe. op.cit., 558, May 9, 1975.

32. Wade, N. op.cit., 45.

33. McKigney, J. I. Economic Aspects of Infant Feeding Practices in the West Indies, J. Trop. Ped., 55-59, June 1968.

34. Berg, A., portions w/R. J. Muscat. op.cit., 229-232.

35. Butz, W. P., et al. Economic Influences on Breastfeeding in a Guatemalan Population. Rand Corporation Report, forthcoming 1977.

36. Newton, N. and M. Newton. op.cit., 1179.

37. Jelliffe, D. B. Breast-Milk and the World Protein Gap. Clin. Ped., 7, 96, February 1968.

38. Gopalan, C. Studies on Lactation in Poor Indian Communities, J. Trop. Ped., 97, Dec. 1958.

39. Jelliffe, D. B. op.cit., 23, January 1962.

40. Gonzalez, N. L. Solien de. op.cit., 873.

41. McGeorge, M. op.cit., 37.

42. _____ ibid, 36, January 1960.

43. Meyer, H. F. op.cit., 119.

44. Jelliffe, D. B. Unique Properties of Human Milk. J. Reproduc. Med., 14, 134, April 1975.

45. Jelliffe, D. B. op.cit., 98-99, February 1968.

46. Wade, N. op.cit., 45-48.

47. Buchanan, R. op.cit., 49, 55.

48. Harfouche, J. K. op.cit., 156-158.

49. Brown, R. E. Breast Feeding in Modern Times. Am.J. Clin. Nut., 26, 556-562, May 1973.

50. Berg, A. op.cit., 103-104.

51. Berry, R. A. and W. R. Cline. Farm Size, Factor Productivity and Technical Change in Developing Countries. Preliminary, January 1976.

52. Bhalla, S. S. Farm Size, Productivity and Technical Change in Indian Agriculture, Appendix A in Berry, R. A. op.cit.

53. Sukhatme, V. Unpublished Ph.D. dissertation, Department of Economics, University of Chicago, 1976.

54. Jelliffe, D. B. Infant Nutrition in the Subtropics and Tropics, 2nd ed., 244. World Health Organization, Geneva, 1968.

55. Jelliffe, D. B. op.cit., 33-34, January 1962.

56. Ford, C. S. A Comparative Study of Human Reproduction, 32, 79. Yale University Publications in Anthropology, 1945.

57. McGeorge, M. op.cit., 37.

58. Popkin, B. M., S. de Jesus. Determinants of Breast-Feeding Behavior Among Rural Filipino Households (revised). Institute

59. Jelliffe, D. B. Breast Feeding in Technically Developing Regions. Courrier, 6, 91, April 1956.

60. Buchanan, G. op.cit., 51.

61. McGeorge, M. op.cit., 37.

62. Jelliffe, D. B. and E.F.P. Jelliffe. op.cit., 558, May 9, 1975.

63. Jelliffe, D. B. and E.F.P. Jelliffe. An Overview, The American J. Clin. Nut., 24, 1017, August 1971.

64. Oomen, H.A.P.C. op.cit., 107-108.

65. Harfouche, J. K. op.cit., 144.

66. Harfouche, J.K. Feeding Practices and Weaning Patterns of Lebanese Infants, Khayats, Beirut, 1965.

67. Welbourn, H. F. Bottle Feeding: A Problem of Modern Civilization. J. Trop. Ped., 4, 157-166, March 1958.

68. Nerlove, S. B. Women's Workload and Infant Feeding Practices: A Relationship with Demographic Implications. Ethnology, 13: 207-214, 1974.

69. Wong, H. B., K. Paramathypathy and N. B. Tham. op.cit., 92.

70. Newton, N. and M. Newton. op.cit., 1184.

71. Chen, L. C., S. Ahmed, M. Gesche and W. H. Mosley. op.cit.,295.

72. Gopalan, D. op.cit., 97.

73. Jelliffe, D. B. op.cit., 24, January 1962.

74. Butz, W. P., et al. Economic Influences on Breastfeeding in A Guatemalan Population. Rand Corporation Report, forthcoming 1977.

75. Schultz, T. W. Fertility and Economic Values in: T. W. Schultz, ed., Economics of the Family, 14-22, National Bureau of Economic Research, New York, 1974.

76. Nerlove, Marc. Toward a New Theory of Population and Economic Growth in: T. W. Schultz, ed. Economics of the Family, op.cit., 527-545.

77. Hill, L. F. Infant Feeding: Historical and Current. The Pediatric Clinics of North America, 14: 255-268, 1967.

78. Butz, W. P. and J.-P. Habicht. The Effects of Nutrition and Health on Fertility: Hypotheses, Evidence, and Interventions in Ronald G. Ridker, ed., Population and Development, The Search for Selective Interventions, 210-238, Resources for the Future, Washington, D.C., 1976.

ANALYTICAL MODELS OF NUTRITION-FERTILITY RELATIONSHIPS

INTRODUCTORY STATEMENT

Robert G. Potter

Brown University

Providence, Rhode Island

In this section, three articles present analytical models that differ greatly in scope, structure, and purpose.

As Menken and Bongaarts point out in their paper, mathematical models of family-building, devised over the past two decades, have helped investigators "to understand which components of the reproductive process are most important in determining fertility, how these components interact, and what the magnitude of the potential effects of changes in these components might be." The principal components considered by the two authors pertain to natural fertility only, with no heed given to contraception, abortion, or sterilization. Hence, the principal components treated are: 1) lengths of pregnancy and subsequent periods of temporary amenorrhea, conditional on outcome of pregnancy; 2) lengths of menstruating intervals between end of amenorrhea and next conception in the absence of contraception; 3) probabilities of pregnancy outcomes unaffected by induced abortion; and 4) length of the reproductive period as framed by the events of entering a first sexual relationship and menopause, without truncation of childbearing by sterilization. In several articles of this Proceedings, and perhaps most explicitly in R. Frisch's paper, influences of nutrition upon all four of these basic components have been posited.

Having defined what is an important size of effect upon natural fertility, one may use models of the type reviewed by Menken and Bongaarts to deduce what change of value in a particular reproductive component is necessary to generate the criterion fertility change; this change of component value then may be compared with its empirical range to test whether such a fertility effect through this mechanism is plausible or not. Using this strategy, Menken and Bongaarts conclude that sizable reductions of natural fertility by malnutrition are not likely through the mechanisms of delaying menarche or increasing the risk of pregnancies ending in spontaneous abortion; but are more plausibly realized through such mechanisms as hastening the onset of secondary sterility, prolonging menstruating intervals, deferring marriage, or lengthening postpartum amenorrhea (at least in cultures featuring prolonged lactation). Of course, demonstrating that a particular reproductive component has an empirical range sufficient to produce significant effects on fertility is not at all the same thing as showing that that empirical range is largely or even in small part accountable by variation in nutritional status. Only cumulative field work, informed by more detailed and specialized models, can hope to achieve a verdict on this second issue and therefore decide what are the quantitative effects of nutrition upon natural fertility through the several possible mechanisms.

As an additional point, Menken and Bongaarts remark that the rather general family-building models reviewed by them can also be used to estimate the minimum size of nutritionally induced change in a particular reproductive component that is necessary to produce a large enough fertility effect to be of interest. One is then in a position to employ standard statistical means for determining the size of sample needed to detect differences of this minimal size with a predesignated degree of confidence. In this fashion models of the type discussed in their paper serve as aids to designing field studies of nutrition and fertility.

In a second paper, Masnick offers a conceptual scheme rather than a formal mathematical model. The reproductive performance of a woman is viewed as a process over time in which the timing of events is crucial. Giving attention to these timing subtleties one can expect to find great variation among women of a single population. Three sets of factors - fecundity, union exposure, and capacity to practice birth control - interact to determine fertility.

Nutrition affects all three. The manifold influences of nutrition upon fecundity have constituted the focus of many of the papers of this Proceedings. Malnutrition can potentially reduce union exposure by delaying menarche and thereby in some societies marriage, as well as by raising widowhood rates. With respect to family planning, it is hypothesized by Masnick that an initial period of unsuccessful contraception, or a period of childbearing without any attempt at fertility regulation at all, conduces to a trained incapacity that makes the later acquisition of anticonception skills difficult to achieve. Efficient birth control practices are most easily acquired through self-reinforcing contraceptive successes early in a reproductive career. It is theorized that malnutrition by prolonging the period of adolescent subfecundity, by protracting postpartum amenorrhea, and by lowering the monthly risks of conception during menstruating intervals widens opportunities for early contraceptive successes.

In a third paper, Wils utilizes systems analysis with respect to the easternmost province of Zaire in order to depict what might happen when mainly subsistence agriculture in combination with rapid population growth are allowed to persist in an easily eroded environment. Increased realism is obtained by replacing a single-region model with a two-region counterpart in which migration motivated by excessive crowding of the land is permitted from the region of best agricultural land to the second, much larger area of adequate but still less favored soils. As local population density mounts, there occurs soil degradation both of a reversible and irreversible nature, together with lowered agricultural output and reduced per capita food. The latter two factors lead to attempts by families to farm more land. Concurrently, lower per capita food leads to lessened work capacity (which ultimately limits the area a family can successfully farm); it leads to longer birth intervals, higher death rates, and forced migration to the less crowded region. This migration being selective of young adults has pronounced effects on the period birth and death rates of the two regions which experience their crises at different times.

The most striking result of the two-region model is the rapidity with which environmental degradation accelerates following early stages of rather slow rates of change that give little hint of what is impending. A special advantage claimed for the systems analysis approach is that its results expressed as graphs can be grasped by a wide audience. On the other hand, its results depend closely on the functional relationships posited between pairs of key variables and these relationships are usually no more than educated guesses drawn from consultants chosen for their local expertise.

REPRODUCTIVE MODELS IN THE STUDY OF NUTRITION-FERTILITY

INTERRELATIONSHIPS

Jane Menken, John Bongaarts

Princeton University, Princeton, New Jersey

The Population Council, New York, New York

INTRODUCTION

Over the past two decades, mathematical models of the human reproductive process have been devised to meet a broad range of needs. First, because of the difficulty of performing meaningful experiments in real populations, investigators have turned to models to understand which components of the reproductive process are most important in determining fertility, how these components interact, and what the magnitude of the potential effect of changes in these components might be. Second, in many cases, accurate data on one or a few components are not available, although an investigator might be able to make an informed guess as to the maximum and minimum values feasible. A model, if sufficiently realistic, could then estimate whether, within the range or ranges given, differences in the component could imply substantial differences in fertility. In this way, models have served as aids in deciding the kinds of studies needed and which measurements were crucial to an understanding of fertility in an actual population. Finally, once a model has been devised and validated, it can also provide a means of indirectly estimating either a specified fertility indicator from the components of reproduction, or a component from knowledge of the other variables and fertility itself.

In this paper, we will first discuss the basic operation of the reproductive process from the demographic model-builder's perspective and review briefly some of the available evidence for relationships between nutrition and components of this process. A description of two existing models will be followed by an analysis of some of the effects of variations in the factors included on

261

fertility, with particular reference to possible mechanisms whereby
nutrition might influence fertility.   The analysis will be limited
to populations with natural fertility, i.e., populations in which
no deliberate fertility control is practiced.*

BASIC OPERATION OF THE REPRODUCTIVE PROCESS

The basic outline of a woman's reproductive career is shown
in Figure 1 (level of analysis B).   The limits of the potential
reproductive years of women are determined by menarche and menopause.   Menarche, the first menstruation in a woman's life, occurs
in the early or mid-teens, with an average age at menarche equal to
about 13 years in the contemporary Western world (1,2) and somewhat
higher in developing countries and in historical populations.
Menopause, the complete cessation of menstruation signals the end
of the reproductive years.   In the U.S. and Europe, mean age at
menopause is about 49 years, with substantial variations among
individuals ranging from below 40 to near 60 (3,4).   Studies of
menopause in developing countries are rare, but menopause apparently
occurs slightly earlier than in the West.   From the mean ages at
menarche and menopause one could, by subtracting, obtain an estimate
of the duration of the potential reproductive years.   Unfortunately,
this procedure is inaccurate because a woman only rarely becomes
fully fecundable (able to conceive) at menarche.   Much more typical
is a period of up to several years with irregular menses and a high
incidence of anovulatory cycles following menarche.   A similar
period of menstrual irregularity precedes menopause and functional
sterility can set in years before menstrual bleeding stops
completely.

Although childbearing could theoretically start at menarche,
reproduction in virtually all societies is limited to women who
are married (marriage is defined here as any stable sexual union,
e.g., consensual unions are included).   In many traditional societies marriage takes place shortly after menarche and the mean age
at first marriage is often under 20 years.   In contrast, the mean
age at first marriage in a number of European countries exceeds

---

* The term <u>natural fertility</u> as defined by demographers, connotes
a population in which none of the determinants of reproductive
behavior are deliberately altered in response to the number of
children already born.   Thus long nursing can occur under conditions of natural fertility if the length of breastfeeding is
intended to be the same for all children.   Abstinence practiced
after the oldest child reaches a certain age is an example of
deliberate fertility control which does not require modern techno-
logical advances in contraceptive methods.

25 years, thus substantially reducing the time available for child bearing.

Within marriage, reproduction can continue until separation, widowhood or permanent sterility intervene. While married and before becoming permanently sterile, women reproduce at a rate which is inversely related to the time between births, i.e., short birth intervals are associated with a large number of births by the end of the reproductive years and vice versa. To get insights into the determinants of fertility rates among married women it is therefore useful to study the various biological and behavioral factors which influence the duration of birth intervals.

As is summarized in Figure 1 (level of analysis B), the birth interval may be divided into the following three principal components (5,6,7):

1) The postpartum amenorrhea interval from birth to the first postpartum menses. During this interval the normal cyclical pattern of menstruation and ovulation is absent. The first postpartum ovulation usually takes place within a few weeks before or after the time of the return of the menses. It

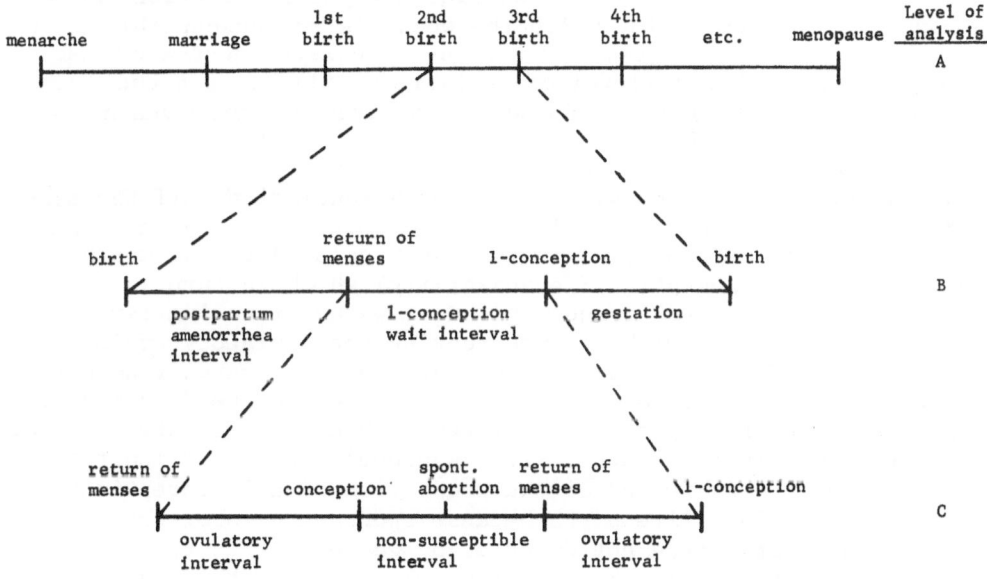

Figure 1. Segmentation of reproductive years into birth intervals and birth interval components.

is now well established that the duration and intensity of
breastfeeding are the principal determinants of the duration
of postpartum amenorrhea (8). Since lactation practices
vary widely among societies, observed mean postpartum
amenorrhea intervals also have a wide range from a few months
or less (U.S., Europe) to more than one and a half years
(Bangladesh).

2) The 1(live)-conception wait interval, defined as the
interval from the first postpartum menses - indicating the
return of ovulation - to the conception that ends in a
live birth. Its determinants will be discussed below.

3) The full term pregnancy interval of 9 months duration.

This basic segmentation of the birth interval is a convenient
one demanding few data and can be done with a relatively high
degree of reliability because it requires the measurement of only
two types of well defined events - the live birth and return of
menses. The conception ending in a live birth can be assumed to
take place 9 months before each birth.

Before a 1-conception terminates the 1-conception wait interval, other conceptions leading to abortions or still births may
occur. In this case, it is possible to subdivide the 1-conception
wait interval into segments during which regular ovulation takes
place and segments during which the woman is non-susceptible as a
result of the aborted pregnancy or the associated post-abortion
amenorrhea. Figure 1 (level of analysis C) illustrates the
sequence of events in the case where one intra-uterine death
precedes the next birth.

An ovulatory interval precedes each conception. If the menstrual cycle is regular and lasts approximately one month, then
the mean ovulatory interval is inversely related to the monthly
probability of conception (fecundability) which in turn is a
function of the coital frequency. Here we are ignoring fertilized
ova which disappear without interrupting the ovulatory cycle.
Typical mean durations of the ovulatory interval range from 6 to 9
months in the absence of contraception. The average duration of
the non-susceptible period associated with each intra-uterine death
is approximately 2.5 months. It has proven rather difficult to
obtain accurate estimates of the proportion of all conceptions
that will end in a live birth because spontaneous abortions early
in pregnancy are often not detected by women. It is tentatively
estimated that of all embryos which are viable at the end of the
conception month about 75-80% will yield a live birth (9). This
percentage is somewhat higher for women in the mid-reproductive
years, but it declines rapidly with advancing age.

NUTRITION-FERTILITY INTERRELATIONSHIPS

In the previous section the behavioral and biological factors affecting birth intervals and fertility were introduced. These so-called intermediate fertility variables (10) are the most immediate determinants of fertility, and through them the socioeconomic and biological environment operates to influence fertility. Nutrition therefore does not affect fertility directly but instead acts by modifying one or more of the intermediate fertility variables.

Figure 2 presents the different possible links between the nutrition of the mother and child on the one hand and fertility on the other. Studies of the effects of nutrition on the various intermediate fertility variables are available in the medical and demographic literature; some of this evidence can be summarized as follows:

Nutrition and Menarche

In an analysis of age at menarche among a group of Alabama girls, Frisch (11) found that malnourished girls reached menarche an average of two years later than their well nourished counterparts. Indirect evidence supporting this finding is provided by the negative correlation between socioeconomic status and age at menarche reported in a variety of societies (12,13,14) and by the secular decline in age at menarche in European populations in the late nineteenth and early twentieth centuries, a decline that has been attributed to improving diets (15).

Nutrition and Menopause

Different studies of this relation are often conflicting. MacMahon (16) reports that lean women reach menopause slightly earlier than average, but Jaszmann (17) is unable to find any relationship between age at menopause and antoropometric measures. In a study of Ceylonese women, it is estimated that urban women attained menopause on average 2.4 years later than rural women (18). Other investigators report no significant effect of socioeconomic status on age at menopause (19,20,21). A rising secular trend in age at menopause is found among Polish women (22) but not among women in England (23). Further study of this topic is clearly necessary before any definite conclusions can be drawn. Nutritional variations in age at menopause affect fertility through changes in the age at which permanent sterility is attained. Since direct measurement of sterility has proven very difficult, virtually no comparative data on age at sterility are available. It will be assumed here that there is a fixed time difference between the ages at sterility and menopause, so that any changes in age at sterility are directly reflected in changes in the age at menopause

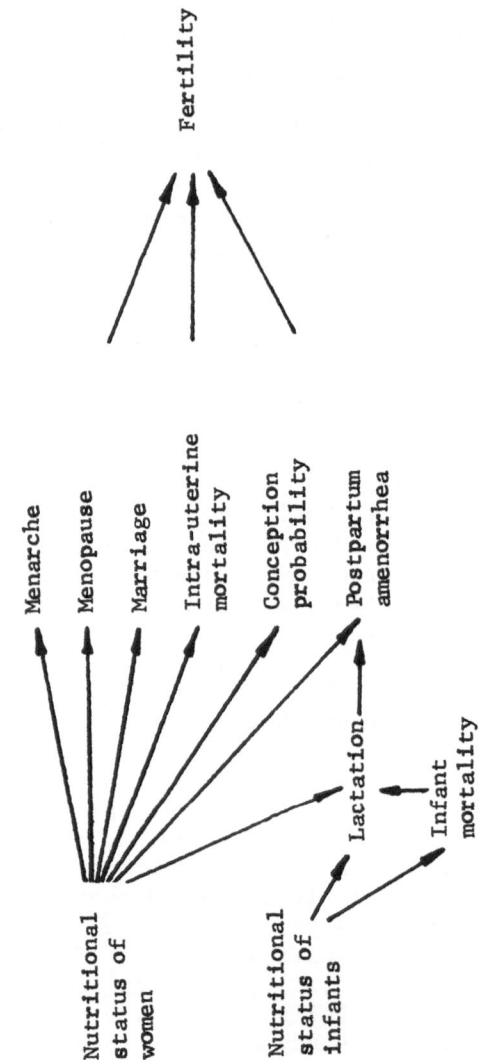

Figure 2.   Nutrition-fertility interrelationships.

Nutrition and Marriage

The potential effect of nutrition on marriage has received virtually no attention. Two links could exist. First, if nutrition affects menarche as seems probable, and if menarche affects age at first marriage as is the case in some traditional societies where menarche indicates that a woman has become marriageable, then the nutritional status of a woman would influence her age at marriage through variations in age at menarche. Secondly, the duration of marriage, which depends on the survival of both spouses, would be affected if nutrition is one of the determinants of mortality.

Nutrition and Intrauterine Mortality

Although caloric intake during pregnancy is known to be one of the determinants of birth weight (24), the effect of current nutrition on intrauterine mortality is less clear. A negative relationship between socioeconomic status and intrauterine and perinatal mortality is now well established (25,26,27,28), but it appears to be unrelated to current maternal nutrition (29). Experimental studies in animals, however, have shown that severe nutritional deprivation does affect the survival of the fetus (30, 31).

Nutrition and Fecundability (Probability of Conception)

Conception is dependent on the production of viable ova and sperm as well as on the occurrence of intercourse. All these factors are apparently affected by severe restrictions in dietary intake. Menstruation and ovulation stop when a woman suffers severe weight loss (32,33) and many women become amenorrheic during famine (34). Chronic severe malnutrition disturbs the function of the endocrine system, resulting in atrophy of the gonads, hypopituitarism, and reduction in urinary gonadotropins (35). In starving males, semen volume, sperm count, and sperm mobility are significantly reduced and interest in sexual activity markedly declines (36). American prisoners of war in a Japanese concentration camp showed universal loss of libido, an absence of nocturnal emissions, and other indications of androgen suppression (37). It should be noted that these findings all relate to severe nutritional deprivation. Under less severe conditions existing studies suggest that there may be no effect of nutrition on ovulation. In Bangladesh, where there are wide monthly fluctuations in the food supply associated with the harvests, no systematic monthly fluctuation in the regularity of menstruation has been observed (38). In rural Guatamala, the 1-conception wait interval was found to be unrelated to the mothers' nutritional status (39).

Nutrition and Postpartum Amenorrhea

The postpartum amenorrhea period is longer for malnourished, lactating women than for their well fed counterparts (40,41,42). Postpartum amenorrhea among lactating women has also been found to be negatively related to socioeconomic status (43,44,45).

On the basis of the above evidence, one can conclude that nutrition has some influence on fertility. However, the magnitude of the overall effect and the importance of each intermediate fertility variable remains uncertain.

SOME MEASUREMENT ISSUES

A detailed study of the relationships between nutrition and fertility involves the measurement of three factors: nutrition, fertility, and the intermediate fertility variables. A complete review of the methodological issues involved is not possible here and the primary objective of this section is therefore to guide the reader to sources in the existing literature.

Nutrition

A number of methods are available for evaluating different aspects of the nutritional status of individuals or of populations. A discussion of this methodology is available in reports by Jellife (46) and WHO (47).

Fertility

Fertility measurement has long been a major concern of demographers and as a result a variety of measures are available (48). The simplest index of fertility is the crude birth rate (CBR), the number of births per 1,000 persons in a population. The CBR is widely used and easily calculated, but it has one drawback: it is influenced by the population's age structure. For this reason, "purer" fertility measures such as the total fertility rate (TFR) are often preferred. The TFR equals the average number of births a woman has by the end of the reproductive years; it can be calculated by adding the age specific fertility rates (the number of births per 1,000 women in each age group) over the entire reproductive period. Although the total fertility rate is considered a more accurate measure of fertility, there is a high degree of correlation between the CBR and TFR of a population and variations in fertility are reflected in both indices.

INTERMEDIATE FERTILITY VARIABLES

For the purpose of measurement, intermediate fertility variables may be divided into two types: a) events, such as menarche, menopause and marriage; and b) intervals such as postpartum amenorrhea, 1-conception and ovulation intervals. (The estimation of the risk of spontaneous abortion is difficult and requires special life table techniques (49) which will not be discussed here). Relatively simple demographic methodology is available for summarizing the incidence and timing of age at first marriage (50,51); these same techniques can also be applied for the analysis of menarche and menopause. The unbiased measurement of intervals, however, is a rather complex topic which is not yet fully explored. Two issues are of particular importance:

1. Truncation bias (52). Since prospective studies of fertility usually terminate at a fixed point in time, many intervals will be incomplete, i.e., their end is not observed. Unfortunately, an analysis based on the intervals whose beginning and end are both observed (closed intervals) leads to a truncation bias, because in that case shorter intervals have a higher probability of being included than longer ones. To avoid this bias, a life table procedure can be applied to all intervals that start during the observation period, regardless of whether they are incomplete or closed. Further details can be found in studies by Potter (53) or Chen et al.(54).

2. Sampling frame (55). A sample of intervals can be obtained in two different ways - by selecting a sample of women who each contribute one interval or by selecting a sample of all intervals starting within a given period of time, in which case a woman may contribute more than one interval. It is important to make a distinction between the two methods, because the former tends to result in longer intervals than the latter as a consequence of the population's heterogeneity. The more fecund women have intervals that tend to be shorter than average; therefore these women have a higher probability of contributing intervals than the less fecund ones if the sampling frame consists of all intervals in a study period. An investigator is free to choose between the two sampling frames; for example, in a retrospective study where women of reproductive age are interviewed, it may be more convenient to limit the analysis to the most recent birth interval, while in a prospective study lasting a few years, all intervals starting during the observation period may be used to maximize sample size. It should be noted, however, that only in the latter case will there be a simple inverse relationship between the fertility rate and the birth interval mean, as will be discussed next.

A SIMPLE MODEL OF THE REPRODUCTIVE PROCESS

Reproductive models summarize the relationship between intermediate fertility variables and fertility in the form of mathematical equations. In the context of nutrition-fertility studies,
reproductive models are useful for estimating the change in fertility that results from nutritionally induced variations in specific
intermediate fertility variables. In recent decades a number of
different types of reproductive models have been developed, ranging
from relatively simple to highly complex ones (56,57). One of the
simplest of these models, based on the work of Henry (58) and
Perrin and Sheps (59) will be summarized here.

Let the fertility rate, expressed in births per 1,000 women be
represented by the variable FR. Since some women are sterile or
not married, FR is less than the fertility rate among women who are
reproducers. To find this rate, the marital fecund fertility rate
MFR, FR is divided by S, the proportion of all women that is both
fecund and married:

$$MFR = \frac{FR}{S} \qquad\qquad [1]$$

From renewal theory, it is known that the equilibrium rate of
occurrence of an event equals the inverse of the mean duration of
the interval between two successive events (60). This finding can
be applied with good approximation to the rate of childbearing
among women in the mid-reproductive years when fertility rates are
close to equilibrium and the intermediate fertility variables are
approximately age-invariant. If B represents the mean birth interval (calculated by using all births in a time interval as the
sampling frame) then

$$MFR = \frac{12000}{B} \qquad\qquad [2]$$

where B is expressed in months and MFR is calculated per 1,000
married fecund women per year. Substitution of [2] in [1] yields

$$FR = \frac{12000\ S}{B} \qquad\qquad [3]$$

Under the assumption that the three principal birth interval components are independently determined, B equals the sum of the mean
durations of each of the sub-components:

$$B = P + L + G \qquad\qquad [4]$$

where   P = mean duration of the postpartum amenorrhea
        interval (months)

        L = mean duration of the 1-conception interval
        (months)

        G = full term pregnancy of 9 months duration

After substitution of [4], equation [3] becomes

$$FR = \frac{12000\ S}{P + L + G} \qquad\qquad [5]$$

This basic version of the model can be refined further by introducing the determinants of the 1-conception interval. It can be shown (61,62) that

$$L = \frac{0}{1-A} + \frac{AI}{1-A} \qquad\qquad [6]$$

where   A = the proportion of all conceptions that ends
        in a spontaneous abortion or still birth

        0 = mean duration of the ovulation interval
        (months)

        I = mean duration of non-susceptability associated
        with a intrauterine death (months)

The first term on the right side of this equation represents the average total time women ovulate during the 1-conception interval and the second term equals the time they are non-susceptible. It can further be demonstrated that 0 equals the inverse of the population's harmonic mean fecundability F:

$$0 = \frac{1}{F} \qquad\qquad [7]$$

Substitution of [7] in [6] and [6] in [5] finally results in the complete version of this reproductive model:

$$FR = \frac{12000\ S}{P + \dfrac{1}{(1-A)\ F} + \dfrac{A\ I}{1-A} + G} \qquad [8]$$

where the denominator of [8] is simply the mean interval between live births. A very rough estimate of the total fertility rate, TFR, can be obtained by multiplying [8] by the number of years women are both fecund and married, the EP or effective reproductive period:

$$TFR \sim FR \times EP \qquad\qquad [9]$$

The following simple example of an application serves to illustrate how the above model can be used in the analysis of the effect of nutrition on fertility. Assume that in a hypothetical group of women the following estimates have been obtained:

- proportion of women
  fecund and married   0.90

- mean postpartum
  amenorrhea duration   10 months

- mean duration of
  1-conception interval   9 months

In that case, the fertility rate for these women is 12000 x 0.9/(10+9+9) or 386 births per 1,000 women per year, as estimated from equation 5 . Assume further that a study of the effect of nutrition on postpartum amenorrhea has demonstrated that a subgroup of undernourished women have a mean postpartum amenorrhea interval 3 months above average, i.e., 13 months. According to the model, fertility in this group of poorly nourished women should be 9.7% below average, or 348 births per 1,000 women per year. If women in both groups all become fecund at age 15 and reach secondary sterility at age 43, then their fecund period lasts 43-15=28 years; if they marry at age 18, their effective reproductive period is 25 years. The TFR will be 25 x (386/1000)=9.6 in the first case and 25 x (348/1000)=8.7 in the second, so that the reduction in TFR attributable to poor nutrition is also 9.7%. Of course, if poor nutrition also decreased the effective reproductive period, an even greater reduction in the TFR would be observed. It is interesting to note that a 30% increase in the postpartum amenorrhea interval results in only a 9.7% decrease in fertility. This finding becomes intuitively clear when one considers that changes in fertility are tied to alterations in the total birth interval. A change in an intermediate fertility which affects one component of the birth interval by a given percentage can only produce a much lower percentage change in the entire birth interval.

MORE COMPLEX MODELS

The model of the reproductive process already presented is a useful descriptive and analytic tool. It highlights the importance, first, of the birth interval and its components as the determinants of fertility rates within the reproductive span and then, of the duration of reproductive life and its influence on total fertility and therefore crude birth rates. Because it leads to analytic expressions for indices such as mean birth interval lengths and fertility rates and because it includes only a limited number of factors, it is relatively easy to study the effects of changes in each of these components. However, as soon as more realism is sought, either by allowing variation among women or with age in each determinant, or by the inclusion of more factors that influence the occurrence of births in real life (e.g., differential age at marriage, widowhood, coital frequency), the mathematics can rapidly become intractable. Researchers have turned to computer models in which results are calculated from specific parameter values and a set of assumptions about the action and interaction of the factors. These models have been of two types, macrosimulation and microsimulation, each useful in a variety of situations (63,64).

Macrosimulation

Macrosimulation models usually generate results month by month, obtaining, for example, the number of conceptions at age 20 years 10 months by multiplying the number of women in the ovulating interval in that month by the fecundability at that age. The fertility rate nine months later is calculated as the number of conceptions multiplied by the proportion leading to live births (1-A) and divided by the total number of women. The number in the ovulating interval at age 20 years 11 months is equal to the number in the previous month, minus the number conceiving the previous month, plus the number of newly married plus the number ending their periods of postpartum amenorrhea following either a live birth or fetal death. Although computer programming of such models can be tedious, the method itself is straightforward.

Microsimulation

Microsimulation differs in that an entire reproductive history is generated for a sample of <u>individuals</u> by using random numbers to determine the occurrence and timing of each successive event for one individual at a time. For example, if a sample woman is in the first month of marriage and her fecundability is .20, a random number between zero and one can be chosen. If the random number is greater than .20, she does not conceive in that month. If it is less than .20, a conception is recorded in her history as occurring in that month. Another random number can be generated to determine whether a live birth or an abortion is the next event. Step by step, the life of this one woman is thus determined. The fertility rate at a particular age can later be found by counting the number of histories in which a record of a birth at that age is recorded and dividing by the number of women, exactly the same procedure one would use on real survey or vital statistics and census data.

Microsimulation models are most useful under two circumstances: either when the number of variables involved is large and their interrelationships complex or when interest is focused upon characteristics of samples. For example, the fertility rate given in [8] is an expected or mean value, but could vary among samples, not because any of the intermediate fertility variables were different, but simply because of random variation. A microsimulation model could be used to draw many samples of a given size so that the values and variations in the birth rate (or any other statistic, for that matter) could be studied. Anthropologists, concerned with the study of very small human groups, have made increasing use of large-scale microsimulation models in recent years (65,66).

For our current purpose, to illustrate how the levels and changes in a number of intermediate variables affect fertility, a macrosimulation model can be employed.

THE MACROSIMULATION MODEL

A recently developed macrosimulation model of the reproductive process which allows intermediate fertility variables to change with the age of a woman will be used here (67). After briefly reviewing the variables included, we will examine the effects on fertility of changes in these reproductive parameters that encompass the range of values speculated for or observed in populations in which fertility-limiting practices have not been adopted.

<u>Fecundability</u>. It is assumed that fecundability is the same for all women of a given age. It is zero until menarche (M) (all women reach menarche at the same age), then rises linearly until

age 20 simulating adolescent sterility, remains at a plateau (F) until age 35, and declines again linearly to zero at age 48. Age at menarche and the maximum, or plateau, are values specified by the researcher. Figure 3 shows fecundability when M = 12 and F = .20.

Intrauterine Mortality. The probability of spontaneous abortion (including still births) varies with age in a J-shaped distribution, the mean value of which, A, is an input parameter. When the mean (ages 20 to 40) is .24, the curve in Figure 4 is generated. The pregnancy plus postabortion non-susceptible period associated with a fetal loss follows a geometric distribution with a mean of 2.5 months.

Live Births. The duration of pregnancy is fixed at nine months. The postpartum amenorrhea period varies randomly according to a Pascal distribution (68) whose mean increases with the age of the mother at the birth of the child. The mean duration at age 30 is the input parameter, P, that determines the distribution of the means and, consequently, the length of the period until both ovulation and intercourse resume. In Figure 5, P is taken equal to 6 months.

Marriage. A distribution of age at marriage proposed by Coale (69) is incorporated into this model and requires the specification of three parameters: the proportion of a cohort that will ever marry (PEM), their mean age at marriage (AAM), and the earliest age at which marriages can occur (FAM). In Figure 6, 90% marry starting at age 15 and the average age at marriage is 25.

Sterility. The proportions nonsterile at each age were estimated from data of Henry (70) and are shown in Figure 7. The mean age at sterility is 41.5 for the 97% of the population who do not have primary sterility.

On the basis of these assumptions and the input parameters selected, the computer program (which is reproduced in Appendix A*) calculates age-and-order specific fertility rates and total fertility rates. The 5-year age specific fertility rates generated by the preceding assumptions are shown in the highest line, labeled "Standard", of Figure 8. They are representative of the age patterns of fertility observed in many late marrying populations with natural fertility.

---

* An extended version of this model and the user's manual are available upon request from J. Bongaarts, The Population Council, New York. In the extended version, allowances are made for heterogeneity and birth control practice.

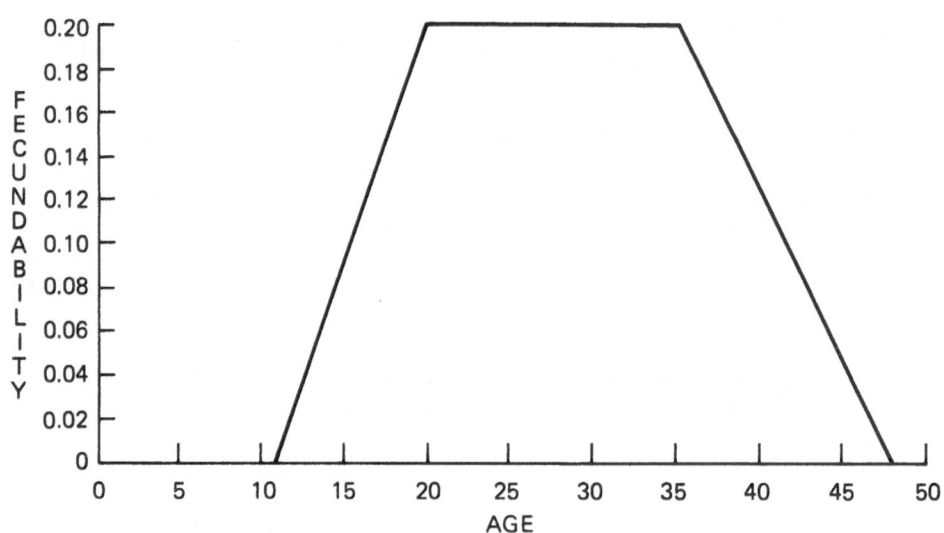

Figure 3. Model fecundability by age when menarche is M = 12
and the plateau level is F = .20.

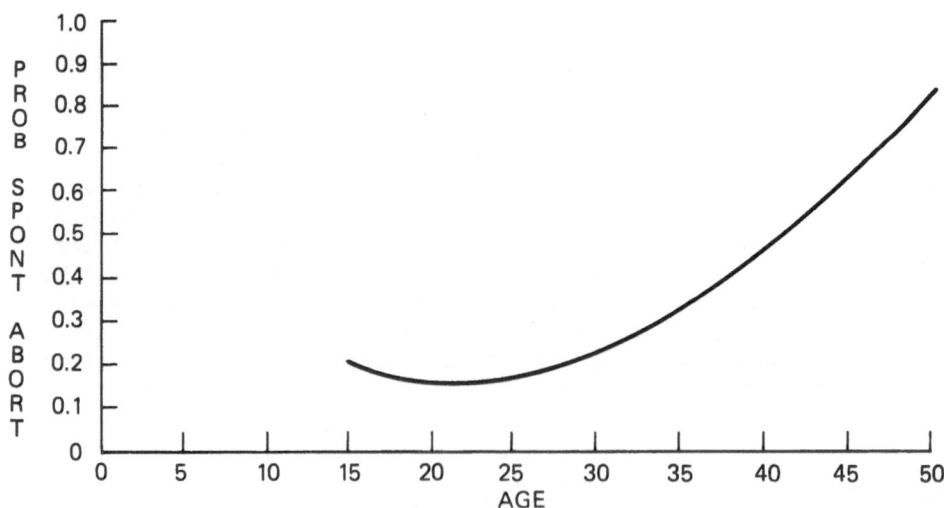

Figure 4. Model spontaneous abortion probabilities by age when
the mean probability is A = .24.

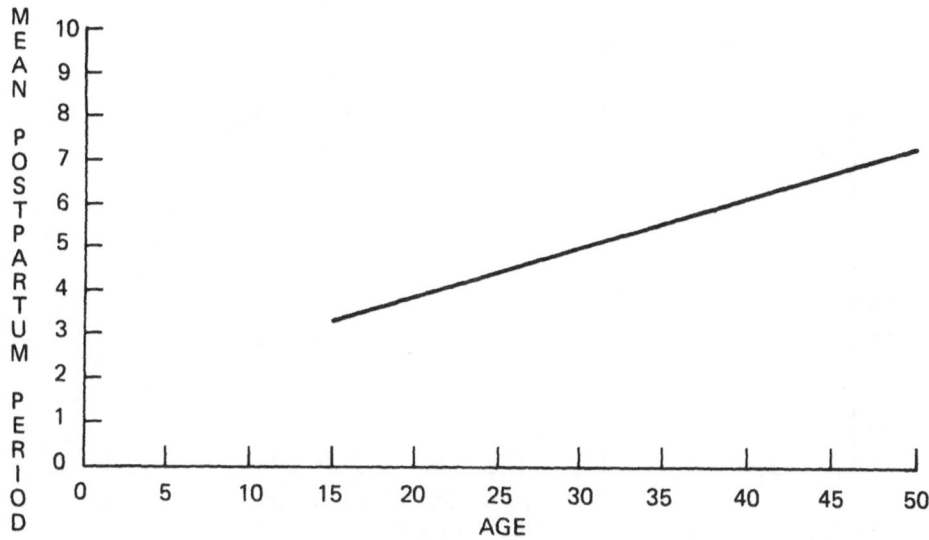

Figure 5. Model mean lengths of postpartum amenorrhea when the mean at age 30 is P = 6 months.

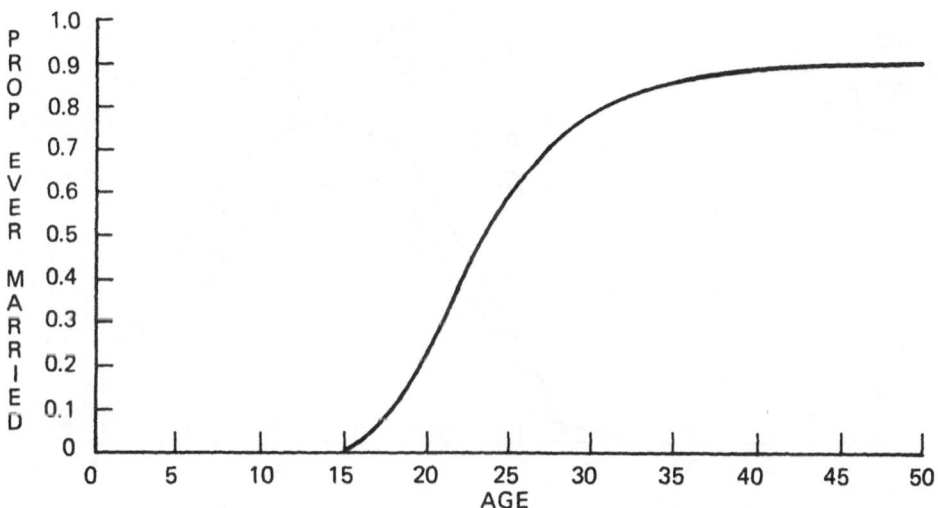

Figure 6. Model Proportions ever married by age: final proportion = PEM = .90, first age at marriage = FAM = 15 years, average age at marriage = AAM = 25 years.

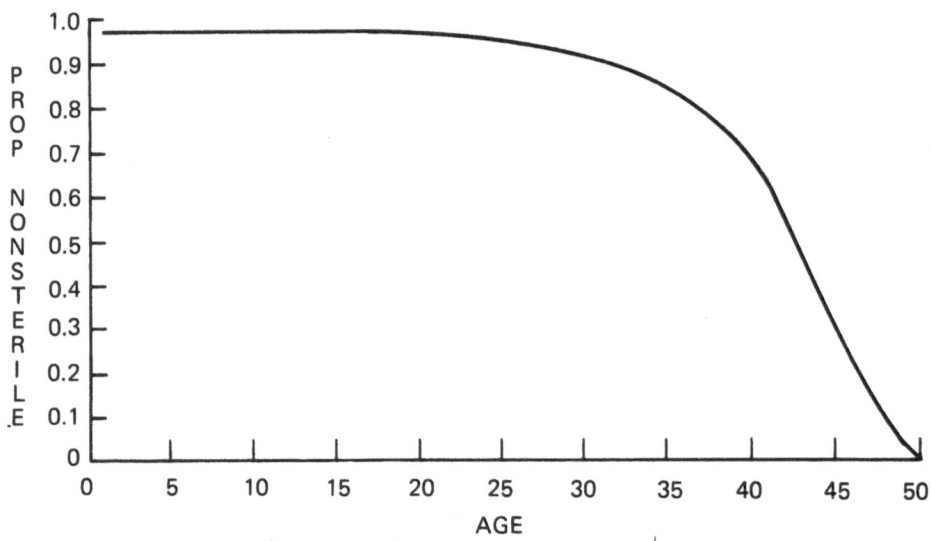

Figure 7. Model proportion of women non-sterile by age, estimated from data of Henry (1961).

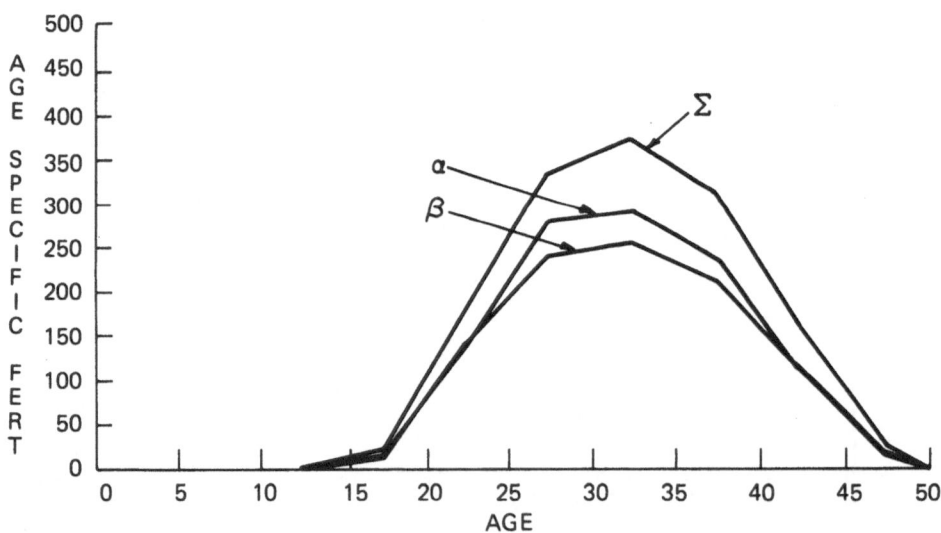

Figure 8. Model fertility rates by age in the standard population. (Σ), when fecundability is reduced to .10 (α), and when the mean length of postpartum amenorrhea is increased to 17 months (β).

The Standard Population

The population with parameters just described has - compared with typical natural fertility populations - early menarche, late marriage and sterility, short postpartum amenorrhea, and a moderate rate of spontaneous abortion. It will be taken as our standard.

With the following average standard parameter values

$$
\begin{aligned}
P &= 6 \text{ months} \\
F &= .2 \text{ per month} \\
A &= .24 \\
I &= 2.5 \text{ months} \\
G &= 9 \text{ months} \\
FAM &= 15 \text{ years} \\
AAM &= 25 \text{ years} \\
PEM &= .9
\end{aligned}
$$

the macro simulation model yields a total fertility rate of 6.97, a value which is close to the fertility levels found in contemporary developing countries where birth control is virtually absent.

Effects of Changes in Intermediate Fertility Variables

We will now examine the effect on fertility of plausible variations in each of the above parameters, using a macrosimulation model which allows age variation in the parameters.

Fecundability Change. Most reported estimates of fecundability lie between .1 and .3, so that we calculated results for these two extreme values. Table 1 shows that reducing fecundability from .2 to .1 lowered the TFR by 25%, from 6.97 to 5.23. Raising fecundability to .30 has less effect (13%) on the TFR. In either case the percentage change in fecundability is much larger than the percentage change in fertility.

The implications of even these simple results for designing studies of nutrition and fertility are significant. If there is any suspicion that nutrition affects fertility through the conception rate, a study which measures fecundability (or the 1-conception wait or ovulation interval) will be more likely to find an effect, if it exists, than one which measures only the birth interval, the fertility rates, or the total fertility rate.

Spontaneous Abortion Change. The non-obvious conclusion we reach from reducing spontaneous abortion rates from .24 to .20 or .15 in the model (shown in Table 1) is that fertility is not very sensitive to changes in fetal wastage. The lowest value, .15, induced only a 7.5% change in fertility. Spontaneous abortion rates have to rise to very high levels or drop to levels far below any valid values ever measured before any easily detectable or very significant change in fertility occurs. One direct consequence is the now well-known fact that many repeated abortions are necessary to prevent births in a society that resorts only to induced abortion, without contraception, to limit fertility (71). We also suspect that a study to determine the effect of nutrition on spontaneous abortion rates should not be given very high priority on any research agenda, first, because so little natural variation in abortion has been observed in populations drastically different nutritionally and, second, because only if the effect is very large could it be detected except in a very large scale study.

Postpartum Amenorrhea Changes. Wide variation in this parameter has been observed in actual populations (72) and the model confirms that plausible large differences in this variable can also strongly affect fertility. In Table 1, it is estimated that increasing the mean length of the period of postpartum amenorrhea to 10 months reduced fertility by about 14%, while when the mean was 17 months the reduction was 30%.

Such results make it easy to see the unfortunate consequences of another kind of nutritional change on fertility. Any population which has been practicing lengthy breastfeeding and which experiences trends away from the traditional practices toward the adoption of supposedly more "modern" bottle substitutes can expect fertility to rise abruptly unless other family limiting practices are adopted concurrently (73).

Although large differences in the postpartum period seem to exert large enough effects on fertility to be easily detectable in real life, rather small differences within a population attributable to differential nutrition may not be easy to find, even when they exist, unless large samples are studied. Table 2, discussed in the next section, furnishes further support for this comment.

Infant Mortality. There are two ways in which infant mortality can affect fertility: indirectly through a psychological effect of making more children desirable, and directly through a biological effect of shortening lactation and thus postpartum amenorrhea, especially in populations which normally continue breastfeeding well into childhood. Although provisions for infant mortality are not explicit in the model we are working with, we can introduce the direct effect implicitly by adjusting the distribution of the length of postpartum amenorrhea when the child survives to reflect the earlier resumption of ovulation that follows an infant death.

The following procedure was adopted: a recent analysis of patterns of timing of infant deaths within the first year of life

Table 1

Model Levels and Changes in the Total Fertility Rate
Resulting from Changes in the
Components of Birth Intervals

	Parameter Change (%)	TFR	Change in TFR	
			Absolute	Percent
Standard*		6.97		
Change in:				
Fecundability				
Standard (.20)				
Low (.10)	-50	5.23	-1.74	-24.5
High (.30)	+50	7.86	.89	12.8
Abortion				
Standard (.24)				
Low (.15)	-37.6	7.49	.52	7.5
Med. (.20)	-16.7	7.21	.24	3.4
Postpartum Amenorrhea				
Standard (6 mos.)				
Mod. (10 mos.)	66.7	6.01	-.96	-13.8
Long (17 mos.)	183.3	4.88	-2.09	-30.0

* In the standard,   menarche = 12 years
                     first age at marriage = 15 years
                     average age at sterility = 25 years
                     proportion ever marrying = .90
                     average age at sterility = 41.5 years

(74) led to a series of model life tables for that year. We selected two: one, with a fairly low infant mortality (IMR = 50/1000)
and a pattern of deaths rather late in the first year, was expected
to have only a very limited effect on the distribution of the postpartum period; the second, with higher infant mortality (140/1000)
concentrated early in life was chosen to produce greater change.
Mortality in the second and third year of life was taken from the
Coale-Demeny model life tables (75) corresponding to the infant
mortality rates above. The monthly death rates were assumed con-

Table 2

Model Fertility Changes Resulting From Infant Mortality
Induced Changes in Postpartum Amenorrhea

Postpartum Amenorrhea	Infant Mortality	Postpartum Amenorrhea			Change in TFR	
		Adjusted Change	%	TFR	Absolute*	Percent*
Short (6 mos.)	None	6.00		6.97		
	Low (50/1000)	5.84	-2.7	7.01	.04	0.6
	High (140/1000)	5.55	-7.5	7.10	.13	1.9
Moderate (10 mos.)	None	10.00		6.01		
	Low (50/1000)	9.65	-3.5	6.08	.07	1.2
	High (140/1000)	9.03	-9.7	6.21	.20	3.3
Long (17 mos.)	None	17.00		4.88		
	Low (50/1000)	15.59	-8.3	5.07	.19	3.9
	High (140/1000)	14.35	-15.6	5.25	.37	7.6

* All changes are calculated relative to the same original mean postpartum period and no mortality.
All other variables were assigned the standard values described in the text.

stant for each of the two years. New distributions of the postpartum period were found by assuming that the period lasted x months
if either the infant survived at least until that month and the
woman resumed ovulating spontaneously, or an infant death in month
x-1 had stopped lactation and triggered ovulation. The adjustments
for infant mortality were carried out for the distributions under
infant survival with postpartum anenorrhea means of 6, 10, and 17
months. The adjusted means are given in Table 2.

Under either regime of infant mortality, the longer the mean
postpartum period was originally, the greater the reduction induced
by increasing infant mortality. Increasing infant mortality thus
produced increases fertility quite independent of any psychological
or motivational change on the part of the parents; however, only
when the original mean postpartum period was quite long (17 months)
was the increase substantial (7.6%).

Sterility Change. The fertility determinants considered thus
far all influence reproduction through their effects on birth
intervals. The final three to be discussed, sterility, menarche,
and age at marriage, are the determinants of the length of the
effective reproductive period during which a woman is both fecund
and sexually active.

To test the effect of accelerated age at sterility on fertility,
we advanced the mean age to 39.5 and then 36.5 by translating the
curve in Figure 7 first two years and then five years to the left.
The results in Table 3 show that the TFR was reduced by 7% and
20%, respectively. These changes would have been even greater if
we had allowed fecundability in the model to be reduced as a woman
approached sterility rather than depending upon age alone until
sterility was reached abruptly. Therefore, if nutritional deprivation hastens sterility by several years, its effect on fertility
may be considerable.

Age at Marriage Change. In our standard population, marriage
always follows menarche by a number of years. Therefore, the
effective reproductive period could be lengthened by earlier
marriage. Keeping the first age at marriage at 15 and the proportion ever-married fixed at 0.90, we lowered the average age at
marriage to 23 and 20 years, increasing the TFR by 13% and 34%,
respectively, as shown in Table 3.

In most nations of Europe, fertility reduction was first
achieved by postponing marriage without reducing the birth rate
within marriage. The simple analysis presented here clearly illustrates just how effective this adaptive behavior is. Not so well
known is the converse: in a population with high birth rates and
very early marriage, it is almost impossible to achieve fertility

Table 3

Model Levels and Changes in the Total Fertility Rate
Resulting from Changes in the Length
of Effective Reproductive Life

	TFR	Change in TFR	
		Absolute	Percent
Standard	6.97		
Change in:			
Sterility			
Mod. (2 years early)	6.48	-.49	-7.0
Early (5 years early)	5.59	-1.38	-19.8
Marriage			
Mod. (AAM = 23 years)	7.85	.88	12.6
Early (AAM = 20 years)	9.31	2.34	33.6
Menarche			
Late marriage (AAM = 25)			
Menarche Early (12)	6.97		
Mod. (15)	6.96	-.01	-0.1
Late (18)	6.92	-.05	-0.7
Early marriage (AAM = 20)			
Menarche Early (12)	9.31		
Mod. (15)	9.28	-.03*	-0.3*
Late (18)	9.10	-.21*	-2.3*

* Compared to the TFR = 9.31 when marriage and menarche are early.

low enough to halt population growth unless either extremely
effective fertility limiting methods are almost universally used
or a considerable rise in age at marriage is introduced (76) concurrently with adoption of only somewhat less effective methods of
control within marriage.

  Menarche Change. The effect of changing age at menarche
depends to a great extent upon the marriage pattern it is associated with. If marriage before age 20 is rare, then altering age
at menarche will have only a very small effect on the length of
the effective reproductive period and fertility will be rather

insensitive to nutritionally induced differences in the timing of puberty. This contention is borne out by the values, given in Table 3, for the TFR when age at menarche was raised from 12 to 15 and 18 in the late marriage case. Reductions of only 0.1% and 0.7% respectively were found. When the early age at marriage distribution was employed, increasing menarche to 15 and 18 reduced the TFR by 0.3% and 2.3% respectively.

We may be underestimating the effect of late menarche slightly. because we allow fecundability to reach its maximum at age 20 in all cases, so that the later menarche occurs, the faster fecundability rises. If the model allowed fecundability to rise gradually for a certain number of years following menarche, slightly larger changes in the TFR would have been calculated. However, it seems clear that age at marriage affects fertility far more than age at menarche does, except under very unusual circumstances such as consummation of marriage regularly preceding menarche.

Combinations of Changes. Appendix B contains tables showing the TFR for all combinations of levels of the parameters specified in this paper. These tables are included for the convenience of the reader who is particularly concerned with the interaction of several simultaneous changes in the parameters, whether or not they are causally linked.

Age Patterns of Fertility. Figures 8 and 9 exemplify the kinds of modifications in fertility by age produced by altering birth interval determinants (Figure 8) and reproductive period determinants (Figure 9), respectively. The former act on the level of fertility without altering the typical shape of the configuration. By contrast, striking differences in the age pattern are introduced by changing either the initiation or termination of the reproductive period.

Table 4 summarizes the effects of all the parameters we have examined on age-specific fertility. Bearing in mind that these results are somewhat dependent upon our assumptions regarding age patterns in the fertility determinants, we can see that fecundability change affects the early and late reproductive years the most percentage-wise but, because these years have the lowest fertility rates, the greatest absolute decline is in the middle years associated with most rapid childbearing. Spontaneous abortion reduces fertility at the older ages by the largest percentage, but also causes the greatest absolute change toward the end of the reproductive years. Since we allowed the length of the postpartum nonsusceptible period to increase with age, it is not surprising that the greatest effects of changes are seen at the older ages percentage-wise, although the middle years are changed most in absolute terms. Sterility change, almost by definition, affects

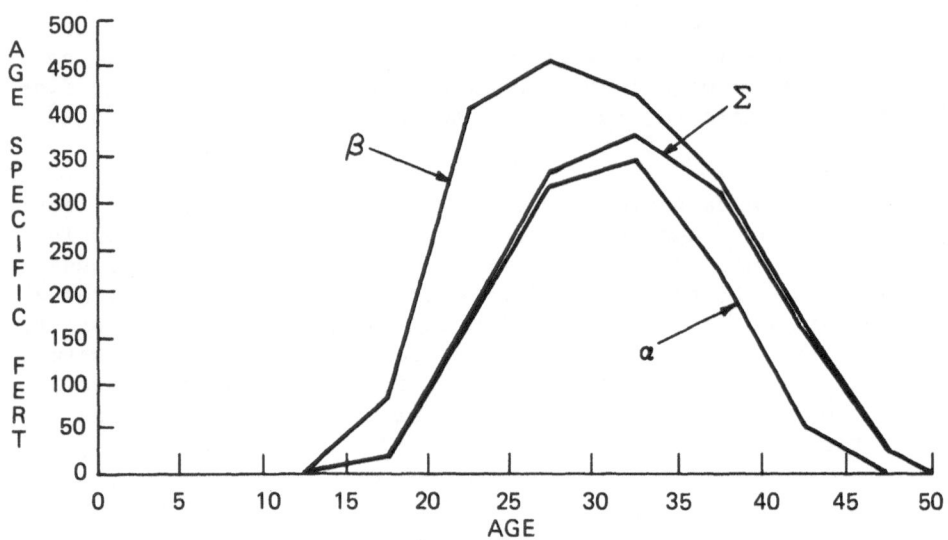

Figure 9. Model fertility rates by age in the standard population
(Σ) when sterility occurs 5 years early (α), and when marriage
occurs 5 years early (β).

the upper end of the age scale, while both marriage and menarche
change are most noticeable at the youngest ages. In fact, menarche
change had no effect beyond age 20.

CONCLUSIONS

Based on the application of the model, the set of intermediate
fertility variables may tentatively be divided into two types
according to the likelihood of their having a sizeable effect on
fertility:

Unlikely   Plausible

spontaneous abortion rates   fecundability
menarche   postpartum period
                                            sterility
                                            marriage

If nutrition has a demographically important effect on fertility, it is most likely to do so through at least one of the first three variables in the second column. We will now briefly consider the mechanisms whereby nutrition or other factors might alter these components of fertility.

Fecundity is a rather catch-all term demographers have invented to refer to the complex of biological and social factors which influence whether or not conception occurs in any given month. Assuming a woman is menstruating, these factors include the frequency of anovulatory cycles in the female and the production of sperm in the male as purely biological factors. Coital frequency can be considered both biologically determined by libido and socially determined through norms with regard to frequency of intercourse. A third variable, biological in nature, is the rate with which a recognizable conception follows intercourse close to the time of ovulation. Fecundability has often been interpreted as reflecting the biological capacity to conceive rather than a combination of capacity and opportunity, although we know from other work on models that each of the factors may alter fecundability considerably (77,78,79). A study which measures only overall fecundability, even if it finds some evidence of variation with nutrition, will not be able to pinpoint the mechanisms by which the effect was produced. Although coital frequency seems to be difficult to measure, its measurement becomes necessary if we want to explain fecundability variation.

As is summarized in Figure 2, there are a number of possible links between the nutrition of mother or child and postpartum amenorrhea: a) a direct physiological effect on the woman's ability to resume menstruation and ovulation; b) a modification in the quantity and quality of breastmilk resulting in variation in lactation behavior and thus in postpartum amenorrhea; c) an effect of supplementation of the infant on the intensity and duration of lactation, and d) a potential change in infant mortality related to the degree of malnutrition among infants. If a detailed understanding is desired of the effect of nutrition on postpartum amenorrhea, then all these factors require measurements, in particular the extent of breastfeeding and the supplementation of the infant.

The third potentially important intermediate fertility variable through which nutrition could modify fertility is sterility. As already mentioned, sterility is very difficult to measure accurately and comparative statistics are lacking. Perhaps the best approach would be to focus on obtaining more detailed information about the timing and determinants of menopause in different societies. At the moment data on menopause, particularly in the developing world, are still scarce.

Table 4

Model Levels and Changes in Age-Specific Fertility Rates

Age	15-19	20-24	25-29	30-34	35-39	40-44	45-49	TFR
Standard	18.5	180.8	333.4	371.6	312.4	155.7	21.3	6.97
Change in:								
Fecundability								
Low (.10)	12.6	136.5	257.0	287.1	233.8	105.8	12.7	5.23
Percent change	(-31.6)	(-24.5)	(-22.9)	(-22.7)	(-25.1)	(-32.1)	(-40.5)	
High (.30)	21.7	202.6	370.1	412.0	352.3	185.6	27.7	7.86
Percent change	(17.6)	(12.1)	(11.0)	(10.9)	(12.8)	(19.1)	(30.2)	
Abortion								
Low (.15)	19.3	186.9	345.6	390.7	340.2	185.0	30.2	7.49
Percent change	(4.5)	(3.4)	(3.6)	(5.1)	(8.9)	(18.8)	(41.9)	
Mod. (20)	18.8	183.6	339.0	380.4	325.4	169.6	25.6	7.21
Percent change	(1.9)	(1.5)	(1.7)	(2.4)	(4.2)	(8.9)	(20.2)	
Postpartum Amenorrhea								
Mod. (10.0)	17.6	161.5	287.6	315.4	264.6	135.2	19.3	6.01
Percent change	(-5.0)	(-10.7)	(-13.7)	(-15.1)	(-15.3)	(-13.1)	(-9.2)	
Long (17.0)	16.6	139.0	234.5	250.4	209.1	109.7	16.5	4.88
Percent change	(-10.3)	(-23.1)	(-29.7)	(-32.6)	(-33.1)	(-29.5)	(-22.4)	

Table 4, Continued

Age	15-19	20-24	-25-29	30-34	35-39	40-44	45-49	TFR
Change in:								
Sterility								
Mod. (2 years early)	18.5	177.9	327.7	360.8	287.4	113.8	9.46	6.48
Percent change	(0)	(-1.6)	(-1.6)	(-1.7)	(-8.0)	(-26.9)	(-55.5)	
Early (5 yrs.early)	18.3	172.7	317.7	345.1	220.1	52.0	0.3	5.59
Percent change	(-1.3)	(-4.5)	(-4.7)	(-7.1)	(-29.6)	(-66.6)	(-98.4)	
Marriage								
Mod. (AAM=23)	28.8	253.1	390.7	397.7	321.5	157.7	21.4	7.85
Percent change	(55.7)	(40.0)	(17.2)	(7.0)	(2.9)	(1.3)	(0.7)	
Early (AAM=20)	83.2	402.1	454.4	416.6	326.3	158.5	21.4	9.31
Percent change	(349.7)	(122.4)	(36.3)	(12.1)	(4.4)	(1.8)	(0.7)	
Menarche								
Late marriage (AAM=25)								
Menarche								
Mod. (15)	16.9	180.8	333.4	371.6	312.4	155.7	21.3	6.96
Percent change	(-8.7)	(0)	(0)	(0)	(0)	(0)	(0)	
Late (18)	9.6	180.5	333.4	371.6	312.4	155.7	21.3	6.92
Percent change	(-48.2)	(-0.1)	(0)	(0)	(0)	(0)	(0)	

Table 4, Continued

Age	15-19	20-24	25-29	30-34	35-39	40-44	45-49	TFR
Early marriage (AAM = 20)								
Menarche								
Early (12)	83.2	402.1	454.4	416.6	326.3	158.5	21.4	9.31
Mod. (15)	75.9	401.9	454.4	416.6	326.3	158.5	21.4	9.28
Percent change*	(-8.7)	(-0.0)	(0)	(0)	(0)	(0)	(0)	
Late (18)	41.3	401.4	454.4	416.6	326.3	158.5	21.4	9.10
Percent change*	(-50.4)	(-0.2)	(0)	(0)	(0)	(0)	(0)	

* Compared to fertility when marriage and menarche are early.

Further practical application of these models can be made in the statistical design of studies of nutrition-fertility relationships or, more generally, of intermediate variable-fertility relationships. In a somewhat different context, models are already being used in the design of family planning programs. For example, models are now available to estimate the number of acceptors of contraceptives the program must enroll in order to produce the reduction in crude birth rates which the policy-makers are aiming to achieve (79,80).

In the discussion thus far, we concentrated on applying models to identify those variables which, over their range of known or speculated variation in human populations, can affect fertility significantly. However, in any specific study, the question we want to address is: Do nutritional differences cause <u>enough difference</u> in fertility or in one of the intermediate fertility variables to consider nutrition an important determinant of fertility rates? The models can serve as a tool for defining what is enough difference leading to the design of studies capable of detecting this critical level of variation. Consider, for specificity, a study to examine the effect of nutritional differences in postpartum amenorrhea. Suppose we decide that a change in fertility must be at least 10% for us to conclude that the nutritional factor, working through postpartum amenorrhea, is really important. From models we can estimate the minimum difference in postpartum amenorrhea in poorly versus well-nourished women necessary to produce fertility change of at least that magnitude. Standard statistical techniques can then be applied to design studies capable of detecting differences in the length of postpartum amenorrhea at least equal to this minimum difference.

Theoretical developments of reproductive models have progressed to the point where validation and wider application are far more imperative than development of successively more sophisticated extensions. One of the objectives of this paper is to stimulate work in this direction.

ACKNOWLEDGEMENTS

We would like to thank Carolyn Lichtenstein for preparing the data for this paper and James Trussell for reading an earlier version and making many pertinent comments.

APPENDIX A

COMPUTER PROGRAM FOR THE AGE-CHANGE MODEL

The program requires one card of input data, the users' specification of seven variables:

Cols.	Example	Variable
1-5	0.20	F = fecundability (plateau level)
6-10	0.24	A = probability of spontaneous abortion (average over ages 20-40)
11-15	6.0	P = mean duration at age 30 of postpartum amenorrhea
16-20	¢¢¢12	M = age at menarche (integer value only)
21-24	¢¢¢15	FAM = first age at marriage (integer value only)
26-30	20.00	AAM = average age at marriage
31-35	0.90	PEM = proportion ever married

¢ indicates a blank space

Note that the last digits of M and FAM must be punched in columns 20 and 25 respectively. For all other input parameters, if no decimal point is punched, it is assumed to lie between the third and fourth column of the field.

In order to change the sterility distribution, DATA cards in the program labeled STER must be changed. STER is a vector of 50 numbers in which the number in position I is the proportion non-sterile at age I.

The program is reproduced in the next three pages and the output corresponding to the input data above is reproduced on the following page. Note that in the program, the variables F,A,P, and M have slightly longer names: FECU, ABOR, PPAM, and MEN.

Appendix A, Continued

```
C     BASIC MODEL
      INTEGER AGE,T,FAM,ORDER
      DIMENSION BI(600),BO(610),AOSBR(20,50),ASBR(50)
      DIMENSION STER(50),FEC(50),ABO(50),PPA(50),FMAR(50),STERIL(50)
      DATA ABO/50*0./,PPA/50*0/,FMAR/50*0./,STERIL/50*0./
      DATA STER/22*.97,.96,.95,.94,.93,.92,.91,
     1 .91,.90,.89,.88,.87,.85,.84,.82,.80,.77,
     2 .74,.69,.62,.55,.46,.38,.30,.22,.15,.09,.04,.0/
C
C
C          MODEL OF REPRODUCTION PROPOSED BY J. BONGAARTS
C
C     DEFINITION OF INPUT VARIABLES:
C     MEN   = AGE AT MENARCHE
C     FECU  = PLATEAU LEVEL OF FECUNDABILITY
C     ABOR  = AVERAGE RATE OF SPONTANEOUS ABORTION
C     PPAM  = MEAN DURATION AT AGE 30 OF POSTPARTUM AMENORRHEA
C     FAM   = FIRST AGE AT MARRIAGE
C     AAM   = MEAN AGE AT MARRIAGE
C     PEM   = PROPORTION EVER MARRIED

    1 READ (5,10,END=99) FECU,ABOR,PPAM,MEN,FAM,AAM,PEM
      TFR=0.
      WRITE (6,5) FECU,MEN,ABOR,AAM,PPAM,PEM,FAM
      CUM=0.
      DO 42 LL=1,610
      BO(LL)=0.
   42 BI (LL)=0.
      DO 41 LM=1,50
      ASBR(LM)=0.
      FEC(LM)=0.
      DO 41 LN=1,20
      AOSBR(LN,LM)=0.
   41 CONTINUE
C     CALCULATE AGE SPECIFIC INTERMEDIATE FERTILITY VARIABLES
      DO 100 AGE=20,34
  100 FEC(AGE)=FECU
      DO 150 AGE=MEN,19
  150 FEC(AGE)=FECU*(AGE-MEN+.5)/(20. - MEN)
      DO 175 AGE=35,48
  175 FEC(AGE)=FECU*(48.5-AGE)/14.0
      DO 200 AGE=10,50
      STERIL(AGE)=STER(AGE)*.75+STER(AGE-1)*.25
      ABO(AGE)=(0.805+0.004*(AGE-21.4)**2)*0.84*ABOR
```

```
200   PPA(AGE)=(1.0+(AGE-29.5)*0.0230)*PPAM
      P=(AAM-FAM)/11.36
      DO 250 AGE=FAM,50
      X=AGE-FAM+0.5-6.06*P
250   FMAR(AGE)=(.19465/P)*EXP((-.174/P)*X-EXP((-.2881/P)*X))*PEM
C     CALCULATE AGE-ORDER SPECIFIC BIRTHS RATES
      S=1.0
      DO 400 ORDER=1,20
      W11=0
      W12=0
      W 2=0
      W 3=0
      DO 300 AGE=FAM,49
      ENTER=S*FMAR(AGE)/12.*1000.
      DO 300 MONTH=1,12
      T=12*AGE+MONTH-1
      R11=W11*2.0/PPA(AGE)
      R12=W12*2./PPA(AGE)
       R2=W2*FEC(AGE)
       R3=W3*0.4
      WN11=W11-R11+BI(T)
      WN12=W12-R12+R11
      WN2=W2-R2+R3+R12+ENTER
      WN3=W3-R3+R2*ABO(AGE)
      BO(T+9)=R2*(1.0-ABO(AGE))
      AOSBR(ORDER,AGE)=AOSBR(ORDER,AGE)+BO(T)*STERIL(AGE)
      W11=WN11
      W12=WN12
      W2=WN2
      W3=WN3
300   BI(T)=BO(T)
400   S=0.0
C     PRINT OUT RESULTS
      WRITE (6,30)
      DO 500 AGE=FAM,50
      DO470 ORDER=1,20
470   ASBR(AGE)=ASBR(AGE)+AOSBR(ORDER,AGE)
      TFR=TFR+ASBR(AGE)/1000.
      CUM=CUM+FMAR(AGE)*1000.
500   WRITE(6,20)AGE,(AOSBR(I,AGE),I=1,10),
     1 ASBR(AGE),CUM,FEC(AGE),ABO(AGE),PPA(AGE)
      WRITE (6,40) TFR
      GO TO 1
5     FORMAT(1H1,'FECUNDABILITY (20-35)',F8.2,
     1 14X,'AGE AT MENARCHE',I5,/,
     2 'SP ABORTION RISK (20-40)',F5.2,9X,
     3 'MEAN AGE F MARRIAGE',F5.2,/,
     4 'POSTPARTUM INFEC (20-40)',F5.2,9X,
     5 'PROP EVER MARRYING ',F5.2/29X, 'FIRST AGE AT MARRIAGE',I5//)
```

```
10    FORMAT(3F5.2,2I5,2F5.2)
20    FORMAT(I4,10F4.0,F6.1,F14.1,F10.2,3F6.2)
30    FORMAT(11X,'AGE-SPECIFIC BIRTH RATES ',
   1       24X, 'EVER',5X,'FECUN SPONT POST ',
   2       /, ' AGE 1  2  3  4  5  6  7  8  9  10  ALL ',
   3       9X, 'MARR ',5X,' DAB ABORT PARTUM ',/)
40    FORMAT(/,' TOTAL FERTILITY RATE= ',F6.2)
   99 STOP
      END
```

Appendix A, Continued

Fecundability (20-35)	0.20	Postpartum Infection (20-40)	6.00	Mean Age of Marriage	25.00
SP Abortion Risk (20-40)	0.24	Age at Menarche	12	Prop Ever Marrying	0.90
		First Age at Marriage	15		

Age	\multicolumn{10}{c}{Age-Specific Birth Rates}	All	Ever Marr	Fecun Dab	Spont Abort	Post Partum
	1	2	3	4	5	6	7	8	9	10					
15	0.	0.	0.	0.	0.	0.	0.	0.	0.	0.	0.1	4.0	0.09	0.20	4.00
16	2.	0.	0.	0.	0.	0.	0.	0.	0.	0.	2.0	16.7	0.11	0.19	4.14
17	9.	1.	0.	0.	0.	0.	0.	0.	0.	0.	9.2	44.5	0.14	0.18	4.27
18	22.	4.	0.	0.	0.	0.	0.	0.	0.	0.	26.0	90.7	0.16	0.17	4.41
19	40.	13.	2.	0.	0.	0.	0.	0.	0.	0.	55.1	153.8	0.19	0.17	4.55
20	58.	29.	7.	1.	0.	0.	0.	0.	0.	0.	94.4	228.5	0.20	0.16	4.69
21	70.	47.	18.	3.	0.	0.	0.	0.	0.	0.	138.5	308.3	0.20	0.16	4.83
22	76.	61.	34.	11.	1.	0.	0.	0.	0.	0.	183.6	387.6	0.20	0.16	4.97
23	76.	70.	50.	23.	6.	1.	0.	0.	0.	0.	225.3	462.3	0.20	0.16	5.10
24	72.	73.	62.	38.	14.	3.	0.	0.	0.	0.	262.2	529.9	0.20	0.17	5.24
25	65.	72.	68.	52.	27.	8.	1.	0.	0.	0.	293.3	589.5	0.20	0.17	5.38
26	57.	67.	70.	61.	40.	17.	4.	0.	0.	0.	318.5	641.0	0.20	0.18	5.52
27	49.	61.	68.	66.	52.	29.	10.	2.	0.	0.	338.0	684.9	0.20	0.19	5.65
28	42.	53.	63.	67.	60.	42.	20.	6.	1.	0.	352.3	721.9	0.20	0.20	5.79
29	35.	46.	57.	65.	64.	52.	31.	12.	3.	0.	365.1	752.8	0.20	0.21	5.93

Appendix A, Continued

Age	Age-Specific Birth Rates										All	Ever Marr	Fecun Dab	Spont Abort	Post Partum
	1	2	3	4	5	6	7	8	9	10					
30	29.	39.	50.	60.	64.	58.	42.	22.	7.	1.	372.1	778.5	0.20	0.22	6.07
31	24.	33.	43.	54.	61.	61.	50.	32.	14.	3.	374.7	799.9	0.20	0.24	6.21
32	20.	27.	37.	47.	56.	60.	55.	41.	22.	8.	374.6	817.5	0.20	0.25	6.34
33	16.	23.	31.	40.	50.	57.	57.	48.	31.	14.	372.1	832.1	0.20	0.27	6.48
34	13.	19.	25.	34.	43.	52.	56.	51.	39.	22.	364.4	844.0	0.20	0.29	6.62
35	11.	15.	21.	28.	37.	46.	52.	52.	44.	29.	354.6	853.9	0.19	0.31	6.76
36	8.	12.	17.	23.	31.	39.	46.	50.	46.	35.	337.3	862.0	0.18	0.33	6.90
37	7.	10.	13.	19.	25.	33.	40.	45.	45.	38.	315.8	868.7	0.16	0.36	7.03
38	5.	7.	11.	15.	20.	27.	34.	39.	42.	38.	290.6	874.2	0.15	0.38	7.17
39	4.	6.	8.	12.	16.	21.	28.	33.	37.	36.	263.6	878.6	0.14	0.41	7.31
40	3.	4.	6.	9.	12.	17.	22.	27.	31.	32.	231.1	882.3	0.12	0.44	7.45
41	2.	3.	5.	7.	9.	12.	17.	21.	25.	27.	192.9	885.4	0.11	0.47	7.59
42	2.	2.	3.	5.	7.	9.	12.	16.	19.	21.	155.3	887.9	0.09	0.50	7.72
43	1.	2.	2.	3.	4.	6.	8.	11.	13.	15.	116.6	889.9	0.08	0.54	7.86
44	1.	1.	1.	2.	3.	4.	5.	7.	9.	11.	82.8	891.6	0.06	0.57	8.00
45	0.	1.	1.	1.	2.	2.	3.	4.	6.	7.	54.3	893.0	0.05	0.61	8.14
46	0.	0.	0.	1.	1.	1.	2.	2.	3.	4.	31.3	894.1	0.04	0.65	8.28
47	0.	0.	0.	0.	0.	1.	1.	1.	1.	2.	15.0	895.0	0.02	0.69	8.41
48	0.	0.	0.	0.	0.	0.	0.	0.	0.	1.	5.1	895.8	0.01	0.73	8.55
49	0.	0.	0.	0.	0.	0.	0.	0.	0.	0.	0.7	896.4	0.0	0.78	8.69
50	0.	0.	0.	0.	0.	0.	0.	0.	0.	0.	0.0	896.9	0.0	0.82	8.83

Total Fertility Rate = 6.97.

APPENDIX B

TOTAL FERTILITY RATES FOR ALL POSSIBLE COMBINATIONS OF
SELECTED VALUES OF PARAMETERS OF THE REPRODUCTIVE PROCESS

Table B1

Model Levels in the Total Fertility Rate*
When Sterility is Late (Standard)

a. Fecundability is Standard (.20)

| Abortion | Marriage | Menarche | Postpartum Amenorrhea | | |
			Stand. 6 Mos.	Mod. 10 Mos.	Long 17 Mos.
Standard(.24)	Early (20)	Stand. (12)	9.31	8.02	6.49
		Mod. (15)	9.28	7.99	6.47
		Late (18)	9.10	7.83	6.34
	Mod. (23)	Stand.	7.87	6.78	5.50
		Mod.	7.86	6.77	5.49
		Late	7.79	6.71	5.44
	Stand.(25)	Stand.	6.97	6.01	4.88
		Mod.	6.96	6.00	4.87
		Late	6.92	5.97	4.85
Mod. (.20)	Early	Stand.	9.60	8.23	6.64
		Mod.	9.56	8.20	6.61
		Late	9.38	8.05	6.49
	Mod.	Stand.	8.13	6.98	5.63
		Mod.	8.12	6.96	5.62
		Late	8.05	6.91	5.58
	Stand.	Stand.	7.21	6.19	5.01
		Mod.	7.20	6.19	5.00
		Late	7.17	6.15	4.97
Low (.15)	Early	Stand.	9.92	8.48	6.80
		Mod.	9.88	8.45	6.78
		Late	9.70	8.29	6.65
	Mod.	Stand.	8.43	7.20	5.78
		Mod.	8.41	7.19	5.77
		Late	8.35	7.13	5.72
	Stand.	Stand.	7.49	6.40	5.15
		Mod.	7.48	6.39	5.14
		Late	7.44	6.36	5.11

* Average age at marriage: Early (20), Mod. (23), Standard (25);
  Age at menarche: Standard (12), Mod. (15), Late (18).

Table B1, continued

b. Fecundability is Low (.10)

Abortion	Marriage	Menarche	Postpartum Amenorrhea Stand. 6 Mos.	Mod. 10 Mos.	Long 17 Mos.
Standard(.24)	Early (20)	Stand. (12)	7.03	6.26	5.28
		Mod. (15)	6.99	6.23	5.25
		Late (18)	6.86	6.10	5.15
	Mod. (23)	Stand.	5.92	5.27	4.45
		Mod.	5.91	5.26	4.45
		Late	5.86	5.22	4.41
	Stand.(25)	Stand.	5.23	4.66	3.94
		Mod.	5.22	4.65	3.94
		Late	5.19	4.63	3.91
Mod. (20)	Early	Stand.	7.28	6.46	5.43
		Mod.	7.25	6.43	5.40
		Late	7.11	6.31	5.30
	Mod.	Stand.	6.15	5.46	4.59
		Mod.	6.14	5.45	4.58
		Late	6.09	5.41	4.54
	Stand.	Stand.	5.44	4.84	4.07
		Mod.	5.44	4.83	4.07
		Late	5.41	4.80	4.04
Low (.15)	Early	Stand.	7.59	6.70	5.60
		Mod.	7.55	6.67	5.58
		Late	7.41	6.55	5.47
	Mod.	Stand.	6.43	5.68	4.75
		Mod.	6.42	5.67	4.74
		Late	6.36	5.62	4.70
	Stand.	Stand.	5.70	5.04	4.22
		Mod.	5.69	5.03	4.22
		Late	5.66	5.01	4.19

Table B1, continued

c. Fecundability is High (.30)

| Abortion | Marriage | Menarche | Postpartum Amenorrhea | | |
			Stand. 6 Mos.	Mod. 10 Mos.	Long 17 Mos.
Standard(.24)	Early (20)	Stand. (12)	10.47	8.87	7.05
		Mod. (15)	10.43	8.84	7.03
		Late (18)	10.24	8.68	6.89
	Mod. (23)	Stand.	8.86	7.51	5.98
		Mod.	8.85	7.50	5.97
		Late	8.78	7.44	5.92
	Stand.(25)	Stand.	7.86	6.67	5.31
		Mod.	7.85	6.66	5.31
		Late	7.81	6.62	5.28
Mod. (.20)	Early	Stand.	10.76	9.08	7.19
		Mod.	10.72	9.05	7.17
		Late	10.52	8.89	7.03
	Mod.	Stand.	9.13	7.70	6.10
		Mod.	9.11	7.69	6.10
		Late	9.04	7.63	6.05
	Stand.	Stand.	8.11	6.85	5.43
		Mod.	8.10	6.84	5.43
		Late	8.06	6.81	5.40
Low (.15)	Early	Stand.	11.08	9.32	7.34
		Mod.	11.04	9.29	7.32
		Late	10.85	9.12	7.18
	Mod.	Stand.	9.42	7.92	6.24
		Mod.	9.41	7.91	6.24
		Late	9.34	7.85	6.19
	Stand.	Stand.	8.39	7.05	5.56
		Mod.	8.38	7.05	5.56
		Late	8.34	7.01	5.53

Table B2

Model Levels in the Total Fertility Rate When
Sterility is 2 Years Earlier than Standard

a. Fecundability is Standard (.20)

| Abortion | Marriage | Menarche | Postpartum Amenorrhea | | |
			Stand. 6 Mos.	Mod. 10 Mos.	Long 17 Mos.
Standard(.24)	Early (20)	Stand. (12)	8.78	7.56	6.12
		Mod. (15)	8.74	7.53	6.10
		Late (18)	8.57	7.38	5.97
	Mod. (23)	Stand.	7.36	6.34	5.14
		Mod.	7.35	6.33	5.13
		Late	7.28	6.27	5.08
	Stand. (25)	Stand.	6.48	5.58	4.53
		Mod.	6.47	5.57	4.53
		Late	6.43	5.54	4.50
Mod.(.20)	Early	Stand.	9.02	7.74	6.25
		Mod.	8.99	7.71	6.22
		Late	8.81	7.55	6.09
	Mod.	Stand.	7.58	6.50	5.25
		Mod.	7.56	6.49	5.24
		Late	7.50	6.43	5.19
	Stand.	Stand.	6.68	5.74	4.64
		Mod.	6.67	5.73	4.63
		Late	6.63	5.69	4.60
Low (.15)	Early	Stand.	9.30	7.95	6.38
		Mod.	9.27	7.92	6.36
		Late	9.08	7.76	6.23
	Mod.	Stand.	7.83	6.69	5.37
		Mod.	7.82	6.68	5.36
		Late	7.75	6.62	5.32
	Stand.	Stand.	6.92	5.91	4.75
		Mod.	6.91	5.90	4.75
		Late	6.87	5.87	4.72

Table B2, Continued

b. Fecundability is Low (.10)

Abortion	Marriage	Menarche	Postpartum Amenorrhea		
			Stand. 6 Mos.	Mod. 10 Mos.	Long 17 Mos.
Standard(.24)	Early (20)	Stand. (12)	6.65	5.92	4.99
		Mod. (15)	6.62	5.89	4.97
		Late (18)	6.48	5.77	4.86
	Mod. (23)	Stand.	5.56	4.95	4.18
		Mod.	5.55	4.94	4.17
		Late	5.50	4.90	4.13
	Stand. (25)	Stand.	4.88	4.35	3.68
		Mod.	4.88	4.35	3.68
		Late	4.85	4.32	3.65
Mod. (.20)	Early	Stand.	6.88	6.10	5.12
		Mod.	6.84	6.07	5.10
		Late	6.70	5.95	4.99
	Mod.	Stand.	5.76	5.11	4.30
		Mod.	5.75	5.10	4.29
		Late	5.70	5.06	4.25
	Stand.	Stand.	5.07	4.50	3.79
		Mod.	5.06	4.50	3.79
		Late	5.03	4.47	3.76
Low (.15)	Early	Stand.	7.14	6.31	5.27
		Mod.	7.11	6.28	5.25
		Late	6.96	6.15	5.14
	Mod.	Stand.	6.00	5.30	4.44
		Mod.	5.99	5.29	4.43
		Late	5.94	5.25	4.39
	Stand.	Stand.	5.29	4.68	3.92
		Mod.	5.28	4.67	3.91
		Late	5.25	4.64	3.89

Table B2, Continued

c. Fecundability is High (.30)

| Abortion | Marriage | Menarche | Postpartum Amenorrhea | | |
			Stand. 6 Mos.	Mod. 10 Mos.	Long 17 Mos.
Standard(.24)	Early (20)	Stand. (12)	9.85	8.34	6.63
		Mod. (15)	9.81	8.31	6.61
		Late (18)	9.62	8.15	6.48
	Mod. (23)	Stand.	8.26	7.00	5.57
		Mod.	8.25	6.99	5.56
		Late	8.18	6.93	5.51
	Stand.(.25)	Stand.	7.28	6.17	4.92
		Mod.	7.28	6.17	4.92
		Late	7.23	6.13	4.89
Mod. (.20)	Early	Stand.	10.09	8.52	6.75
		Mod.	10.05	8.49	6.72
		Late	9.86	8.32	6.59
	Mod.	Stand.	8.48	7.16	5.67
		Mod.	8.47	7.15	5.67
		Late	8.40	7.09	5.62
	Stand.	Stand.	7.49	6.32	5.02
		Mod.	7.48	6.32	5.01
		Late	7.44	6.28	4.98
Low (.15)	Early	Stand.	10.36	8.72	6.87
		Mod.	10.33	8.69	6.85
		Late	10.13	8.52	6.71
	Mod.	Stand.	8.73	7.34	5.79
		Mod.	8.72	7.33	5.78
		Late	8.65	7.27	5.73
	Stand.	Stand.	7.72	6.49	5.13
		Mod.	7.71	6.48	5.12
		Late	7.67	6.45	5.09

Table B3

Model Levels in the Total Fertility Rate When
Sterility is 5 Years Earlier than Standard

a. Fecundability is Standard (.20)

Abortion	Marriage	Menarche	Postpartum Amenorrhea		
			Stand. 6 Mos.	Mod. 10 Mos.	Long 17 Mos.
Standard(.24)	Early (20)	Stand. (12)	7.81	6.73	5.45
		Mod. (15)	7.77	6.69	5.43
		Late (18)	7.60	6.54	5.30
	Mod. (23)	Stand.	6.43	5.54	4.50
		Mod.	6.42	5.53	4.49
		Late	6.35	5.47	4.44
	Stand.(25)	Stand.	5.59	4.82	3.92
		Mod.	5.58	4.81	3.91
		Late	5.55	4.78	3.89
Mod. (.20)	Early	Stand.	7.99	6.86	5.54
		Mod.	7.96	6.83	5.52
		Late	7.78	6.68	5.39
	Mod.	Stand.	6.59	5.66	4.58
		Mod.	6.58	5.65	4.57
		Late	6.52	5.59	4.52
	Stand.	Stand.	5.74	4.93	3.99
		Mod.	5.73	4.92	3.99
		Late	5.69	4.89	3.96
Low (.15)	Early	Stand.	8.21	7.02	5.65
		Mod.	8.17	6.99	5.62
		Late	7.99	6.83	5.49
	Mod.	Stand.	6.78	5.80	4.67
		Mod.	6.77	5.79	4.66
		Late	6.70	5.73	4.61
	Stand.	Stand.	5.91	5.06	4.08
		Mod.	5.90	5.05	4.07
		Late	5.86	5.01	4.04

Table B3, Continued

b. Fecundability is Low (.10)

| Abortion | Marriage | Menarche | Postpartum Amenorrhea | | |
			Stand. 6 Mos.	Mod. 10 Mos.	Long 17 Mos.
Standard(.24)	Early (20)	Stand. (12)	5.95	5.30	4.47
		Mod. (15)	5.92	5.27	4.44
		Late (18)	5.78	5.14	4.34
	Mod. (23)	Stand.	4.89	4.36	3.68
		Mod.	4.88	4.35	3.67
		Late	4.83	4.30	3.63
	Stand.(25)	Stand.	4.25	3.78	3.20
		Mod.	4.24	3.78	3.20
		Late	4.21	3.75	3.17
Mod. (.20)	Early	Stand.	6.13	5.44	4.57
		Mod.	6.09	5.41	4.54
		Late	5.95	5.28	4.44
	Mod.	Stand.	5.05	4.48	3.77
		Mod.	5.04	4.47	3.76
		Late	4.99	4.42	3.72
	Stand.	Stand.	4.39	3.90	3.28
		Mod.	4.38	3.89	3.28
		Late	4.35	3.86	3.26
Low (.15)	Early	Stand.	6.33	5.60	4.69
		Mod.	6.30	5.57	4.66
		Late	6.16	5.44	4.55
	Mod.	Stand.	5.23	4.62	3.87
		Mod.	5.22	4.61	3.86
		Late	5.17	4.57	3.82
	Stand.	Stand.	4.55	4.03	3.38
		Mod.	4.55	4.02	3.37
		Late	4.51	3.99	3.35

Table B3, Continued

c. Fecundability is High(.30)

Abortion	Marriage	Menarche	Postpartum Amenorrhea		
			Stand. 6 Mos.	Mod. 10 Mos.	Long 17 Mos.
Standard(.24)	Early (20)	Stand. (12)	8.73	7.40	5.89
		Mod. (15)	8.69	7.37	5.87
		Late (18)	8.50	7.20	5.73
	Mod. (23)	Stand.	7.19	6.10	4.86
		Mod.	7.18	6.09	4.85
		Late	7.11	6.03	4.80
	Stand. (25)	Stand.	6.26	5.31	4.24
		Mod.	6.25	5.30	4.23
		Late	6.21	5.27	4.20
Mod. (.20)	Early	Stand.	8.90	7.53	5.97
		Mod.	8.87	7.50	5.95
		Late	8.68	7.33	5.81
	Mod.	Stand.	7.35	6.21	4.93
		Mod.	7.34	6.20	4.92
		Late	7.27	6.14	4.88
	Stand.	Stand.	6.40	5.41	4.30
		Mod.	6.39	5.40	4.30
		Late	6.35	5.37	4.27
Low (.15)	Early	Stand.	9.11	7.68	6.07
		Mod.	9.08	7.65	6.04
		Late	8.88	7.48	5.91
	Mod.	Stand.	7.53	6.34	5.02
		Mod.	7.52	6.33	5.01
		Late	7.45	6.27	4.96
	Stand.	Stand.	6.57	5.53	4.38
		Mod.	6.56	5.52	4.37
		Late	6.52	5.49	4.35

References

1. Johnston, F. E. Control of Age at Menarche. Human Biology 46: 159, 1974.

2. Zacharias, L. Age at Menarche. New England J. Med. 280: 868, 1969.

3. Leridon, H. Aspects Biometriques de la Fecondite Humaine. Presses Universitaires de France, Traveaux et Documents de INED, Cahier No. 65: 1973.

4. MacMahon, B. et al. Age at Menopause, U. S. 1960-1962. Vital and Health Statistics, National Center for Health Statistics, Series 11, 19: 1966.

5. Leridon, op. cit.

6. Sheps, M. C. and Menken, J. Mathematical Models of Conception and Birth. University of Chicago Press, Chicago, 1973.

7. Bongaarts, J. Intermediate Fertility Variables and Marital Fertility Rates. Population Studies 30: 227, 1976.

8. Perez, A., Potter, R., and Masnick, G. Timing and Sequence of Resuming Ovulation and Menstruation after Childbirth. Population Studies 25: 491, 1971.

9. Leridon, op. cit.

10. Davis, K. and Blake, J. Social Structure and Fertility: An Analytic Framework. Economic Development and Cultural Change 4: 21, 1956.

11. Frisch, R. Weight at Menarche: Similarity for Well-nourished and Under-nourished Girls at Different Ages, and Evidence for Historical Constancy. Pediatrics 50: 445, 1972.

12. Chinnatamby, S. Fertility Trends in Ceylonese Women. J. Reproduc. and Fertility 3: 342, 1962.

13. Laska-Mierzejewska, T. Effect of Ecological and Socio-economic Factors on the Age at Menarche, Body Height and Weight of Rural Girls in Poland. Human Biology 42: 284, 1970.

14. Zacharias, op. cit.

15. Tanner, J. Earlier Maturation in Man. Scientific American 218: 21, 1968.

16. MacMahon, op. cit.

17. Jaszmann, L. et al. Age at Menopause in the Netherlands.
    International J. Fertility 14: 106, 1969.

18. Chinnatamby, op. cit.

19. Jaszmann, op. cit.

20. McKinley, S. et al. An Investigation of Age at Menopause.
    J. Biosocial Science 4: 161, 1972.

21. MacMahon, op. cit.

22. Wolanksy, N. Current Anthropology 13: 255, 1972.

23. McKinley, op. cit.

24. Lechtig, A. et al. Effect of Food Supplementation during
    Pregnancy on Birth Weight. Pediatrics 56: 508, 1975.

25. Agualimpia, C. Demographic Facts of Colombia: The National
    Investigation of Morbidity. Milbank Memorial Quarterly, 47:
    255, 1969.

26. Baird, D. Variations in Fertility Associated with Changes in
    Health Status. In: M. C. Sheps and J. C. Ridley, eds., Public
    Health and Population Change: Current Research Issues,
    University of Pittsburgh Press, Pittsburgh, 1966.

27. Nortman, D. Parental Age as a Factor in Pregnancy Outcome and
    Child Development. Reports on Population/Family Planning 16:
    1974.

28. Soangra, M. R. et al. Socio-economic and Environmental Factors
    Affecting Stillbirths, Indian J. Medical Sciences 29: 5, 1975.

29. Baird, op. cit.

30. Moustgaard, J. Nutritive Influences upon Reproduction.
    J. Reproductive Medicine 8: 1, 1972.

31. Nelson, M. et al. Journal of Nutrition 51: 71, 1953.

32. Frisch, R. Menstrual Cycles: Fatness as a Determinant of
    Minimum Weight for Height Necessary for their Maintenance or
    Onset. Science 185: 949, 1974.

33. Lev Ran, A. Secondary Amenorrhea Resulting from Uncontrolled
    Weight Reducing Diets. Fertility and Sterility 25: 459, 1974.

34. LeRoy Ladurie, E. L'amenorrhee de Famine (XVII-SS siecles).
    Annales 24: 1589, 1969.

35. Zubiran, E. et al. Endocrine Disturbances in Chronic Human
    Malnutrition. Vitamins and Hormones 4: 97, 1953.

36. Keys, A. et al. The Biology of Human Starvation. University
    of Minnesota Press, Minneapolis, 1950.

37. Jacobs, E. Effect of Starvation on Sex Hormones in the Male.
    J. Clin. Endocrin. 8: 1946.

38. Menken, J. Estimating Fecundability. Ph.D. Thesis,
    Princeton University, 1975.

39. Bongaarts, J. and Delgado. H. Effects of Nutritional Status
    on Fertility. In: Proceedings of IUSSP 1977 General Confer-
    ence, Mexico, 1977 (in press).

40. Chavez, A. et al. Nutrition and Development of Infants from
    Poor Rural Area, III. Maternal Nutrition and Its Consequences
    on Fertility. Nutrition Reports International 7: 1, 1973.

41. Delgado, H. et al. Effect of Improved Nutrition on the Dura-
    tion of Postpartum Amenorrhea in Moderate Malnourished
    Populations. Abstracts of the Xth International Congress of
    Nutrition, Kyoto, Japan (in press).

42. Saxton, G. Human Birth Interval in East Africa. J. Reproduc.
    and Fertility (Supplement) 6: 83, 1969.

43. Mayer, G. Undernutrition, Prolonged Lactation, and Female
    Infertility. J. Trop. Ped. 12: 58, 1966.

44. Bonte, M. et al. Influence of the Socio-economic Level on the
    Conception Rate During Lactation. International J. Fertility
    19: 97, 1974.

45. Gonzalez, Solien de N. Lactation and Pregnancy: A Hypothesis.
    American Anthropologist 68: 873, 1964.

46. Jelliffe, D. et al. The Assessment of the Nutritional Status
    of the Community, W.H.O., Geneva, 1966.

47. W.H.O., Expert Committee on Medical Assessment of Nutritional
    Status. W.H.O. Technical Report Series No. 258, 1963.

48. Shryock, H. S. and Siegel, J. S. The Methods and Materials of
    Demography. U.S.G.P.D., Washington, 1973.

49. Leridon, op. cit.

50. Coale, A. J. Age-patterns of Marriage. Population Studies 25: 193, 1971.

51. Hajnal, J. Age at Marriage and Proportions Marrying. Population Studies 7: 111, 1953.

52. Sheps, M. C., Menken, J., Ridley, J. C. and Linger, J. The Truncation Effect in Closed and Open Birth Interval Data. J. Am. Stat. Assoc. 65: 678, 1970.

53. Potter, R. et al. Application of Field Studies to Research on the Physiology of Human Reproduction. J. Chron. Dis. 18: 1125, 1965.

54. Chen, L. et al. A Prospective Study of Birth Interval Dynamics in Rural Bangladesh. Population Studies 28: 277, 1974.

55. Wolfers, D. Determinants of Birth Intervals and Their Means. Population Studies 22: 252, 1968.

56. Sheps and Menken, op. cit.

57. Menken, J. A. Biometric Models of Fertility. Social Forces 54: 52, 1975.

58. Henry, L. On the Measurement of Human Fertility (translated by M. Sheps and E. Lapierre-Adamcyk). Elsevier Publishing Company: New York, 1972.

59. Perrin, E. B. and Sheps, M. C. Human Reproduction: A Stochastic Process. Biometrics 20: 28, 1964.

60. Sheps and Menken, op. cit.

61. Bongaarts, op. cit.

62. Sheps and Menken, op. cit.

63. Sheps, M. C. A Review of Models for Population Change. Review of the International Statistical Institute 39: 185, 1971.

64. Menken, op. cit.

65. Dyke, B. and MacCluer, J. Computer Simulation in Human Population Studies. Academic Press, 1973.

66. Hamel, E. A. et al. SOCSIM, Demographic-Sociological Micro-simulation Program. University of California Research Series, 27: Berkeley, 1976.

67. Bongaarts, J. A Dynamic Model of the Reproduction Process. Population Studies, 1977 (in press).

68. Barrett, J. C. A Monte Carlo Simulation of Human Reproduction. Genus 25: 1969.

69. Coale, op. cit.

70. Henry, L. Some Data on Natural Fertility. Eugenics Quarterly 8: 81, 1961.

71. Potter, R. G. Births Averted by Induced Abortion, an Application of Renewal Theory. Theoretical Population Biology 3: 19, 1972.

72. Potter, R. C. Changes of Natural Fertility and Contraceptive Equivalents. Social Forces 54: 36, 1975.

73. Potter, op. cit. 1975.

74. Hogan, H. R. Age Patterns of Infant Mortality. Ph.D. Thesis, Princeton University, 1976.

75. Coale, A. J. and Demeny, P. Regional Model Life Tables and Stable Populations. Princeton University Press: Princeton, 1966.

76. Lesthaeghe, R. Nuptiality and Population Growth. Population Studies 25: 415, 1971.

77. Leridon, op. cit.

78. Bongaarts, op. cit. 1976.

79. Barrett, J. and Marshall, J. The Risk of Conception on Different Days of the Menstrual Cycle. Population Studies 23: 455, 1969.

80. United Nations, ESCAP region, Report of the Multinational Study in Methodologies for Setting Family Planning Targets in the ESCAP Region, Asian Population Studies Series, No. 31 (under preparation).

81. Nortman, D. and Bongaarts, J. Contraceptive Practice Required to Meet a Prescribed Crude Birth Rate Target: A Proposed Macro-Model and Hypothetical Illustrations. Demography 21: 471, 1975.

FECUNDABILITY AND CONTRACEPTIVE OPPORTUNITIES

George S. Masnick

Harvard University

Boston, Massachusetts

INTRODUCTION

The paper by Menken and Bongaarts in this volume demonstrates how nutrition can affect fertility in non-contracepting populations through its impact on the length of the reproductive period and on the several components of birth intervals, including the length of the period of temporary postpartum amenorrhea, the waiting time to conception once menstruation resumes, and the proportion of conceptions that go to term. The nutritional status and the pattern of food intake of both mothers and infants are hypothesized to be important. Ages at menarche and menopause are clearly related to the growth, and therefore the nutritional history, of the woman (Frisch in this volume), whereas the large variability observed in postpartum amenorrhea can perhaps be better explained by the frequency, duration and intensity of nursing, independent of the nutritional status of the mother. The potential impact of secular trends or of temporal fluctuations in nutrition on the probability of conception once ovulation resumes is more difficult to evaluate, and is the subject of discussion in this paper.

It is generally assumed that the levels of fecundability, or monthly probabilities of conception, for a sexually active, non-pregnant, non-amenorrheic woman range between 0.1 and 0.3, with 0.2 frequently taken as a "medium" value (1). These values can be estimated by observing the waiting times to conception in non-contracepting populations in the period immediately following marriage, where the assumption of sufficient sexual activity is not in question and where postpartum anovulation does not complicate observations. Similarly, couples can be observed when they deliberately stop practicing contraception in order to conceive.

313

Assuming that these probabilities remain constant from month to month, they yield mean delays to conception of between three to ten months, which corresponds to the range in mean waiting times observed in many "natural fertility" studies.

On the basis of these figures we might be led to conclude that the potential direct impact on fertility of change in nutrition working through conception probabilities is modest at best. If, for example, a highly fecund woman (0.3 fecundability) has her monthly probability of conception reduced by 50% through nutritional stress, the birth interval will only be increased by 3.4 months, from 3.3 to 6.7 months. Such an increase amounts to about ten or fifteen percent of the total length of average birth intervals, and as such can be projected to account for only that much of a reduction in total fertility over the reproductive life of a woman. With these figures in mind, it is understandable why demographers have turned more attention toward the relationship between nutrition and the period of temporary postpartum sterility. Not only is amenorrhea as an indicator of anovulation easier to observe than conception, but the apparent direct impact of variation in nutrition is far greater, with mean durations of amenorrhea having been observed to range between four and twenty months (2). Such figures have led some observers to comment that breastfeeding has been the world's most effective contraceptive in terms of births averted by long postpartum delays.

The assumptions that permit one to give relatively less weight to the importance of nutritional variation on fecundability are two. First, the assumption about the baseline or "normal" level of fecundability is important. If mean fecundability is set at 0.1, yielding a ten-month mean delay to conception, and then reduced to 0.05 or raised to 0.15 by variations in nutrition that affect the probability by 50 percent in either direction, the mean waiting time to conception would range from 7 to 20 months. Such figures are then comparable to those for variation in temporary postpartum sterility.

The second assumption that becomes important when judging the impact on fertility of nutritionally derived variation in fecundability is whether or not the population under consideration is contracepting. It is not only plausible that a mean fecundability level of 0.1 might be a more realistic figure for a population which finds itself on the margin of adequate nutrition during normal times, and where patterns of temporary separation of spouses combine with periodic abstinence and occasional use of other measures to prevent conception in order to postpone or space births; it is also likely that most populations in which we are interested are contracepting populations. Furthermore, I suggest that the ability of a couple to develop the necessary skills at birth control will depend upon the existence of critical "learning"

periods where motivation to practice fertility regulation is high
and where fecundability is low enough to delay a pregnancy from
quickly intervening to short-circuit the learning process. In
other words, we perhaps ought to give more weight to the interaction effects between natural fecundity and use of birth control in
our attempts to evaluate the impact of nutrition on fertility.
This is the theme I would like to develop more fully in the
remainder of the present paper.

LEARNING TO REGULATE FERTILITY

Birth control involves a complex set of actions with subtle
interactions between mind and body which we often tend to overlook.
Ansley Coale (3) has nicely captured much of this complexity in
his statement of the conditions that must be present in any population which effectively regulates fertility through the use of
birth control:
(1) Potential parents must consider it an acceptable mode of
thought and form of behavior to balance advantages and disadvantages before deciding to have another child.
(2) Perceived social and economic circumstances must make
reduced fertility seem an advantage to individual couples.
(3) Procedures that will in fact prevent births must be known,
and there must be sufficient communication between spouses and
sufficient sustained will, in both, to employ them successfully.

Although these three dimensions of birth control do not give
enough weight to the importance of birth control behavior during
the early reproductive ages for the development of these prerequisites, the symbolic and perceptual substructures necessary
for effective contraception are given their due recognition.
Birth control is not something that is simply "switched on" by a
couple deciding to adopt some method to stop childbearing
altogether. Successful family planners are not individuals who
do nothing about birth control until they have reached their
desired family size at which time they begin to effectively "use"
something. Rather, effective birth control depends importantly on
the development of appropriate orientations toward one's self as a
fertility planner, familiarity with procedures and communication
skills, all of which require time to be internalized.

An important element of the effectiveness with which birth
control comes to be used is the degree to which attitudes and
behavior are sustained for sufficiently long periods of time for
the Coale prerequisites to become learned. The early reproductive
ages, the postpartum period and periods of economic and social
stress are conducive for the learning process because of the
combination of high motivation to avoid pregnancy, reduced fecund-

ability and the perception that whatever the physical and emotional
costs of contraception, they are only temporary. Under these
conditions, it is more likely that individuals and couples will
strive to find those procedures acceptable in preventing pregnancy
and be rewarded for their effort. In contemporary populations
birth control in the early reproductive ages is particularly
critical. As we have stated elsewhere:

> Learning to regulate reproduction effectively is best
> done during the months following the onset of regular
> sexual activity. An individual that does not learn
> birth control early will be less able to achieve con-
> trol of fertility later in the reproductive period. A
> late start at birth control requires one to overcome the
> inertia of established self-perceptions and roles geared
> to expectations of continued parenthood, break with
> familiar and comfortable patterns of non-contracepting
> sexual activity, embark on new patterns of communication
> with one's sexual partner regarding the measures to be
> taken to avoid pregnancy, and perhaps to be confronted
> with a new form of behavior at a stage in family build-
> ing when the motivation to avoid an accidental pregnancy
> might not be the strongest, all while fecundity is
> peaking (4).

SOME REINTERPRETATIONS THAT FOLLOW FROM THE LEARNING PERSPECTIVE

According to our perspective, a large part of the "excess"
childbearing that has been revealed in KAP surveys in the developing world can be explained by a high fraction of women reaching
desired family size while still at peak fecundability, when the
lack of previous contraceptive experiences makes the "adoption" of
birth control extremely difficult (5). Likewise, the high amount
of unwanted and unplanned fertility characteristic of the mothers
of the baby boom generation in post WW II United States can be
explained by trained incapacities to contracept brought about by
an unusually long succession of cohorts accelerating their household formation and family building without making an effort to
control the timing of early pregnancies.

Motivation to accelerate the childbearing process, which
undermines contraceptive capacity, is likely to be present especially during periods of rapid social change where there is a clash
between the traditional and the modern as embodied in the values
of middle age parents and their young adult children. The post
WW II period was just such a social setting in much of the world
where urbanization, education, communications and other forces of
modernization served to strain the continuity between generations.
With most young people the final hurdle to adulthood and "independ-

ence" is parenthood, for only in this way can one begin to put their status as dependent child into the background. Parenthood is a universal mechanism accepted as legitimate in all societies by which young couples can "put distance" between the generations in a culturally acceptable manner. The high prevalence of nuclear households in most non-industrial societies argues strongly for the view that adulthood is supported by independence of residential units and a certain degree of independence of domestic activities including parenting (6). We might alter our view of the role of extended kinship networks in structuring childbearing behavior by challenging the conventional wisdom that propinquity of kin make it _easy_ for young couples to bear children without having to bear the full costs. Instead, I suggest that the presence of extended kin makes it _hard_ for the young couple not to bear children quickly. Once the inertia of the childbearing process has been started, large families will be difficult to stave off, and the kin network may certainly be called upon to assist in childrearing, although it is more likely that older siblings will take on the child care responsibilities even when other adult relatives are nearby.

Furthermore, we should also re-evaluate the reasons behind the high discontinuation rates that have been observed in many family planning programs as having less to do with lack of motivation to practice birth control or with problems in the methods themselves (although there is certainly room for much improvement on the latter count), but with trained incapacities for couples to sustain birth control behavior in spite of the costs, inconvenience or of side effects. Family planning programs will be more successful both in acceptance and continuation rates when social changes permit couples to use birth control to delay the timing of early pregnancies, and thus to develop their skills as contraceptors at a time when learning opportunities can be maximized.

HISTORICAL USE OF BIRTH CONTROL IN THE UNITED STATES

In Europe and America during the 19th century and before, when marital union patterns, extended breastfeeding practices and overall levels of fecundability that might have been lower than in today's better nourished populations combined to produce mean numbers of live born children on the order of six or seven, the question of contraceptive use to achieve a certain desired family size might have been less salient than the need to behave in a way to insure proper spacing and a satisfactory age distribution of children in the household. Large families, where living children were spaced three years apart, would not be problematical for parents because teenage children would leave the parental household and enter the labor force earlier than today's youth, and older siblings would be in a better position to lend a hand with caring for the younger. More problematical for the family would

be several children born in rapid succession. Five children under
the age of 10 would provide a household size/childrearing/labor
force dynamic in marked contrast to five children spread in ages
from infancy to age 15 or so.

Even a cursory review of the available literature pertaining
to early 19th century childbearing in the United States reveals
that contraception was a theme well before the small family norm
could be said to have become established. Writing in 1850, one
physician succinctly summed up the case for open discussion of
birth control in the following way:

> To say that there _are_ means of preventing conception, is
> only stating what every person has already heard, or
> believes, and is, therefore, nothing new. Even if such
> information was likely to be productive of great evil,
> it is now impossible to prevent its dissemination, and
> it is, therefore, useless to avoid the topic (7).

He goes on to discuss the advantages and disadvantages of various
methods of birth control including abortion, coitus interruptus,
ejaculation with only partial penetration, condoms, douching with
and without spermatic inhibitors, sponges to block the uterine
passage and rhythm. In his discussion of the various methods he
attempts to weigh the tradeoffs among safety, contraceptive
efficiency and effect in reducing sexual pleasure, in what amounts
to a very sensitive and sensible understanding of the problems in
practicing birth control. On douching, for example, he comments:

> In all cases it is necessary for them to be used
> _immediately_ after emission and the too early sepa-
> ration, together with the anxiety and revulsion of
> feeling attendant upon the preventive act are both
> agitating and injurious, to say nothing of
> inconvenience (8).

On variations of coitus interruptus he adds:

> ...this plan, therefore, diminishes the liability,
> but does not totally prevent (9).

On rhythm the author observes:

> In every instance it may be confidently relied upon -
> conception takes place within sixteen days after a
> menstrual period, and usually within eight or nine days,
> though it may be often difficult to ascertain the period,
> and other phenomenon may be mistaken for it (10).

Of all methods, rhythm is most strongly recommended because of its relative effectiveness, least interference with the pleasure of intercourse and complete safety. It also is interesting to note that nowhere does the author proselytize for small families, but he does argue that at least three years is recommended between every two births as "it is better for both mother and child."

I have perhaps digressed too much on the subject of use of birth control in the first half of the 19th century in order to make a simple point. We should not be too quick to label a population as "non-contracepting" in attempting to evaluate the relative importance of one set of factors, such as nutrition, on fertility. The postpartum period is especially important as a time when couples might move in and out of contracepting behavior: low practice during pregnancy, high degree of abstinence in the immediate postpartum period, followed by a period of high sexual activity, with increasing motivation to practice contraception later in the postpartum period once menstruation resumes, especially if the youngest child is still being breastfed both because of the popular belief that pregnancy will poison or dry up the breast milk (11) and the desire to insure adequate spacing.

The distinction between the population and the individual is important, and it cannot be stressed enough that unwanted fertility at the individual level is consistent with any level of desired completed family size at the individual level and with any level of aggregate fertility at the societal level. The dimension of unwanted fertility relating to excess over small desired completed family size may be a relatively modern concept as applied to a majority of individuals in a population, but the dimension of motivation to control the timing of one's pregnancies in an appropriate fashion undoubtedly has roots much deeper in human history. Once contraception becomes a factor, it leads to the difficulty in sorting out the effects of nutritional stress on fecundity, such as in the Dutch famine of 1943 (Stein and Susser in this volume) or the Bangladesh famine of 1974, where both disrupted unions and high motivation to postpone pregnancy by practicing birth control are added to whatever the impact is on the biological capacity to reproduce.

THE FECUNDABILITY MATRIX

In the above paragraphs I have been emphasizing the importance of a critical learning period early in the reproductive ages in order for individuals to effectively use birth control, especially methods that have side effects or diminish sexual spontaneity, or have both liabilities. In this section I will tentatively offer some hypotheses about the length of this critical learning period and how shifts in fecundability could serve to either enhance or undermine the chances of the learning period being effective.

At the outset, it is worth making an explicit recognition
that the term "fecundability" as used by demographers has both a
biological and behavioral dimension. Biologically, the probability
of conception could be affected by the frequency of anovulatory
menstrual cycles, the production of non-viable ova or sperm, sperm
count and motility, adequacy of tubal function, unknown factors
related to sperm penetration, and the fraction of fertilized ova
that successfully nidate. Behaviorally, the factors that vary
include the fraction of time individuals are in unions, the timing
and frequency of intercourse within unions, type of intercourse
and perhaps variations in the fraction of time that ejaculation
occurs. Many of these factors, both biological and behavioral,
could be related in theory to health, growth, and nutrition,
although the evidence to date is sparse. Let us, in the absence
of firm figures, hypothesize three levels of biological capacity
(under "adequate" levels of coital activity) that range from a
high of 0.30 to a low of 0.10 per month. That is, under the
assumption of all behavioral factors being favorable, conception
delays would range from about three to ten months on average. Call
this range the biological dimension. Next, let us superimpose a
range of variability in the behavioral dimension that will reduce
baseline fecundability by 25 and 50 percent, respectively, and
label these values of coital frequency high, medium and low. Such
a decomposition of fecundability into the biological and behavioral dimensions can be represented by the matrix given in Table 1.

The fecundability matrix can be used to characterize shifts
in expected conception waiting times in several ways. The reader
should keep in mind that the actual values in the matrix have been
selected for illustrative purposes only, and while they are within

Table 1

Monthly Probabilities of Conception
and Mean Conception Delays (in Parentheses)

Biological Capacity

		High	Medium	Low
Coital Frequency	High	.30 (3.3 mo.)	.20 (5.0 mo.)	.10 (10 mo.)
	Medium	.225 (4.4 mo.)	.15 (6.7 mo.)	.075 (13.3 mo.)
	Low	.15 (6.7 mo.)	.10 (10 mo.)	.05 (20 mo.)

the range of values normally assumed in many analytical models of reproduction, they are not empirically derived.

First, I have connected the cells with arrows that move on the diagonal to indicate that we can expect shifts in fecundability, whether it is over the reproductive age range of individuals, or as a response to temporary period effects such as famine or as a result of long term secular shifts in nutritional status, to be brought about by simultaneous shifts in biological capacity and union exposure that reinforce each other. For example, a woman moves from the teenage years with reduced biological capacity and low premarital sexual activity to the twenties with increased biological capacity and higher coital frequency in the early years of marriage, and once again to lower values on both the biological and behavioral dimensions in the later reproductive ages.

The case of temporary period effects is straightforward. Longer term secular changes in the biological dimension could be brought about by first the movement from hunting and gathering to settled agriculture as a source of food, then to the market economy, where each successive shift results in food supplies that are more stable and with a greater share of fats and carbohydrates added to the diet. Such secular shifts are also likely to be accompanied by enhanced opportunities for earlier and more continuous marital unions as women become more dependent on the labor force participation of their husbands to provide household income, and men are better able to maintain continuous employment near their families with less hours spent at the work site. As long as such shifts in the biological and behavioral dimensions are simultaneous and reinforcing, and I merely state this as an hypothesis, then it can be seen from the above matrix that significant changes in the waiting times to conception can result.

The second point to be illustrated by the matrix is that certain values of fecundability may lead to conception delays too short to provide an adequate learning period. If allowed to make an educated guess on minimum length of the learning period, I would suggest a period of at least six months. I have enclosed those elements of the matrix that provide such a margin of delay. As one moves from medium levels of union exposure and biological capacity toward high levels of both, the learning period is undermined. If it is the case that fecundability during the teenage years has increased, as one might reasonably infer from evidence on declining age at menarche, then we face the possibility that erosion of teenage subfecundity is a factor operating to buoy up fertility rates, not so much through direct impact by extending the reproductive age range, but through diminising the availability of the teenage premarital period as a time to learn to use traditional methods of birth control. New and more efficient methods of contraception must be substituted to lower effective fecundability during this period so that even their imperfect use would provide a margin of protection of more than six months for the sexually active teenager. However, the IUD is not a method well suited to the nulliparous, and intermittent sexual activity may not be regular enough to sustain motivation to take oral contraceptives each and every day.

CONCLUSION

In an earlier paper we argued that those women most in need of birth control, namely, those that are highly fecund and non-contracepting, who are therefore likely to achieve large families while still in the middle of their reproductive ages, are the very women for whom freestanding clinic type family planning programs are bound to fail (12). Such women will only be "eligible" for accepting the pill during a relatively brief time when they are not pregnant or lactating, and when they enter the fecund state once again. Only a vigorous effort to recruit them as program acceptors could compete successfully with the high risk of a pregnancy that would quickly render them ineligible. Acceptance of the pill early in the postpartum period interferes with lactation, and the period of use that overlaps with natural temporary postpartum sterility is superfluous. Under conditions of high termination rates for first segment of use, this period of overlap would strongly reduce the demographic impact of acceptance. The situation with the IUD is somewhat more favorable provided that early postpartum acceptance does not interfere with lactation and that use is long enough to extend into the period after ovulation has resumed. The key to the success of the pill or IUD program, then, is an ability to reach a highly fecund woman before she has resumed full fecundability. This is the principle that I now see as being of general importance for all contracepting behavior to be learned. Traditional methods of birth control, in particular, require such a learning period. In order for contracepting trials to be rewarded, effective fecundability must be reduced to levels which yield significant conception delays.

I shall resist, for now, the temptation to continue with my speculation about how reduced fecundability increases contraceptive opportunities. If my point has not already been brought home, then it can only be better made on the basis of more data and convincing calculations. Perhaps this discussion will serve as a stimulus to that further work.

References

1. Henry, L. French Statistical Research in Natural Fertility, in M. C. Sheps and J. C. Ridley, eds. _Public Health and Population Change_, University of Pittsburgh Press, Pittsburgh, 33-350, 1965.

2. Masnick, G. S. The Demographic Impact of Breastfeeding, paper presented at Symposium on Biosocial Aspects of Breast-feeding, annual meetings of the American Association for the Advancement of Science, Boston, February 18-21, 1976.

3. Coale, A. J. The Demographic Transition, _IUSSP Proceedings_, Liege, Belgium: 65, 1973.

4. Masnick, G. S. and McFalls, J. A., Jr. A New Perspective on the 20th Century American Fertility Swing, _J. Fam. Hist_. 1: 223-224, 1976.

5. Masnick, G. S. and Potter, R. G. Contraceptive Acceptance and Pregnancy: A Matrix Approach to the Analysis of Competing Risks, _Pop. Stud_. 23: 267-277, 1969.

6. Burch, T. K. The Size and Structure of Families: A Comparative Analysis of Census Data, _Am. Soc. Rev_. 32: 347-363; also, Laslett, P. (ed.), _Household and Family in Past Time_, Cambridge Univ. Press, Cambridge, 1972.

7. Hollick, F. _The Marriage Guide, or, Natural History of Generation: A Private Instructor for Married Persons and Those About to Marry both Male and Female; In Everything Concerning the Physiology and Relations of the Sexual System and the Production or Prevention of Offspring_, W. T. Strong, New York, 332, 1850.

8. _Ibid._ 338

9. _Ibid._ 337

10. Ibid. 217

11. vande Walle, E. and vande Walle, F. Allaitement, Sterilité et Contraception: les Opinions Jusqu'an XIX Siecle, _Population_, 4-5, 685-701, 1973.

12. Masnick and Potter, _op. cit._

MALNUTRITION IN CENTRAL AFRICA

W. Wils

Foundation for Business Administration

Delft, Netherlands

INTRODUCTION

Detailed analyses by the Centre for Scientific and Medical Studies in Central Africa of the Free University at Brussels, (CEMUBAC) showed that 10-15% of the population of Kivu, the easternmost province of Zaire, is affected by protein malnutrition. The CEMUBAC programme covered medical, demographic and nutritional aspects of the problem and such relations as between nutrition, lactation and birth intervals. It became clear that the prospects were rather alarming and that public health programmes could not alleviate the malnutrition. The difficulties were rooted in a situation where a rapidly growing population, practicing mostly subsistance agriculture in a fragile environment, reaches the carrying capacity of its region. Thus the CEMUBAC sponsored in 1975 a general socio-economic study which should lead to an integrating frame work for describing and analyzing the problem, and which could offer insights in the gravity of the situation and the feasibility of proposed policies. This paper contains a brief report of this analysis. After a short description of the problem area, an outline will be given of the constructed models and resulting conclusions (1).

DESCRIPTION OF THE PROBLEM AREA

The analysis concerned the mountainous part of Kivu, a province in the east of Zaire, bordering Uganda, Rwanda and Burundi. It is a hilly area straddling the equator and at altitudes from 1,000 to 2,000 meters. Its surface area is about 34,000

km^2. Roughly 20% of the soils is very fertile; the rest is average.
Half of the land is arable and, although the situation varies, all
of it is erodable. There are two rainy periods, from September to
December and from March to May. Annual rainfall is 1200 $\pm$ 300 mm
and the temperature is 20°C $\pm$5°. The conditions are particularly
heterogeneous so that there are many micro climates and local
agricultural pecularities.

The population, mostly of Bantou and Hamite origin, belongs
to the interlacustrine culture of Central Africa. The estimated
number of inhabitants of the area has increased from 750,000 in
1920 to almost 2,000,000 in 1970. The present annual rate of
natural increase is 2.5 - 3%. The birth-rate went up from some
40 per 1000 in 1920 to around 50 per 1000 in 1970. Practically
all women marry. Primary sterility is of the order of 5%. Birth
intervals are 34-36 months on the average and average completed
fertility is 7-8 children. The women practice natural lactation
during periods up to 24 months. The postpartum amenorrhea varies
from 19 months in rural areas to 9 months in the cities. Due to
various factors, such as strong seasonal fluctuations in food
availability, famines and taboos, birth intervals used to be
longer - up to 4 years - in precolonial times.

Mountainous Kivu is a relatively healthy area. The death
rate was 22-24 per 1000 in 1955. The infant mortality is 100-130
per 1000. The death rate used to be around 30 per 1000 mostly due
to famines and large seasonal fluctuations in availability of food.

Urbanization is a low 5%, and has been increasing at 10 to 20%
annually over the last 20 years. The average density is of the
order of 50 persons/km^2. Migration from the eastern neighbours -
Uganda, Rwanda and Burundi - is not unimportant but very uncertain
and is expected to be more restricted in the future. In first
instance it has not been included in the analysis.

Agriculture in Kivu is semi-intensive. Banana trees and
little vegetable gardens are well tended and manured. Annual
crops are cultivated on a rotational basis with a fallow period
to restore losses of productivity. The main products are - next
to bananas - sweet potatoes, cassave, beans, sorghum and corn.
Also some cash crops like coffee, tea, and pyrethrum or quinine
can be found. The bananas are used to make banana beer and have a
high social and economic importance: 80-90% of the income stems
from the sale of banana beer. Nutritionally bananas account for
about 13% of the energy intake, yet 25-50% of the cultivated area
is taken up by bananas, i.e. $\pm$ 25 ares* per family of 4-5 persons.

---

*100 ares = 1 hectare = 2,47 acres.

The yield is a low: 1,000,000 cal/hectare. The annual food crops
occupy on the average some 50 ares and yield 7,000,000 cal/
hectare.

      Cattle are particularly important socially. They have a low
economic and nutritional value. They graze on fallow fields and
so contribute some manure. By now fallow periods have declined
so much that the density of cattle is too high to do anything but
damage the fields. There is about the equivalent of 1 cow per 6
persons. In the fifties typically one third of the fields was
used for cattle, which produced only 4% of the income.

      The small family is the production unit. Women do most of
the work: if a woman counts for 1, her husband contributes only
0.3. There are the usual bottle-necks in agriculture: preparing
the fields for sowing, distance. In addition to cultivating, the
women do the cooking, gather wood and get and feed the children.
The land ownership is very complicated and does not contribute
to proper husbandry.

      Many improvements of agriculture are possible, technically
seen. The heterogeneous conditions, however, make the situation
difficult. Also the area is rather isolated so that transport
of fertilizers and products is costly. Of all technical improvements mostly only cultivation of cassave has been maintained.

      Pressure on land has increased greatly. Fallow periods are
shorter, so productivity falls. Fields of less quality - and often
on steeper slopes - are being cultivated. Cassave substitutes
beans, keeping up the energy intake but causing an unfavourable
balance for proteins. Wood in reforestated areas is being cut
and erosion prevention is virtually nonexistent anymore.

      In the pre-colonial period a reasonably balanced diet probably
prevailed; however, there were large seasonal fluctuations and
occasional famines. The obligatory cultivation of cassave attenu-
ated the fluctuations and famines diminished, also because transportation facilities improved. However, in 1951 - for the first
time - 51 cases of malnutrition were reported. Again 15 years
later it was shown that 2-5% of the population suffered from malnutrition. Since independence there has been a recurrence of
shortages.

      The prevalent combination of global denutrition and protein
malnutrition affects particularly 3-4 year olds. Everybody is
liable to relative malnutrition as evidenced by the low average
weight - 50 kg for women and 55 kg for men - and length - 1.54 m
and 1.64 m respectively. Indeed energetically food per capita is
5 - 15% below FAO/OMS norms. Protein intake is 50-90% of the

norm and fluctuates strongly with the seasons.

About the economics of Kivu we can be short. The regional
per capita product is estimated at $40. The few existing indus-
tries are declining or closed down. The same is true for the
plantations. Ninety-two percent of the agricultural production
is used for auto-subsistence.

BASIC HYPOTHESES

The above data, gathered mostly in Belgium and during a
series of interviews at Kivu, made clear that the situation in
Kivu could be quite grave. How grave was not certain, because,
for example, large areas a little farther away were still under-
populated and would migration to these areas not occur spontaneously? Erosion was serious but cultivation still went on with
good yields. Economically there seemed to be possibilities, e.g.,
with natural gas in lake Kivu. Would the country not slowly recover after a transition period from the grave set-backs since
obtaining independence? There were enough blue patches in the
dark sky for an optimist to believe in good weather to come and to
have faith that the sliding down would be stopped.

Yet few of the possibilities worked out practically. In
reality no progress was being made. Agriculture did not improve
and virtually had not changed since 1920. The questions to ask
seemed to be: How long can this go on, before major disasters
occur? How much time is available to implement proposed programs?
How could time be gained? Thus, four months into the project, it
was decided not to consider: "What could possibly happen in Kivu
if all kinds of uncertain changes would occur?", but rather "What
could possibly happen in Kivu if no change occurred?" The idea
was to establish a base line and see how much stretch there was in
the existing system. The resulting model would be purely
Malthusian.

In Figure 1 various behaviour modes are represented for a
growing population with a constant technology and in a finite
environment. Carrying capacity equals the maximum number of
persons which can live permanently in a region without degrading
it and at a given level of technology. In principle one can
imagine S-shaped population growth to occur and no degradation of
soils as indicated by the dotted lines in Figure 1. The soils in
Kivu, however, are very susceptible to erosion and it is more
likely that evolution will be as shown by the solid lines.

The main elements of a model corresponding to the developments pictured in Figure 1 are related to each other as in Figure 2.

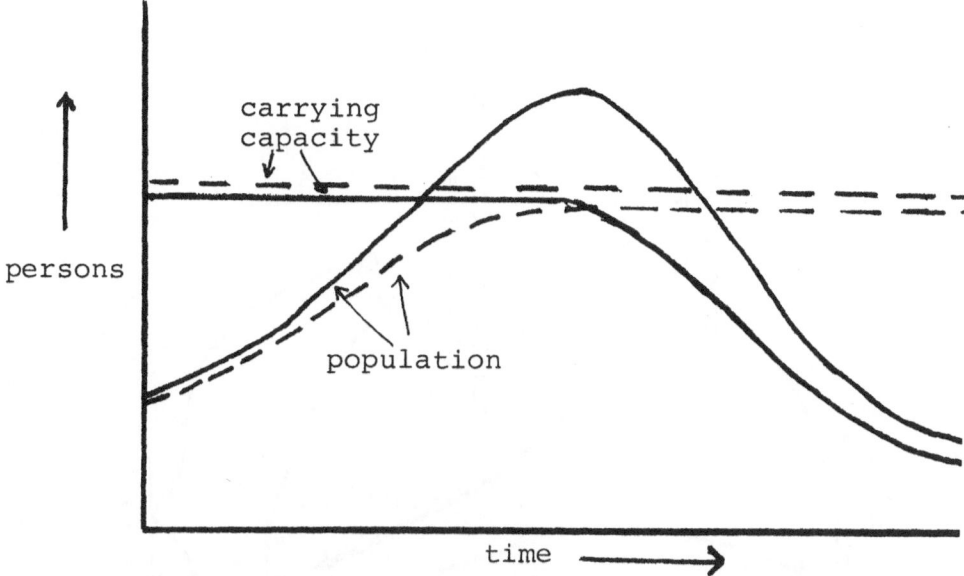

Figure 1. Alternative basic behavior modes for a growing population with finite carrying capacity.

The arrows indicate influences. A + [-] sign at the tip of an
arrow means that the final quantity changes in the same [opposite]
direction as the initial quantity. The (+) [(-)] signs in
Figure 2 refer to positive [negative] feedback loops i.e. closed
chains of influences which reinforce themselves [are goal seeking].
We believe that the interaction of such feedback loops constitutes
the most important determinant of the behaviour of complex social
systems. The diagram in Figure 2 gives only the outlines for a
model. A more detailed description will be given later on, but
first we shall discuss the various feedback loops.

    The first feedback loop connects population and annual popu-
lation growth. It is a positive - self-reinforcing - loop leading
to exponential growth or decline - given that all other conditions
do not change. The loop contains delays since the new children
take a while to grow up and to contribute to the reproductive
process of the population. The second loop from population to food
per capita to population growth and back to population is goal
seeking (and hence negative). It controls the first process in
that an increasing population leads to less food per capita -
everything else being equal - and hence to a decrease of the rate
of growth.

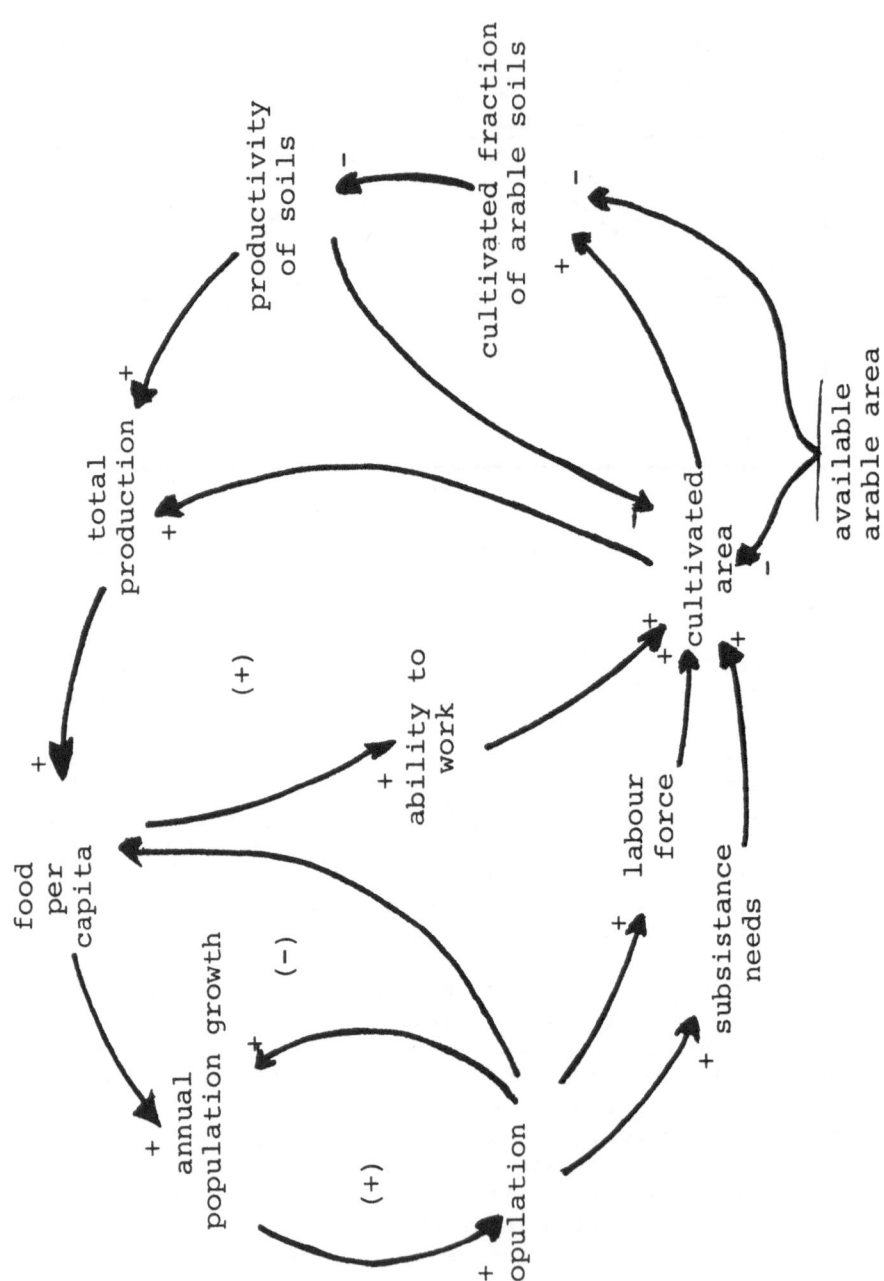

Figure 2.   The main elements of the model and their interactions.

The loss in food per capita is, however, compensated for by an increase of production. This mechanism operates through labor force and subsistance needs, cultivated area and total production. It represents a positive loop. When more land is cultivated, fallow periods shorten, productivity of the soils falls and hence total production increases less than expected. This fourth loop - a negative one - operates slower than the previous loop. Together they produce a behaviour where an increase in cultivated area firstly leads to a proportional increase in total production which subsequently diminishes again somewhat because of a degradation of the soils.

This process of degradation is accelerated because a farmer tries to compensate for the loss of productivity by farming even more land which in time leads to even more degradation, etc. This fifth loop is positive and particularly treacherous in combination with the fourth one. Once degradation starts in earnest it builds up momentum all by itself and leads to a sudden collapse.

We have built in a last mechanism which could play: when people are consistently undernourished their ability to work diminishes. The physical limit to what a person can cultivate drops when he or she is severely undernourished. Hence, less will be produced and malnutrition will increase. This last loop is well known as: the rich get richer and the poor get poorer.

These six processes are all well-known and are the main ones to take place in Kivu. There are theories, of course, which hold that when people get in difficulties automatic corrective actions take place or jumps in technology will occur. As we have remarked earlier, such processes have not been taken into consideration here. We will see later on, however, that if such processes do exist they have to operate very fast to avert a decline.

The conceptual model of Figure 2 had to be quantified and documented as well as possible in order to make a convincing case. This turned out to be a difficult task. Most studies concern special cases and it is hard to deduce more general relations. In this case, three areas had to be dealt with: (1) demographics, (2) production, and (3) degradation of soils. In my opinion, the strength of modelling lies in the possibility of integrating in one consistent framework the knowledge of persons with different backgrounds. For the present study, the CEMBAC team, especially Mr. Caraël, provided the demographic inputs, whereas, in particular, Mr. Tondeur guided the agricultural part. In the next section we shall discuss the model structure in more detail. Special emphasis will be given to demographics.

MODEL STRUCTURE

Given that our main interest is in nutrition, we have choosen
the composition of the population and the productivity of the soil
as the two variables which can usetully characterize the situation
of a people with a constant technology and living in a fixed
finite area. From these two (classes of) data one can calculate
what the needs of the population are and how much land will be
cultivated. Once this is known, we can find out how much will be
produced and what the rate of change of the productivity is.
Then food per capita and therefore also birth- and death- rates
can be calculated. If we assume for the moment that it will not
be necessary to consider subregions, a model with a build up as
above will have three natural parts. The first one concerns the
influence of food per capita on the demography, the second one the
calculation of the cultivated areas, and the third one the effect
of cultivation on productivity.

Demography

Population is divided in 4 age classes: 0-4, 5-14, 15-45,
45+. People mature from one age class to the next. For each class
there is an age specific mortality directly dependent on life expectancy at birth as in the Coale-Demeny tables, model West.
Births enter into the 0-4 class. The birth rate is a simple quoti-
ent of the number of exposed women and the average birth interval.
In determining the average birth interval, we have distinguished
between cases where the previous child died and where this did
not happen. When a baby dies, the mother, of necessity, stops
breastfeeding earlier than normal. In the circumstances of Kivu
this means that the mother's postpartum amenorrhea is shortened
and that she is fertile quicker. Since sexual taboos hardly
exist, the next baby will be so much earlier in coming. Hence,
in this case, birth interval is the sum of the (average) time
before a baby dies (if it dies before lactation is halted
at 1.5 years) plus the conception and pregnancy delays (2.2 years).
When the child lives, there is a longer amenorrhea due to prolonged
lactation.

Given the practice in Kivu of natural lactation, the only
variable affecting length of amenorrhea is food per capita. When
nutrition drops below 80% of the present values both amenorrhea
become much longer. Eventually amenorrhea is practically
permanent. The numerical assumptions are represented in Figure 3.
It is clear that the birth intervals in the two cases differ most
when the nutritional situation is best. The weight, being used
to calculate the average birth interval is proportional to the age
specific mortality for the 0-4 class.

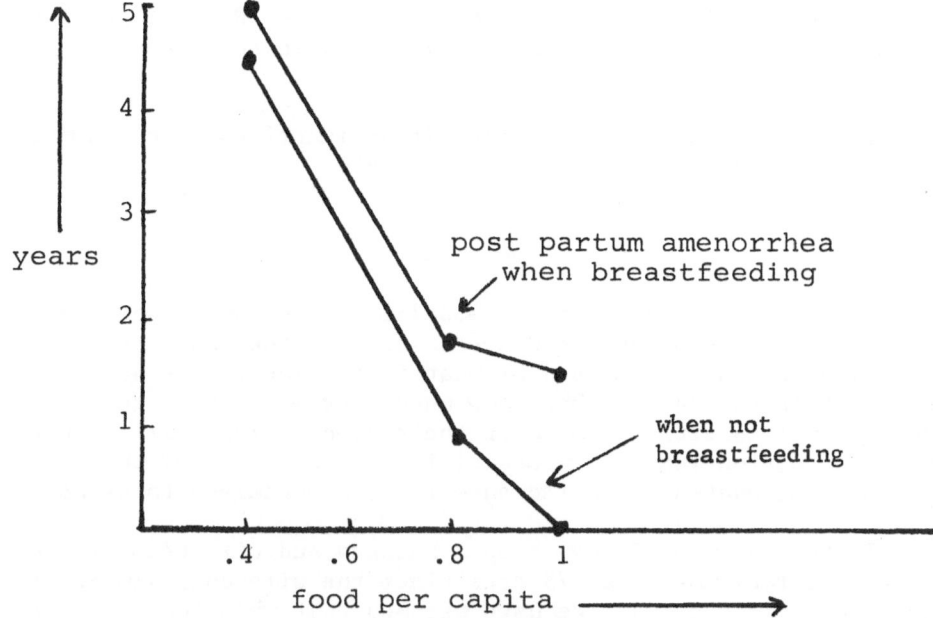

Figure 3. Assumed duration of postpartum amenorrhea as a function of food per capita (expressed as a proportion of requirement).

The number of exposed women is proportional to the population in the 15-44 class. The proportionality factor depends linearly on the age of marriage. Women over 25 form 30% of the population class 15-44. Seventy-five percent of those are still in the reproductive process. Below 25 the only obstacles to having children are not being married or having primary sterility. The latter concerns about 6% and we have assumed that all women over the average age of marriage and below 25 are married. The present age of marriage is about 18.

The death rates depend in an age specific manner on life expectancy at birth. This life expectancy is - in the model - a fixed function of food per capita and some external influence - only of importance before 1960 - representing the introduction of cassave. Given the problem definition, it is sufficient to express food per capita only in calories relative to a daily norm of 2000. Indeed when caloric intake falls, proteins will follow or have preceded in diminishing. It was very difficult to express life expectancy as a function of food per capita. We have assumed that at 80% of the present caloric intake - i.e. about 1600 cal/day/person - life expectancy would fall only to 38 years from the

present 40. At 60% it would be on the average 30 years and for
40% it would be 20 years. Graphically this is represented in
Figure 4.

    The labour force is a simple linear function of the numbers
of people in the age classes 15-44 and 45+.

Production

    The cultivated area in the model is a minimum of what the
inhabitants perceive as their needs, of what they physically
maximally can cultivate, and of what is available. We have
assumed that the farmers know how much they would have to farm
under normal conditions to cover their needs. They will adjust
their perception when the productivity drops. Part of the loss
will be compensated by an increase in area perceived to be needed.

    In the absence of cash crop a husband and wife team will not
be able to farm more than 75 ares since the wife does almost all
the work on food crops. We have assumed that when the food per
capita has been low for some years that this surface area of 75
ares diminished first a little, then more. The precise form is
shown in Figure 5. Because we have distinguished between bananas
and other food crops and we have taken the area used for bananas
by each family of 5 to be constant and equal to 25 ares, food crop
can only grow on arable land which is not used for bananas. A few
simple accounting equations keep track of this. The reason for

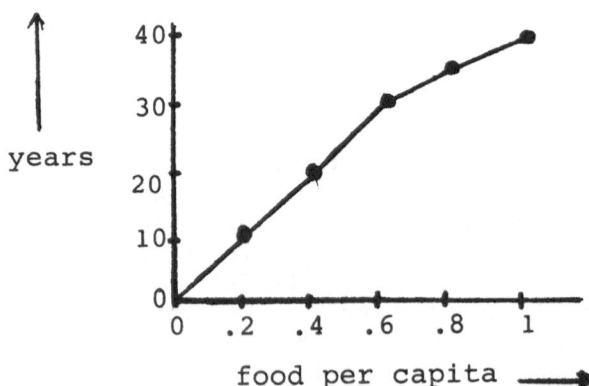

Figure 4. Life expectancy at birth as a function of food per
           capita (expressed as proportion of requirement).

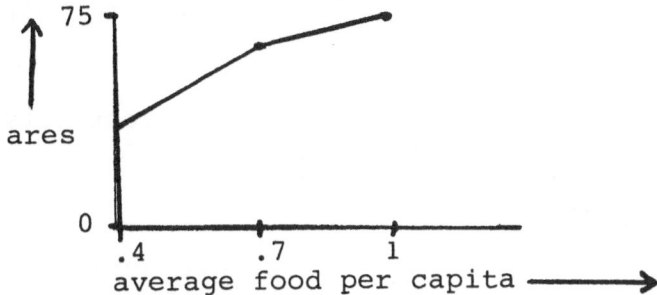

Figure 5. Maximal surface area (in ares) a husband and wife team can cultivate, as a function of food per capita (expressed as a proportion of requirement).

considering separately bananas and other food crop is that the productivity of bananas is only 1,000,000 cal/ha and of other food crop on the average 7,000,000 cal/ha. Also banana trees are cultivated quite differently. They have a high economic value and thus occupy a relatively large fraction of land.

Degradation of Land

This is a relatively complicated part of the model. Only a few general remarks will be made. Degradation of land is particularly important for food crops which are cultivated on an annual basis and for which only fallow periods are used to restore the productivity of the fields. In the model we have taken the fraction of available arable land which is cultivated with annual crops as a measure for the ratio between the periods that soils are being cultivated and lie fallow. This cultivated fraction, for short, is the "motor" of this part of the model.

Two kinds of degradation have been distinguished: on the one hand irreversible degradation or erosion and on the other reversible degradation referring mostly to exhaustion of the soils. Thus at any moment there are two kinds of productivities (see Figure 6). First there is the actual productivity of a field. Next, if this field would be fallow for a long period, its productivity would increase to a certain maximal productivity. This last productivity is lower than the productivity in 1920. The difference represents the irreversible degradation. The difference between actual and maximal productivity corresponds to reversible degradation.

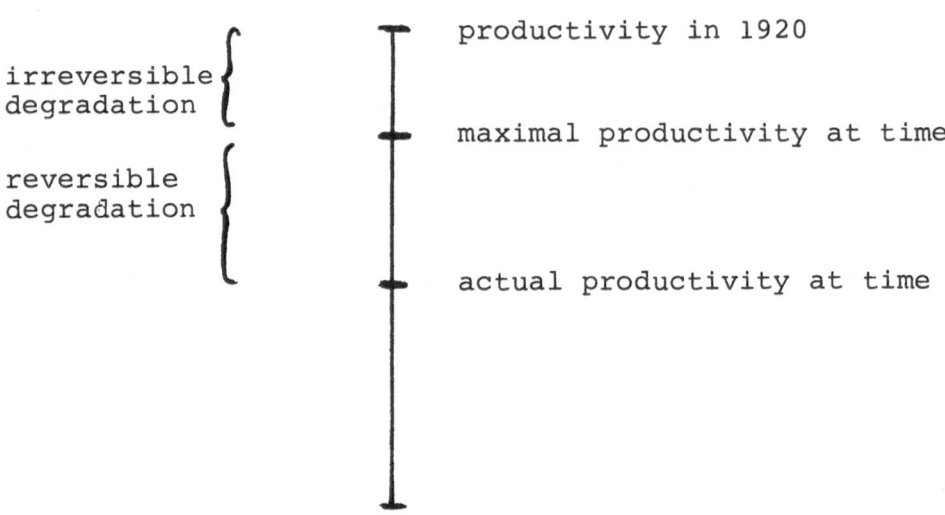

Figure 6.   Productivities and degradation.

It was estimated by the experts that the reversible degradation on the fertile soils of Kivu was not so important - at the
most 20% of the maximal productivity. The irreversible degradation,
however, could be several percentages annually of the maximal productivity. Figure 7 represents an average assumption. Different
rates of irreversible degradation were used for various kinds of
soils. The sensitivity of the model to the precise form of the
rates turned out not to be strong.

SIMULATIONS

At first we have simulated the developments in Kivu with the
model as presented here where all of Kivu is taken as one large
region with homogeneous conditions concerning agriculture and
demography. In Figure 8 the first result is shown. The horizontal
axis in Figure 8 represents time, from 1920 to 2050. On the
vertical axis are scales of 0 to 10,000,000 for the population,
and of 0 to 1 for food per capita, which is expressed in multiples
of 7,000,000 cal/year/person or about 2000 cal/day/person.

Apparently it follows from the assumption in the model that
the nutritional situation in Kivu would not alter significantly
for the worse within the next 20 years. After 2000 an accelerating

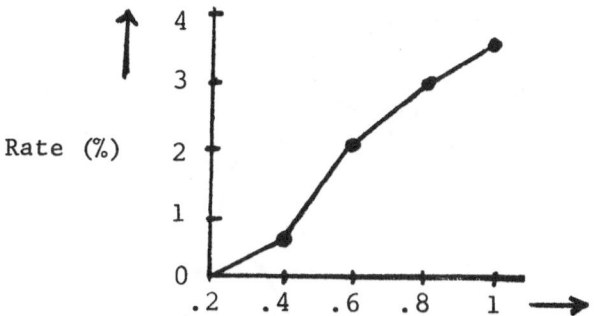

Fraction of arable land being cultivated
with annual crops

Figure 7. Annual rate of irreversible degradation with
increasingly intensive cultivation.

decline would set in. The population would peak around 2020 at
7,500,000, almost 4 times the present value.

     This result does not seem right. There are problems already
now in the more densely populated parts of Kivu. Simulations
with a simpler model show strong sensitivity to population density
and quality of the soil. About 2/3 of the population lives in the
20% of the region where the soils are best. Hence it seems worthwhile to disaggregate Kivu in two regions G and L, where G
represents the best 20% of the soils and L the rest. The G and L
submodels have the same structure as the model described so far.
The parameters and other numerical assumptions are different in
the model. Migration from G to L is possible. On the one hand
young farmers and their wives can migrate to L when there is no
more soil available for them on G and as long as they can still
build on L. On the other hand large scale migration of whole
groups of the population takes place when famines in G force
people to leave.

     In Figure 9 the first simulation with the disaggregated
model of food and population is shown. The scales are the same
as before. The migration of young adults indicates which percentage - from 0 to 100 - of them moves out of C. We have
neglected migration (of adults) due to famines. We see that food
per capita in G starts deteriorating around 1970 and has fallen
to .75, i.e. 1500 cal/day/person, by 2000. The population in G
levels off at about 2,000,000 around 1990, due to a worsening
nutrition and a drastic migration of young adults. This migration

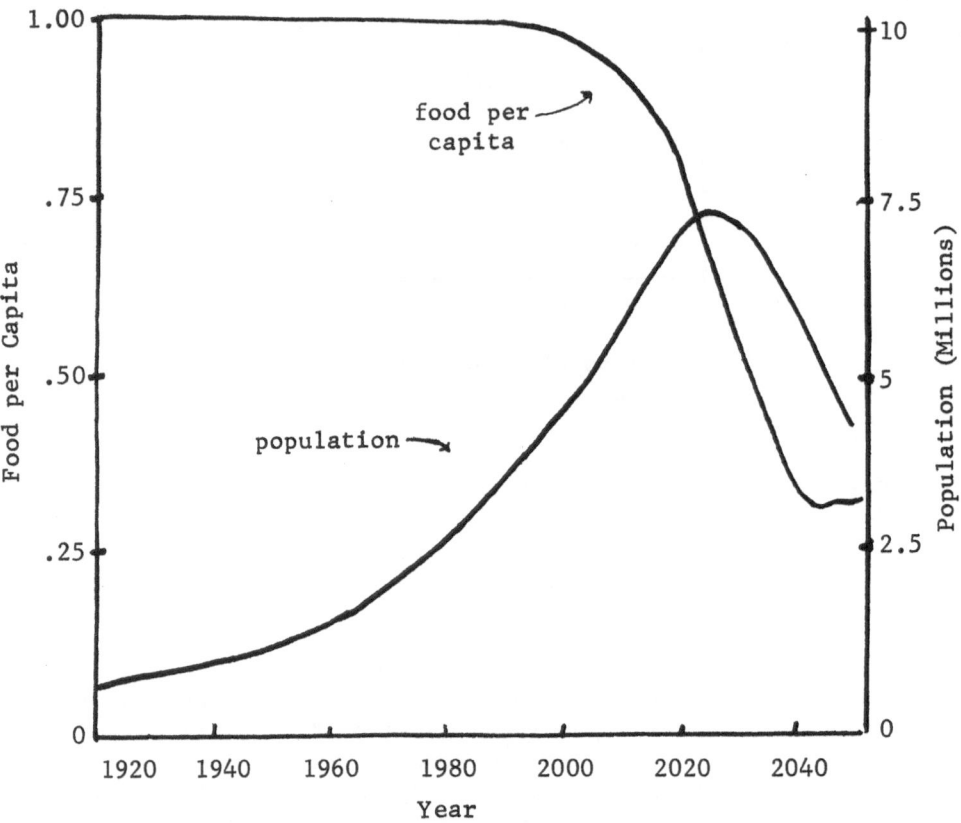

Figure 8. Simulation of population and food per capita in
Kivu considered as one homogeneous region.

declines again when also L is filled up. In L nothing happens
until after 2010. Then decline is very steep because erodability
is bigger in L and all young migrants from G have boosted L's
population.

    In Figure 10 we show the behaviour of birth and death rates
of the same scenario. From 1920 to 1960 mortality falls and birth
rates increase because of exogenous influences. From 1960-1980
they are constant in both G and L. Then food per capita decreases
strongly in G; also G is filling up and critical values of soil
occupation are reached. Hence young adults move in large numbers
to L. The composition of the population on L changes in such a
way that the birth rate increases.

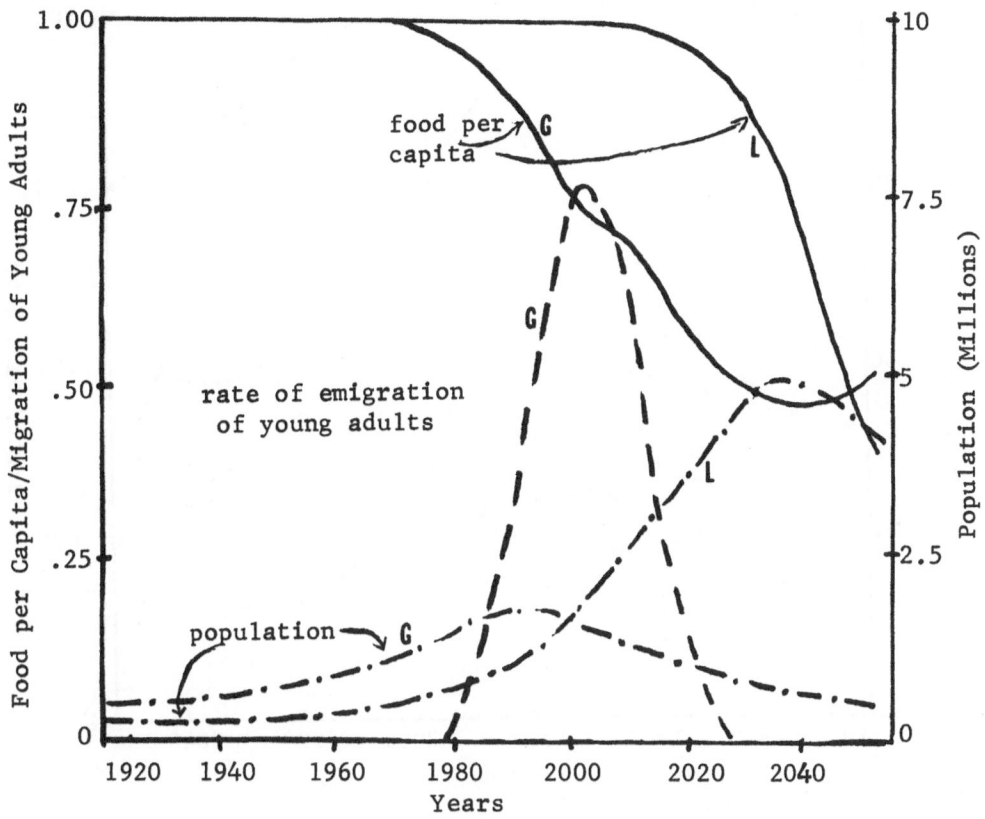

Figure 9. Simulation of population, migration and food per capita in zones G and L of Kivu.

On G the population looses young people. Initially only because of this reason the birth rate on G declines; but then nutrition deteriorates so that birth intervals get longer and the deep drop from around 40 per 1000 to 20 per 1000 must be due to this - assumed - cause. A similar development occurs 40 years later on L except that there migration plays no role.

It is also remarkable to see that death rate increases only slowly and not to such high values. This is due to the gradual onset of the famine: first the weak members of the population die and, so to say, the age composition changes as to maximize life expectancy, even at such low values of food per capita.

The fourth set of graphs of the same scenario show in Figure 11 the development of productivity and cultivated fraction. The same suddeness in the developments appears: the cultivated fraction

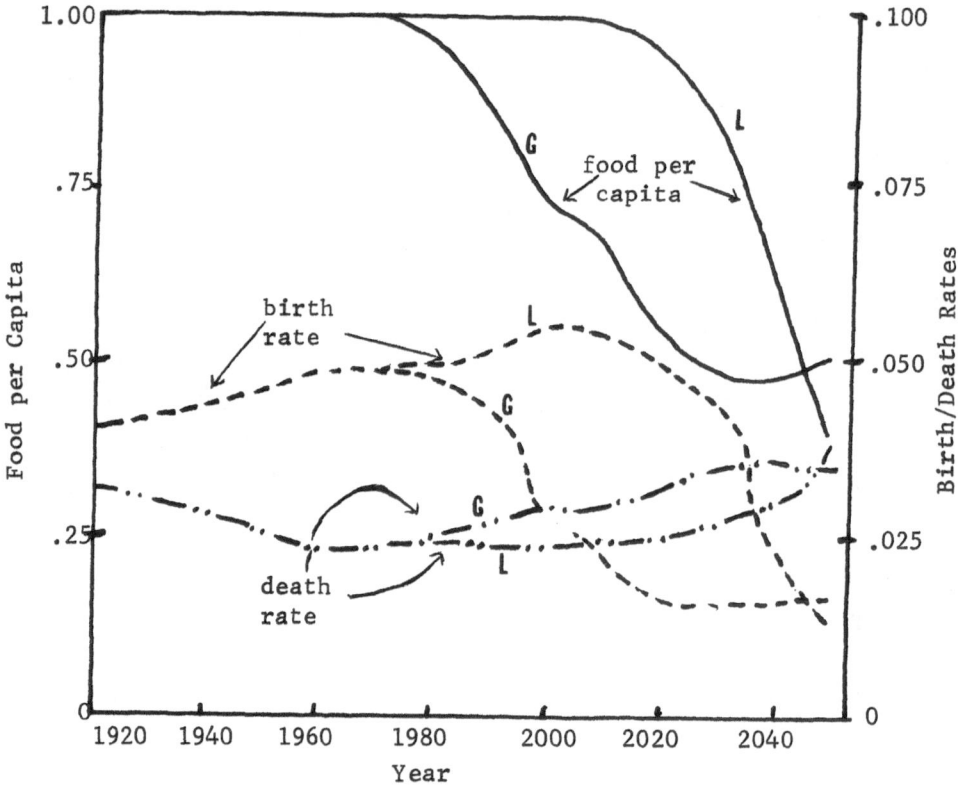

Figure 10. Simulation of birth and death rates in zones G and L in Kivu as a function of food per capita.

on G increases from 30% in 1960 to 50% by 1976, to 80% by 1985, and 100% by 1994. The years are of course only indicative. This is a 3 fold increase within 30 years. The productivity falls from 100% to 50% also in 30 years. In the same period of 1970 to 2000 the population on G doubles, so that food per capita falls anyway, even though the farmers compensate much of the loss in productivity by cultivating more.

The fifth and last figure (Figure 12) of this scenario presents the evolution of the bounds to the cultivated area. It is interesting to see that at least in Kivu - according to the present assumptions of 74 ares maximally per couple - much less is cultivated than is physically possible. Also, there is free land available for cultivation. The reason that there is food shortage in the model from 1970 on is that the farmers compensate only partly for the loss in fertility, which they don't perceive fully. The decline in fertility also would be so much faster if

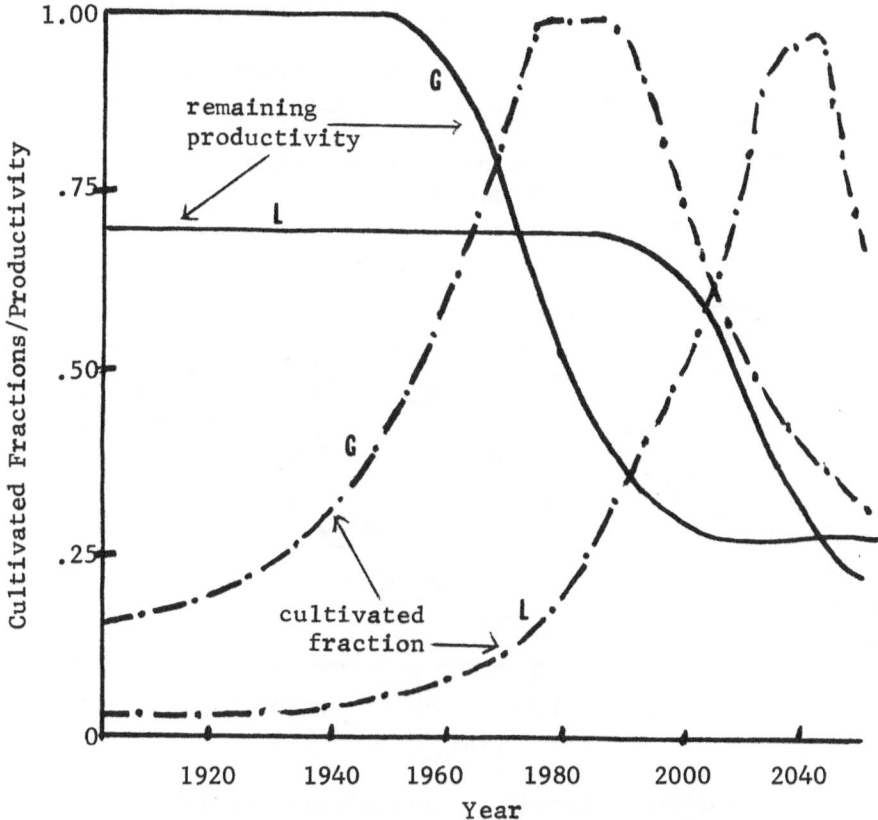

Figure 11. Simulation of agricultural productivity as a function of the cultivated fraction of available land.

compensation for it would be total. Because of low food per capita, the ability to work also diminishes. Hence the maximal physically possible cultivable area declines rapidly after 1990. Also, many people die or leave the area, the strongest young men and women among them. Only after 2010 is the physical ability the operating limit to cultivation.

CONCLUSIONS

It would be possible to show many more simulations. The sensitivity of the model behaviour to reasonable changes in parameters has been tested; erosion-prevention and fertility maintenance programmes have been implemented. Also, assumptions on migration have been varied. It turns out that most programmes just take too long a time to implement to effectively prevent a drastic

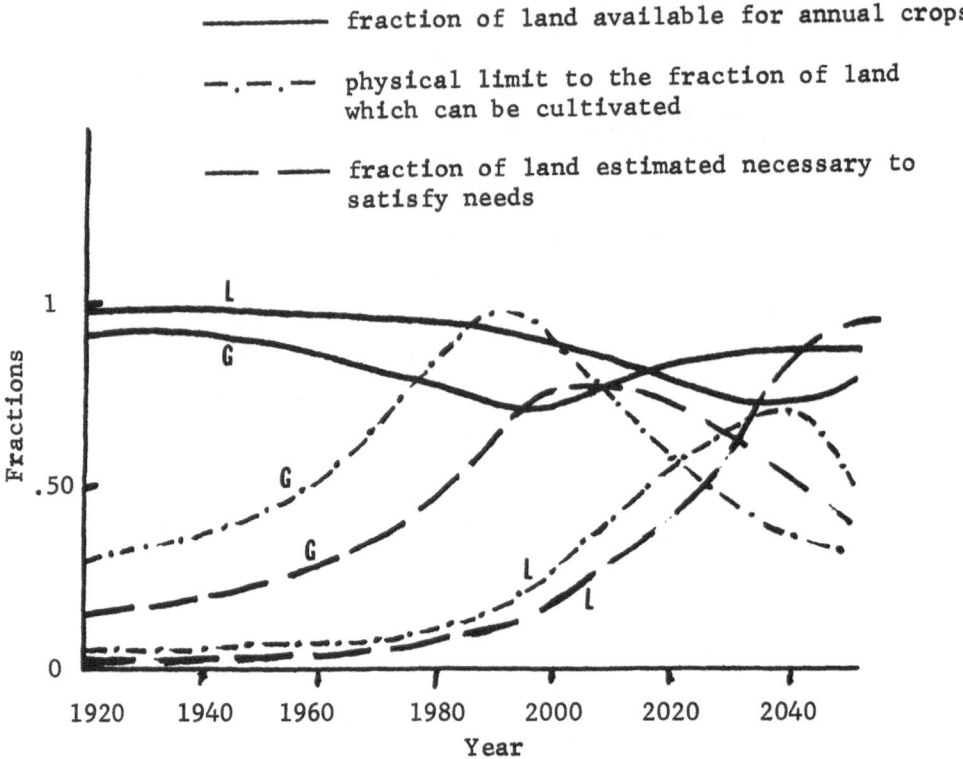

——————— fraction of land available for annual crops

—.—.— physical limit to the fraction of land
which can be cultivated

—— —— fraction of land estimated necessary to
satisfy needs

Figure 12. Simulation of trends in agricultural variables in Kivu.

deterioration of the situation in G. The most effective policy
seems to be to try to gain some time by making it attractive for
the Kivu population to migrate to now under-populated areas
further to the west where there is still an economic potential.
When the population pressure in Kivu can be diminished, it makes
sense to try to improve the situation there also. Programmes
directly aimed at Kivu seem to generate their own undoing by
further pushing up population density.

One of the clearest conclusions of the modeling attempts is
the suddeness with which deterioration sets in and accelerates.
In reality, because of stochastic differences and the relative
unimportance of the first signs of the decline, it is unlikely that
the situation will become clear until Kivu is well on its way to
desertification. Given also the political and economic situation
it will be nearly impossible to implement successfully any project
aimed at resolving the situation.

From a modeling point of view, one could conclude that it seems worthwhile to distinguish between reversible and irreversible degradation ; the interaction between demographic and agricultural processes produces sudden collapses which cannot be predicted by separate sub-models; and the effects of nutrition on birth intervals and on ability to work are potentially very important - but are not well documented.

Bibliography

1. Wils, W., Caraël, M. and Tondeur, G. Le Kivu montagneux, surpopulation, sous-nutrition, érosion du sol. (Etude prospective par simulations mathématiques). Preliminary version available from CEMUBAC, c/o Prof. Dr. H. L. Vis, Hôpital St. Pierre, Rue Haute 320, Brussel 1000, Belgium.

FIELD STUDIES

INTRODUCTORY STATEMENT

Jean-Pierre Habicht

National Center for Health Statistics

Rockville, Maryland

The papers in this section present data on recent and ongoing field studies which seek to define the relationships between nutrition, particularly maternal nutrition and reproductive performance. These field studies from countries in Asia, Africa and Latin America reflect various study designs; however, they share certain fundamental features in their conceptualization of the problems.

Figure 1 provides a general analytical framework illustrating the biological interrelationships between maternal and infant nutrition, breast-feeding and reproduction which is common to all of the studies reported here. This figure identifies quite simply certain known relationships; for example, breast-feeding is known to promote lactation which will lead to improved infant nutrition. Supplemental feeding can improve infant nutrition directly, but it is likely to suppress breast-feeding. Since breast-feeding promotes post partum amenorrhea as well, it is possible that supplementation by reducing breast-feeding will lead to a shortening of post partum amenorrhea and accelerate the onset of the next pregnancy.

Good maternal nutrition is important for a favorable pregnancy outcome and is related to the volume of milk produced during lactation. Both pregnancy and lactation, however, do create a nutritional drain on the mother. The questions that are of major importance to this Conference, are: what is the effect of maternal nutritional status on the duration of post partum amenorrhea and what is its effect on fecundity once menstruation reappears? These questions are important since the durations of these two states determine the timing of the next pregnancy and ultimately the fertility rate.

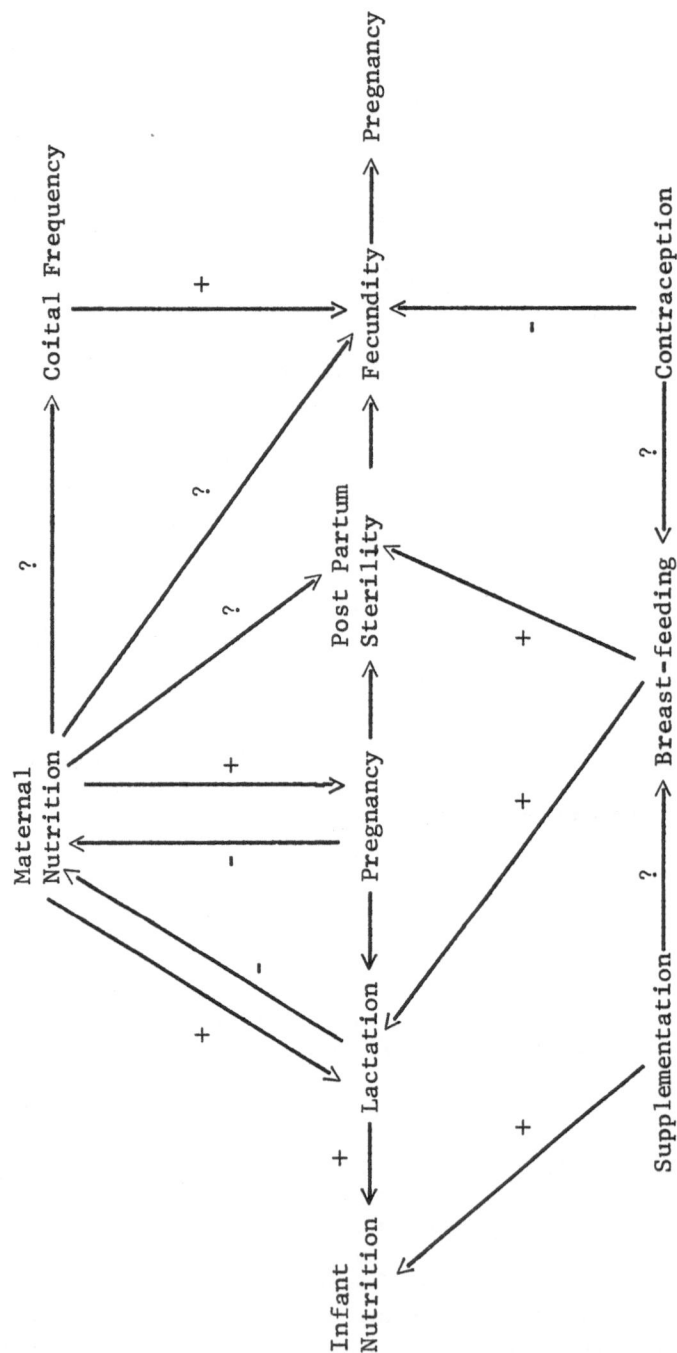

Figure 1. A general analytical framework illustrating some of the biological interrelationships between maternal and infant nutrition, breast-feeding, infant supplementation, lactation, and reproduction. The (+) and (-) with the arrows represent generally recognized positive or negative relationships. The (?) represents uncertain relationships.

The hypothesis supported by Frisch elsewhere in this volume is
that maternal malnutrition suppresses reproductive performance
both by prolonging post partum amenorrhea, and also by suppressing
fecundity. Figure 1 which shows only a few basic biological relationships illustrates some of the variables that must be controlled
in order to test this hypothesis. For example, since the pattern
of breast-feeding influences post partum amenorrhea, and since it
in turn is influenced by supplementation practices, these variables
must be controlled in order to determine if there is an independent effect of maternal nutrition on post partum amenorrhea.
Similarly, in order to assess an effect of maternal nutritional
status on fecundability one must control for variations in contraceptive usage, or the practice of abstinence by identifying the
social factors influencing coital frequency.

The reports in this section provide considerable information
on these questions although each is subject to certain limitations.
The paper by Cantrelle and Ferry looks for nutrition-fertility
relationships in data from Senegal. They seek to extract relationships on the basis of findings from different large scale surveys.
Their analysis, however, is subjected to rather severe limitations
which they clearly identify: the nutrition surveys typically
include nothing on fertility; and fertility surveys generally have
no data on nutrition. Their data do illustrate variations in
breast-feeding between urban and rural areas which are strongly
correlated with variations in postpartum amenorrhea. Independent
studies show variations and calorie and protein consumption
between the rural and urban areas as well as within these areas by
season; however, the data are inadequate to correlate these with
variations in amenorrhea. Subject to the limitations of data,
the authors can only conclude that if nutritional status determines fertility, this influence appears to be minor.

Carael in his report contrasts the variation of lactational
amenorrhea in three Central African communities and seeks to
relate this to rather impressive dietary differences between these
communities. His data indicate that a Highland community with a
high carbohydrate diet deficient in protein had the longest duration of post partum amenorrhea even after controlling for equivalent
durations of breast-feeding. These results are strengthened by
further comparisions between rural and urban communities. The
weakness in the approach is that there were many social and
cultural differences between the communities since they represented
different tribal groups, and it remains possible that some of these
differences could have accounted for the variations in post partum
amenorrhea.

Delgado and others present a secondary analysis of data
obtained from four communities in Guatemala which were partici-
pating in feeding programs designed primarily to study physical

and mental development of infants and young children. Their
analysis reveals a small but consistent reduction in length of
post partum amenorrhea among mothers who took the largest nutritional supplementation during pregnancy. Also there was a small
but not significant negative correlation between mothers' weight
and length of post partum amenorrhea among 160 mothers. All these
data again suggest some effect of maternal nutrition on the duration of lactational amenorrhea. The results are difficult to
interpret, however, since the mothers were self-selected in the
use of the nutritional supplement, and there were no data available
on maternal breast-feeding practices or infant supplementation
during the period of lactation.

Coming to Asia, Chowdhury presents some early results being
generated from a prospective followup of over 2000 women in rural
Bangladesh. In his report he searches for correlates on the duration of the menstruating interval as well as post partum amenorrhea.
The two strongest associations are those that had been reported
elsewhere, that is, with increasing age of the woman both the
length of post partum amenorrhea and the waiting time to conception
are prolonged, and, after controlling for the age effect in a
multiple regression analysis, he finds parity negatively related
to the length of both amenorrhea and menstruating intervals. This
latter finding is not surprising since a woman must have short
intervals in order to reach high parity. Not surprisingly,
husbands' absences are associated with conception delays. The
nutritional indicators he uses (height, weight, and arm circumference) were not significantly associated with either the length of
post partum amenorrhea or the menstruating interval.

Osteria presents the results of a prospective study in urban
Philippines which is undergoing a substantial transition in breastfeeding practices and use of contraception. She shows for a group
of women having recently delivered in one hospital that the duration
of breast-feeding declined sharply with the woman's education and
her employment status. The shorter durations of breast-feeding
were directly correlated with short durations of post partum
amenorrhea. A high percentage of the women accepted contraception.
She undertook an interesting analysis to determine how well contraceptive usage compensated for the expected shortening of birth
intervals due to declines in breast-feeding practice. IUD acceptors
appeared to be quite well protected; by contrast, women who accepted
the pill had very poor continuation rates and thus ultimately got
pregnant as rapidly as women who had used no contraceptives whatso-
ever.

The most comprehensive examination of the multiple factors
linking nutrition to fertility is the study currently underway by
Hall in Indonesia. Only preliminary data are available in her
report; however, she outlines a rather comprehensive analysis

identifying the multiplicity of factors that must be considered, including, for breast-feeding mothers, frequency and duration of suckling, suckling substitutes, use of supplementary foods, arrangement for breast-feeding by working mothers and weaning patterns. Also of importance in this locality is the widespread practice of post partum sexual abstinence. Numerous measurements of nutritional indicators have been taken on infants and mothers although these data are not yet available. This study is the only one of the group reported that not only takes a comprehensive look at most of the important variables but also recognizes the importance of qualitative as well as quantitative variations. For example, she is seeking to define the actual quantity, quality, frequency and timing of supplementary feedings, as well as looking at the timing, duration and intensity of suckling by the infant.

Given that the actual practice of breast-feeding is such a critical component of any analysis of nutrition fertility interrelationships, it is important that the social and cultural factors determining this behavior be dissected out. Popkin has approached this problem in the rural Philippines by seeking to analyze the economic determinants of breast-feeding behavior within a multivariate framework. He focuses to a considerable degree on factors indigenous to the household such as family composition, wage rates and income of family members. The single factor having the strongest effect, both in breast-feeding participation as well as duration of breast-feeding, was actually not an economic variable per se but the mother's belief regarding whether breast-feeding was better than bottle feeding. Lack of sufficient variability in breast-feeding patterns in this rural area resulted in small and mostly insignificant correlations with the economic determinants. As the author suggests, however, these economic models may be useful in the situation where there is a wider range of behavior, such as occurs in the urban areas.

In the discussions following this session, a number of general points particularly relating to methodological considerations were identified. For example, the more explicitly the assumptions are identified, and the experimental design and data collection procedure standardized, the more likely it is that inferences about cause and effect can be drawn from the results. This is true because interrelationships such as those depicted in Figure 1 are extremely complex in field situations. The attempt by Cantrelle to relate aggregate indicators of nutritional status in the population to fertility change was not successful because such aggregates are not sensitive enough at the levels of nutrition which prevailed. The specificity of these indicators is also difficult to ascertain, so that even when they can be related to fertility, as in famine situations, the contributions of biological changes in nutrition status as opposed to accompanying changes in psychological behavior cannot be elucidated.

All field study designs also have measurement problems in that variables that can be measured are often only indirect indicators of the underlying facts that cannot be directly measured. For example, the state of amenorrhea with lactation is taken as an indicator of sterility. In fact, in most cases the first ovulation will occur in the amenorrheac state preceding the first menstruation. Similarly, menstruation is taken as an indicator of ovulatory cycles that are susceptible to successful fertilization and pregnancy. This, of course, may not always be the case.

Ideally, variables that are measured should reflect accurately changes in the underlying facts that one wishes to describe. A clear definition of the underlying fact and its relation to the indicator variable can often help to correct for inevitable deficiencies in the sensitivity and specificity of the indicators.

These studies reveal several types of problems in nutrition-fertility research. For example, measurement and interpretation of indicators of the maternal nutritional status may be quite different if the mother's lactational performance and her reproductive performance depend on different nutritional factors. Several papers in this volume suggest that a woman's fecundability may depend on body fat while her lactation performance may depend on adequacy of protein intake. If this is the case, it is then clear that appropriate indicators of nutritional status that relate to these functions would be different.

With reference to fecundity, reproductive performance cannot be adequately described without some estimate of the timing of insemination as well as the woman's fecundability. Coital frequency is thus important, but reported coital frequency may reflect social norms rather than actual practice. Similarly, separation of the spouses may not be an adequate indicator of no coital activity.

Another area where clarity of terminology is important relates to the distinction between lactation which is a physiological function of the mother and breast-feeding which is a pattern of behavior involving the mother and the child. These inter-relationships are shown in Figure 1. Recognizing this distinction makes it clear that the measurement of breast-feeding should reflect the combination of suckling intensity, frequency, and duration, since these appear to be the factors that promote both lactation and post partum sterility. Thus, while "partial" breast-feeding is indicative of a behavior pattern involving providing other nutritional supplements to the child, it may or may not be associated with any variation in the physiological responses of the mother in terms of lactation and infecundity.

Two examples can clarify the situation. A supplemental

feeding which is calorically inadequate but contains important
nutrients such as protein, vitamins and minerals may be vitally
important for maintaining growth and development of a nine month
old child. At the same time, this supplement may not depress at
all the suckling characteristics that promote maternal lactation
and amenorrhea. We thus have a situation where in the context of
the child this supplementary feeding is critical and thus the
child would be considered as partially breast-feeding. On the
other hand, in the context of maternal physiology, the supplementary feeding is negligible so that the mother is fully lactating.

The opposite situation could exist if sugar water or similar
food is ingested by the suckling child. This sugar water may
provide only negligible nutrients to the child but will likely
markedly reduce the suckling vital for maintaining lactation and
infecundity. From the standpoint of the mother we would have to
say that there is only partial lactation and possibly resumption
of menses. From the standpoint of the nutrition of the child, for
all practical purposes, the child should be considered as fully
breast-feeding since most of the vital nutrients would be provided
by breast milk.

In addition to problems relating to definition of appropriate
indicators, there are problems with imperfect measurements. Differing levels of measurement error will result in differing
strengths of statistical association between independent and
dependent variables even though the true associations are the
same. Therefore different strengths of statistical association
between independent and dependent variables cannot be used to infer
true differences in association unless the statistical parameters
of association are corrected by estimates of measurement error (1).
The error to be estimated must be the error of the indicator in
estimating the underlying mechanism of concern (2).

A number of the studies utilized life tables which permit the
analyzing of open intervals. Life table techniques are required
in order to avoid bias that will occur in utilizing only closed
interval data which are collected over relatively short sampling
times, since a short study will over sample for short intervals.
A disadvantage of life table methods is that they only permit comparison from the large groups and are not amenable to multi-
variant regression analysis. Anderson, et al. (3) has presented a
regression with "open" interval data.

The most frequent reason for incorrect inferences about cause
and effect is not the confusion of cause with effect. The false
inferences about causality that usually occur because of a statistical association between two variables are due to not recognizing
this association as being caused solely by a third unexpected

variable, a "confounding" variable. This is important in considering the possible association between maternal nutrition and shortened post partum amenorrhea. The confounding variable may be the
nutrition of the suckling child. Better nourished mothers may
have better nourished children because the children are better
supplemented; the supplemented child suckles less vigorously so
that the post partum interval is shortened. Similarly, if a
study shows mothers who receive extra food ration having shortened
post partum amenorrhea, this may not be due to improved maternal
nutrition but may well be due to concurrent ingestion of extra
food rations by the suckling child.

While it is clear that such a confounding variable should
enter into all analysis, it is usually not possible in field
studies to measure all imaginable much less unimaginable confounding variables. Therefore, inferences as to causality must depend
upon how consistently an effect, such as shortened post partum
amenorrhea, is associated with the presumed cause, in this case
improved maternal nutrition, across many different circumstances.
These differing circumstances must be so chosen that the possibility of similar inadvertent confoundings are excluded. Feeding
trials can be useful in this context.

References

1. Duncan, O. D. Introduction to Structural Equation Models.
   1975, Academic Press, New York.

2. Habicht, J. P., Yarbrough, C. Y., and Martorell, R. (In
   preparation). Criteria for Selection of Anthropometric
   Indicators of Nutritional Status. In: Nutrition and Growth,
   Jelliff, D. B. and Jelliff, E. F. (eds.). To be published.

3. Anderson, B. A. and McCabe, J. L. Nutrition and the Fertility
   of Younger Women in Kinshasa, Zaire. To be published.

THE INFLUENCE OF NUTRITION ON FERTILITY

THE CASE OF SENEGAL

Pierre Cantrelle and Benoit Ferry

Office de la Recherche Scientifique et Technique

Outre-mer, Paris, France

INTRODUCTION: THE THEORETICAL FRAMEWORK

We can consider the relationship between nutrition and fertility as having a double direction: numerous or closely-spaced pregnancies can have an effect upon the nutritional status of the mother; and, conversely, the woman's nutritional status can have an effect upon her risk of conceiving and upon the outcome of the pregnancy. We will limit ourselves here to the latter case, that is, the influence of nutrition upon fertility.

In order to identify the relationships that may exist between two factors, both a careful description of the factors and a specification of the analytical framework are necessary. Nutrition can be assessed directly or indirectly: directly, by the nutritional status of an individual, measured according to clinical, anthropometric or biochemical criteria; indirectly, by consumption, rarely determinable on an individual level because of measurement difficulties, and therefore most often measured at the household level, and, less precisely, by measuring production and the flow of foodstuffs at the level of the overall population.

As far as fertility is concerned, different measures are applicable: at the individual level, measures based on number of children, at any given age, or on birth intervals; at the global level, measures of current fertility rates. It should be clear that the actual number of children is a result of a past situation and therefore cannot be related to the present nutritional status. On the other hand, birth intervals are a good indicator, provided

that the nutritional status has been evaluated for the corresponding periods.

The relation between nutrition and fertility can only be
explained if the intermediate mechanisms of the relationship have
been taken into account. Dietary deficiencies can be considered
to intervene in several different ways:

1. by acting directly upon the frequency of sexual relations;

2. by creating a climate favorable to the occurrence and
    persistence of infectious diseases, which would, in
    turn, affect the subject's risk of exposure to sexual
    relations and to conception;

3. by prolonging the period of postpartum amenorrhea, or,
    indirectly, by shortening the duration of breast-feeding
    and, therefore, of postpartum amenorrhea;

4. by increasing the risk of spontaneous abortion;

5. by any influence that the mother's nutritional status
    might have on infant and child mortality which would
    have a direct repercussion on the birth interval.

Needless to say, any relationship can only hold true in the
absence of contraception and of non-nutritionally-caused sterility
or infertility.

It should be noted that a less favorable nutritional status
can have either a positive or a negative effect on fertility
according to the intermediate mechanism invoked. While the first
three imply a lengthening of the interval between conceptions, the
fourth tends to shorten it; however, in all of these cases, the
interval between live births would be lengthened. The fifth, on
the other hand, would imply the shortening of the birth interval
and, consequently, an increase in fertility.

Among the different lines of reasoning suggested above, there
is one which would appear to be particularly interesting to pursue:
that is, to compare, for different nutritional levels, the length
of postpartum amenorrhea, which is an essential factor in determining the birth interval under the conditions we have in mind. It
has been found that the length of postpartum amenorrhea after a
stillbirth or the death of an infant in its first week remains
approximately the same, that is 40-60 days, in observations based
on what is probably a wide range of nutritional situations (1).
Prolonged breastfeeding, bringing with it increased nutritional
needs, would tend to cause more noticeable differences in length
of amenorrhea.

It is rare to have available at the same time data on nutrition and fertility, as well as on the intermediate variables, and this is even rarer on the individual level. Detailed data exist, to be sure, but, for the most part, they relate only to one element of the relationship: often nutritional surveys will include numerous parameters but none on fertility; and, conversely, fertility surveys most often have no nutrition input. This state of affairs is due to the generally different aims of these respective types of study, as well as to the research teams in charge of carrying them out. To this can be added the constraints imposed by comparing different sample sizes.

THE CASE OF SENEGAL

The case of Senegal is, no doubt, not an exceptional one in respect to data limitations and will thus be taken here as an example. We will first briefly discuss the various possible sources of data and indicate which seem to be the most solid.

National and Regional Survey Data

Several nationwide surveys were carried out at about the same time, some providing fertility levels (1960-61) and others nutritional levels (CINAM survey 1960). However, the results of the demographic survey were unreliable and the size of the sample in the nutritional survey only provided average indications (clinical and anthropometric) at the regional level; a correlation at this level (seven regions) would, therefore, hardly be worthwhile.

Let us cite as an example a regional survey in the Senegal river valley (MISOES 1957-58), practically the only multiple-objective survey in Senegal, during which observations were made, for the same period and on the same samples, on demography, budgets, consumption, production, and health status. In this case, however, the nutritional investigation, which was clinical and anthropometric, was only carried out on children of less than 15 years, and not on the women. It is still possible, then, to set up a comparison of the different fertility levels according to different categories for which food consumption levels have been calculated, but the data were not tabulated with this in mind, and it is doubtful that we could go back to the original archives.

Longitudinal Surveys

It is known that the exceptional Sahelian drought of recent years affected parts of Senegal, but precise demographic data for

the afflicted regions are, unfortunately, few and far between.
Observations have, however, been carried out over a 10-year period
in an area situated at the edge of the zone touched by the drought.
This area is composed of a group of villages surrounding Ngayorhem,
in the Sine region. A multiple-round survey carried out annually
from 1963 to 1972 permitted the keeping of a population register,
and thus the entire population of the villages (about 4400 inhabitants) was the object of follow-up observation (2,3).

      The series of data on rainfall, natality, infant mortality
and child mortality (1-3 years) are presented in parallel in
Table 1 and illustrate the precariousness of this approach to the
subject. We do not have at our disposal data on variations in
food production and even less on variations in consumption. The
indicator tied here to production is rainfall. The recent years
of marked drought in Africa have been 1968, 1970 and 1972, with
the subsistence crisis being felt especially in the years following
the bad harvest, i.e., in 1969, 1971 and 1973. But measures of
rainfall are not available for 1968; in addition, the small size
of the demographic sample diminishes the significance of the
results.

      As far as natality is concerned, a drop from 55 to 43 per
thousand can be noted after the dry year of 1968; but this rate of
43 does not seem to be exceptional, and there is no significant
drop after the dry year of 1970. In addition, we should emphasize
that a household's expectation of a subsistence crisis following
upon a bad harvest can have an effect on its fertility behavior,
without the actual nutritional status coming into cause. On the
other hand, it is probable that the highest mortality observed
during the famine of 1969 (infant mortality of 388 per thousand
and child mortality of 246 per thousand) is closely related to the
food crisis.

                 Breastfeeding, Amenorrhea, and Nutrition

      Two other surveys offer somewhat more solid data about the
nutrition-fertility relationship by taking into account the variables of postpartum amenorrhea and breastfeeding. In the first
survey, observations were carried out on three groups of about 700
women, one an urban group in Pikine, suburb of Dakar, one semi-
urban in Khombole, a small market town located 100 km from Dakar,
and one rural, in villages of the arrondissement of Thienaba,
neighboring the locality of Khombole.

      The method followed is of the same type as described above,
i.e., longitudinal observations, by even more frequent rounds,
every four months, but only over a two-year period (1968-69). At

each round, the female investigators took note of the situation
with regard to breastfeeding, amenorrhea and postpartum abstinence.

The second survey (4) was carried out in 1972 on an urban
sample, representative of the whole of the city of Dakar. The
national demographic survey provided the basis for the sample of
1460 women. In a retrospective interview each woman was asked
questions about the length of breastfeeding and postpartum amenorrhea corresponding to her last childbirth.

While these two surveys contribute precise data on fertility
in the form of information on birth intervals, postpartum amenorrhea
and breastfeeding, their objective was not centered on the nutrition-fertility relationship. Thus, there were no observations
on the nutrition or health status of the mothers. Nevertheless,
certain global data on the nutrition of the populations in the
areas concerned can be used.

A comparison between the two urban surveys (Table 2) shows a
rather close concordance of fertility related variables. This is
also the case for the rural zone (Table 3). The area of Thienaba,
whose inhabitants belong to the Wolof and Serer ethnic groups,
compares similarly with other rural observations made in 1963-68
in the Sine-Saloum region which were carried out, to a great
extent, on the same ethnic groups. These similarities in results
increase the credibility of the studies.

Table 1

Observations in Rural Ngayorhem,
Sine Region, Senegal, 1962-1972

Year	Rainfall (mm)	Birth Rate (per 1000)	Infant Mortality (per 1000)	Child Mortality Rate 1-3 Years (per 1000)
1962	485	---	---	---
1963	740	51	206	119
1964	850	52	366	173
1965	562	45	193	144
1966	807	49	341	162
1967	729	44	194	70
1968	---	55	192	81
1969	742	43	388	246
1970	422	54	194	113
1971	681	50	---	---
1972	227	52	---	---

Table 2

Comparison of Fertility Related Variables in
an Urban Setting, Dakar, Senegal

	Dakar-Pikine 1968 (Months)	Whole Dakar 1972 (4) (Months)
Breastfeeding mean	18.9	18.9
median	19.3	17.6
Postpartum amenorrhea	12.3	9.8
Mean birth interval	32.5	31.8
Mean age at menarche	14.5 years	14.3 years

Table 3

Comparison of Fertility Related Variables
in Rural Settings, Senegal

	Thienaba 1968-69 (Months)	Sine 1963-68 (Months)	Saloum 1963-68 (Months)
Breastfeeding mean	23.2	24.3	24.5
median	23.7	24.8	24.3
Mean birth interval	32.6	30.9	31.3

If we now compare the three samples, urban, semi-urban and
rural, observed according to the same methodology, we notice
appreciable differences from one milieu to the other (Table 4).
The difference between the median lengths of breastfeeding and
amenorrhea is slightly greater in the urban than the rural setting,
6.9 months as against 5.8 months. In other words, the length of
amenorrhea is relatively longer in the rural setting. This difference is somewhat longer in the Dakar survey, where it reaches
7.6 months (Table 2).

Table 5 relates the duration of amenorrhea to the length of

Table 4

Comparison of Fertility in Related Variables in Three
Different Settings of Senegal 1968-69

		Urban Dakar-Pikine (Months)	Semi-Urban Khombol (Months)	Rural Thienaba (Months)
Breastfeeding	mean	18.9	19.7	23.2
	median	19.3	19.9	23.7
	S.D.	4.3	3.8	3.8
Complete breast- feeding	mean	7.4	5.7	6.1
PP Amenorrhea	mean	12.3	15.4	17.3
	median	12.4	14.4	17.9
Differences between medians		6.9	5.5	5.8
Correlation (r) between breastfeeding and amenorrhea		0.34	0.32	0.29

Table 5

Mean Duration of Postpartum Amenorrhea by Duration of
Breastfeeding in Three Different Settings of Senegal

Breast Feeding Duration (Months)	Whole Daker * Months	N	Dakar Pilkine Months	N	Khombole Months	N	Thienabe Months	N
1-8	3.8	17	4.2	9		2		-
9-14	6.1	53	7.8	24	12.8	13		3
15-20	10.6	367	11.8	180	14.4	164	15.2	44
21-26	13.2	154	16.1	80	16.6	111	18.5	160
26 +			17.9	11	18.9	5	20.0	38
			12.3	304	15.4	295	17.3	275

* The categories of breastfeeding duration are not exactly the
  same, 1-9, 10-14, 15-19, 20-24 months.

breastfeeding. This also reveals the tendency towards a relative lengthening of postpartum amenorrhea for a given length of breast-feeding when passing from an urban to a rural environment.

What is the situation relating to nutritional levels in these respective settings? The clinical data are too heterogeneous to have much comparative value. For Dakar, the report of the Medina Center for Maternal and Child Health, the most important of the city, indicates that the proportion of cases of kwashiorkor noted among the patients between 1969 and 1972 was, year by year, 0.3, 0.4, 0.1, 0.5 and 0.4%, while in one of the villages in the rural sample, M'Bourwaye, only 1% was noted in 1965 and none in 1966 (5).

Measures on food consumption, on the other hand, are more precise. A balance sheet done for all of Senegal in 1974 (6) shows an appreciable difference between urban and rural settings (Table 6). Per capita calorie and protein intake appears higher in urban areas, as does the proportion of animal proteins in the diet, even though the theoretical needs are, no doubt, very simil-ar in the two settings. However, these are only estimates based on an evaluation of available food supplies.

Again for the city of Dakar, a budget sample survey carried out in March 1974 (7) gives only the monetary value of the products consumed, and the quantities consumed are estimated from a price list (6): 2594 calories and 71.9 grams of protein per person and per day, figures which agree with the evaluation for urban areas previously mentioned.

In the semi-urban area under consideration, Khombole, a nutritional sample survey was carried out in early 1967, covering 56 households (512 persons) (8). This was a survey done by weigh-ing foods for four days in each household and was carried out by investigators under the supervision of a doctor/nutritionist. In the rural setting, a nutritional survey was also made in one of the villages, M'Bourwaye, on the same sample used for the fertil-ity survey (5). This, too, was a weighing survey for five days in each household, carried out in 1965 and then one year later, in 1966, in the same households. Table 7 gives the results of these observations in Khombole and M'Bourwaye.

In spite of the interest of weighing surveys in evaluating consumption levels, their limits are apparent in the present case, for they are confined to a particular moment of time, whereas important seasonal variations exist in the rural milieu, as is shown by the results (Table 8) of a 1958 survey in three villages located 30 km from M'Bourwaye, in the Sine region (9). In addition, the period of the fertility survey and that of the nutrition survey do not coincide, thus limiting even further the implications of their conclusions.

Table 6

Food Consumption Levels-Quantities/Person/Day
1974 Evaluations

| | Senegal | |
	Rural	Urban
Total calories	2068	2495
of which: cereals	1549	1363
animal products	68	367
Total proteins (gm)	57.8	87.3
of which: cereals (gm)	39.4	37.3
: leguminous plants (gm)	7.1	3.4
: animal products (gm)	10.1	45.9
(%)	17.5	52.6

Table 7

Results of Consumption Surveys, Semi-urban
and Rural Settings, Senegal

Period	Khombol Jan.-Apr. 1967	(Arr. Thienaba) May 1965	June 1966
Daily diets, number	2049	444	552
Calories			
N/pers./day	2257	2190	1790
Theoretical needs	2038	2120	2105
Difference (%)	+ 10	+ 3	- 15
Proteins Total (gm)	52.8	69.4	62.0
of which: animal (gm)	17.8	5.7	4.2
(%)	33.7	8.2	6.8
Theoretical needs	63.6	63.1	64.9
Difference (%)	- 17	+ 10	- 4

Table 8

Calorie and Protein Consumption (gm) per Capita by
Village, Sine, Senegal, 1968, Illustrating Seasonal Variations

Period	Ngayokhem		Ngane Fissel		Sob	
	Cal-ories	Pro-teins	Cal-ories	Pro-teins	Cal-ories	Pro-teins
January-February	2230	72.6	2191	73.4	2093	67.0
May-June	1933	59.4	1856	57.0	2023	59.3
September-October	1911	56.2	1654	48.0	1801	56.3

We can only note that, as a general rule, the diet is more abundant in the urban setting, and better balanced with regard to the proportion of animal proteins. These findings go along with those concerning the differential urban and rural mortality observed in Senegal, as in a number of countries: a higher child mortality in rural areas, a phenomenon no doubt tied, in part, to the state of nutrition. However, this excess child mortality does not necessarily prove the unfavorable nutritional status of the mothers: this is only another presumption.

CONCLUSION

An epidemiological study with the specific object of measuring the effects of nutrition on fertility would no doubt be more conclusive than the data available in the present case. This requires individual correlations of a woman's fertility and her nutrititional status, in particular with biochemical tests for latent deficiencies. At present we have only general correlations between populations. Nevertheless, the impression we are left with is that, if the nutritional status partially determines fertility, this influence appears very minor.

References

1. Cantrelle, P., Ferry, B., Mondot, J. Relations entre fécondité et mortalité en Afrique Tropicale. In: Seminar on Infant Mortality in Relation to the Level of Fertility, Bangkok, CICRED, Paris, 185-202, 1975.

2. Gendreau, F., Vaugelade, J. A Population Laboratory in Senegal. In: Population in African Development, Liège, ORDINA ed., 231-

236, 1974.

3. Waltisperger, D. Le fichier de population de N'Gayokheme
    (Sénégal). Analyse des données 1963-70. ORSTOM, Centre de
    Dakar, 109 p., 1974.

4. Ferry, B. Données récentes sur la fécondité à Dakar (Sénégal).
    Population, 717-722, 1976.

5. Lariviere, M., Cros, J., Debroise, A., Diallo, S. Anémie,
    parasitose intestinale et nutrition. In: Conditions de vie
    de l'enfant en milieu rural en Afrique. Centre International
    de l"Enfance, Paris, 201-205, 1968.

6. Anonyme - Rapport de mission. Travaux de groupe mixte
    Sénégal/FAO. Rome, Sept.-Oct. Ministere de Plan et de la
    Coopération, CANAS, Dakar, multigr., 1976.

7. Anonyme - Etude: budget consommation. II-Enquête budgets
    familiaux. Universite de Dakar, Institut Universitaire de
    Technologie, Division tertiaire, Juin 1976.

8. Cros, J., Quenum, C. Enquête alimentaire a Khombole (Sénégal)
    Janvier-Avril 1967. Bull. Soc. Med. Afr. Noire (langue fr.),
    70-78, 1968.

9. Hellegouarch, R., Giorgi, R., Monjour, L. and Toury, J.
    Enquête de consommation alimentaire dans une zone pilote du
    Sénégal (1968). ORANA, Dakar, 1970, 22 p. multigr.

RELATIONS BETWEEN BIRTH INTERVALS AND NUTRITION

IN THREE CENTRAL AFRICAN POPULATIONS (ZAIRE)

Michel Caraël

Medical and Scientific Center, University of Brussels,
Central Africa (CEMUBAC); Institute of Scientific
Research in Central Africa (IRS), Lwiro, Kivu, Zaire

INTRODUCTION

The importance of postpartum amenorrhea in natural fertility
no longer requires demonstration. Various authors (1,2,3) have
shown that postpartum amenorrhea is the major factor determining
the differences in birth intervals. The end of amenorrhea is
usually considered to coincide with the resumption of ovulation
(4,7).

Until recently, the common theory was that the non-susceptible
period - postpartum amenorrhea and 9 months childbearing - equalled
$\pm$ 20 months for a live birth when breastfeeding was natural, i.e.,
on demand, and that postpartum amenorrhea lengths longer than one
year were unusual (4). Now observations conducted in rural
classes, generally living on subsistence diets, provide us
with examples of longer postpartum amenorrhea: Baroda, India, 18
months; Kivu, Zaire, 18.7 months (5-8).

Paradoxically enough, knowledge on the causes of postpartum
amenorrhea is still fragmentary (9). Three causes seem to be
important: duration of breastfeeding, nursing state (natural or
not), and nutrition and health level.

The duration of lactation - full and partial nursing - is very
often mentioned as the only factor determining the length of postpartum amenorrhea. The expression "lactational amenorrhea" is
often used, although the correlation between the duration of postpartum amenorrhea and of lactation is not higher than 0.4 or 0.5
(10,11).

The observations, conducted mainly in industrialized countries, show a regular increase of the duration of postpartum amenorrhea with the duration of lactation. With breastfeeding up to 3 months duration, the amenorrhea length may exceed lactation; when breastfeeding is longer, amenorrhea is shorter than the lactation period. In comparisons between countries or between various social classes, explanations had to be provided for the occurrence of amenorrhea of similar durations together with lactation of different lengths. For instance: Taiwan (12) and the Punjab (3) both present an 11 month median duration of postpartum amenorrhea, but the respective durations of lactation are 14 and 21 months. Further, 14 months of breastfeeding is coupled to 11 months of postpartum amenorrhea in Taiwan (12) but only 7 months in France in the year 1900 (13).

Among other factors acting upon the duration of postpartum amenorrhea are age and, to a slighter extent, parity. Both are reported to delay ovulation resumption (2).

Several investigators have observed that breastfeeding practices, full or partial, have an influence on the length of postpartum amenorrhea (14). For example, the introduction of dietary supplements shortens the duration of postpartum amenorrhea. The frequency of lactation could also be important since each suckling is known to trigger the release of the hormone prolactin from the anterior pituary. This hormone stimulates the secretion of milk; antigonadotropin effects are also proposed. Recently, Delvoye et al. (15) observed in Central Africa that the basal prolactin concentrations were lower in menstruating nursing mothers than in amenorrheic nursing mothers and that the basal prolactin level did not increase significantly before and after breastfeeding. During 15 months postpartum, the basal prolactin level stays high.

The hypothesis that malnutrition of the mother induces prolonged postpartum amenorrhea has been suggested in several studies (7,8,12,16-19). Difficulties in identifying and measuring the degree of malnutrition, however, have made investigations uncertain. The criteria used are often quite imprecise: "poor or upper class, well or poorly nourished, poor diet." Monetary income is sometimes used as an indicator for nutrition. Comparisons between populations are difficult; in urban areas of Africa, for instance, even a very low monetary income may lead to a balanced diet. Nutritional status may concern the investigated population as a whole, the group of women only, or each breastfeeding mother individually (20).

The most detailed surveys on nutrition-amenorrhea relations have been done in European countries in two circumstances: during the first and second world war famine periods, and in women in malnutrition due to anorexia nervosa. Secondary amenorrhea in

women is linked to the intensity of the famine; this considerably
decreases when diet returns to normal again. In anorexia nervosa,
amenorrhea is associated with a loss of 15-20% of body weight. In
famine, amenorrhea appears when the diet is reduced to 1500 cal.
intake (21-24). Almost no information relating amenorrhea to
protein and lipid supplies is available. In both war starvation
and anorexia nervosa, psychological factors interfere with a clear
interpretation of the fertility effects of food deficiency (25).

In considering how relevant is the comparison between famine
amenorrhea and postpartum amenorrhea in developing countries, the
following points should be considered: In addition to psychological
stress appearing with famine in Europe, amenorrhea occurs suddenly
in relatively well nourished women showing fat reserves; also,
highly varying methods and durations of breastfeeding make comparisons difficult; finally, famine amenorrhea is secondary and not
postpartum.

INTERACTIONS IN NUTRITION-AMENORRHEA RELATIONSHIPS

The Additional "Stress" of Lactation

Breast milk of poorly or better fed women has a similar protein content (26). The amount of vitamins and fatty acids in
breast milk decreases when the mother is severely undernourished
(26), but we generally observed that there is no close relationship
between diet and lactational performance (27). Thus, lactation
means a considerable consumption of energy for the mother (28).

If the diet does not supply sufficient energy, the consumption
required by lactation is made at the expense of maternal stores,
and the pre-existant malnutrition is therefore aggravated. With
successive pregnancies and prolonged lactation, this nutritional
stress could lead to the syndrome of "maternal depletion" (29).
Indeed, severe malnutrition in breastfeeding women has been
observed in India and New Guinea (30,31). The situation could be
closely related to that frequently described in Europe during the
famines which appeared in both world wars. It should be kept in
mind, however, that in areas with moderate protein-calorie malnutrition like India (32), Gambia (33), Guatemala (34), and Mexico
(35), clinical investigations and biological analysis did not
identify a nutritional stress peculiar to breastfeeding women (33),
nor a significant difference between well or poorly nourished lactating women (34), or between primipara or multipara (35).

Recently, the metabolic efficiency of lactation has been shown
to attain 90% instead of 60% as previously estimated (36). The

energy required by lactation is therefore less important than
previously thought; maternal dietary recommendations have thus
been reduced to 500 additional calories. The energy cost of breastfeeding may also be partially compensated for by using the body
fatness stores which have been accumulated during pregnancy, or
even during the post-puberty period (37).

Protracted lactation may not induce malnutrition but play a
role of homeostasis, thanks to the duration of postpartum amenorrhea.
In fact, birth intervals can extend up to 33-37 months in women of
poorly nourished rural areas, precisely because of a long postpartum amenorrhea (8).

Seasonal Dietary Deficiencies

In rural areas, where the populations live in a self-subsistence economy, the alternation of dry and rainy seasons frequently
induces important fluctuations in food supplies, mainly in proteins
and lipids. According to the seasons, dietary intakes range from
1,600 to 1,200 Cal. in Ethiopia (39), from 2,000 to 1,000 Cal. in
Rwanda (40). In times of scarcity, the nutrient intake of these
populations can be compared to the famine rations reported in
Europe during 1940-45: from 1,000 to 1,500 Cal. (41). In such
situations in Europe, secondary amenorrhea from malnutrition was
frequently observed (22).

If seasonal fluctuations of the body weight are carefully observed in populations living in a self-subsistence economy, we
observe that the mean weight has a smaller amplitude than that
observed in famines: 5 to 8% (33) compared to 15 to 20% during
famines (42). In non-lactating women, secondary amenorrhea due to
malnutrition has scarcely been noticed in areas with chronic
protein-calorie malnutrition, although a 15% loss in body weight
is enough to induce it (43). These facts could be explained by a
better adjustment to the changes in food supplies of the organisms
of these populations.

THE STUDY DESIGN

The purpose of this paper is to compare the relation between
lactation and postpartum amenorrhea in two ecological areas in the
Republic of Zaire. The first area is the Tropical Equatorial
Forest with two tribes, one of them in the lake Tumba area (the
Ntomba) and the other in the Maniéma - Kivu (the Tembo). The
second area is the Highlands with the people of Kivu (the Havu)
suffering from moderate protein-calorie malnutrition. The results
of a retrospective and cross-sectional study of the main components

of birth intervals in rural populations of Zaire are described
below. These populations have been selected in two highly different ecological areas, the Tropical Forest and the Highlands.
These environments induce distinctly different diets in fat and
animal protein. The first area enjoys a well balanced diet, while
the second suffers from a moderate protein-calorie malnutrition.

This comparative analysis is limited by other factors which
also differ - social and sanitary mainly - in addition to dietary
differences. The inclusion in the study of two populations
geographically removed from each other but with the same dietary
patterns helps to resolve this difficulty.

The investigated populations present a large number of common
socioeconomic aspects: self-subsistence dominating the economy with
a weak part played by the monetary transactions; natural lactation;
natural fertility.

All the observations and especially those concerning durations
of postpartum amenorrhea and of lactation have been collected
between 1974 and 1975, by retrospective and cross-sectional investigations in both the studied areas. Each married and assumed fertile
woman has been questioned individually. Defects inherent to
inquiries could not be avoided: omissions, inaccuracy, and digit
preference in numerical responses. The mean durations of lactation
and postpartum amenorrhea were estimated by life-table methods (44)
based on the fully retrospective and retrospective-truncated
events.

Concerning the length of postpartum amenorrhea, any bleedings
have probably been interpreted as menstruation resumption. Women
who conceived before the first menses postpartum were withdrawn
from the sample (less than 1 percent).

The nutritional guides are inquiries on food consumption from
three different sources (45,46,47); they are complemented by clinical data when available. The choice of the investigated populations
has been previously determined by earlier results obtained during
inquiries on food consumption. In the Equatorial Forest, observations were conducted in Ntomba (Province of the Equator), where
285 women from 11 villages were interviewed, and in Tembo (Province
of Kivu) where 148 women from three villages were questioned. In
the Eastern Highlands, in Havu (Province of Kivu) 316 women from
4 hills constituted the sample.

THE ECOLOGICAL AREAS

The Equatorial Forest

Ecology. The Equatorial Forest enjoys a constant rain level of 1,800 to 2,000 mm a year. Temperature fluctuates from 25° to 27°C. Annual variations are slight. The population density is 5-10 inhabitants per square km. Most of these groups live off agriculture, hunting, and fishing. The work distribution is strict: most field work is done by women. Agriculture is itinerant (shifting cultivation). Each family deforests a 1-hectare plot and the vegetation is burnt. Land is cultivated from 1 to 3 years and then left to the forest for 15 to 20 years.

Dietary Pattern. The basic crops are cassava combined with maize or plantain banana for Tembo. Beans, ground-nuts and vegatables are subsidiary food products. Palm oil and ground-nuts provide the largest part of the lipid supplies. Hunting products are scarce but regular thanks to exchanges with Pygmean groups. River fishing is seasonal.

Nutritional Supplies. Ntomba. The mean supply of energy is 100% of the theoretical needs defined by the FAO-WHO Committee (48). Proteins represent 15% of the energy supply, of which 4% are animal proteins. Lipids amount to 30% of the energy supply (45).

Tembo. Their average daily dietary intake is 2,000 Cal. per inhabitant, which is probably slightly below theoretical minimal needs. The Tembo derive 13% of their calories from proteins (2% from animal proteins), 38% from lipids, and 49% from carbohydrates (46). These data are summarized in Figure 1.

Health Situation. Deficiency diseases like kwashiorkor or avitaminosis are rare. The prevalence of infectious and parasitic diseases is high. The serum albumin level in women is below the normal range. The mean weight for adult women is 49.9 ± 5.5 kg in Tembo and 53.4 kg in Ntomba (45) for respective heights of 159.0 and 159.2 cm. Goiter is palpable in 15-20% of the Tembo women; in Ntomba there is no goiter. Primary or secondary sterility, assumed due to venereal infections, affect respectively 15 and 25% of the adult Tembo and Ntomba women. No relation between goiter and sterility has been observed.

The mean age at first marriage generally follows puberty, which takes place around the age of 13-14. Fifty percent of adult women live in monogamy.

The Highlands

Ecology. The Eastern Highlands in Zaire (1500-2000 m) enjoy a rainfall level of 1,200 mm a year and a mean temperature around

18°C. Two rainy seasons and two dry seasons from June to August
and from January to February do not provoke real breaks in the
agricultural activity. These seasonal fluctuations do result in
a deficiency from July to September in protein supplies. The densities of population are the highest in Zaire: an average of 50
inhabitants per square km and densities of 100-200 inhabitants per
square km. The dwellings are scattered on deforested hills. All
field work is done by women. Generally, each family owns 1 hectare
of cultivable land, of which 30 ares are devoted to bananas. Agriculture is semi-intensive. Cattle, although an essential factor
in the social system, are hardly used for food.

   Dietary Pattern. Beans and sweet potatoes cover half the

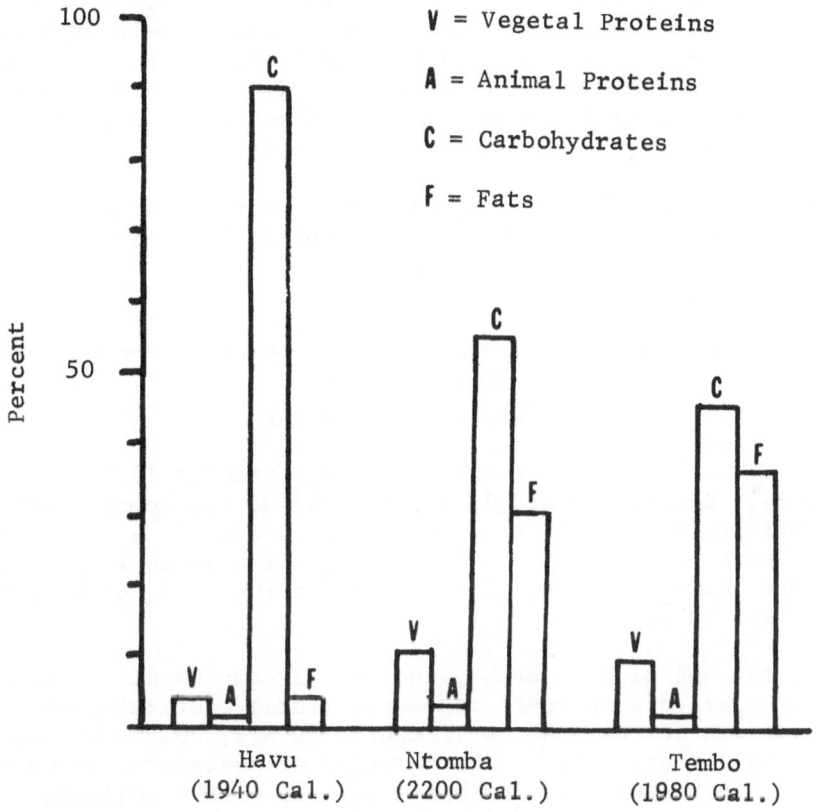

Figure 1. Average daily dietary intake of carbohydrates, proteins,
and fats, as percent of total caloric intake, for Highlands (Havu)
and Equatorial Forest (Ntomba and Tembo).

Source: Vis, et al. (45); Vis and Pagézy (46); Leurquin, et al.
         (47).

supply of energy and 70% of the protein. Cassava, bananas, and ground-nuts are also grown. At higher altitudes, sorghum and maize are most important. Milk is prized but plays only an incidental role. The absence of meat, fish, and palm oil explains the paucity of the protein and fat supplies.

Nutritional Supplies. The supply of energy is at the minimum recommended limit of 2,000-2,200 cal. The supply of protein is 6% of the energy supply: 1% is animal protein. The protein supply covers 85-90% of the theoretical needs. The supply of lipids represents 5% of the energy supplies, although 15% is desirable. Havu is compared with the Tropical forest area in Figure 1.

Health Situation. Relative protein-calorie malnutrition affects 15-20% of the children aged 0 to 5 years (46). The prevalence of the kwashiorkor is high. Women suffer from general endemic malnutrition. The mean weight of adult women is 50.0 kgs for a height of 153.0 cm. Avitaminosis A affects 0.5 to 1% of the adults. The prevalence of goiter ranges from 20 to 30% (49). Secondary sterility is an exception; primary sterility only affects 5% of adult married women aged 25 to 44 years.

Mean age at first marriage is 18-19 years. Puberty occurs late: 17 years. Sixty to seventy percent of the women live in monogamy.

DURATION OF LACTATION AND POSTPARTUM AMENORRHEA

The Tropical Forest

Ntomba. The median duration of lactation is 16.9 months (Table 1). Between 15 and 18 months, 54% of the women completely wean their children. As a matter of fact, according to custom, the child is weaned at about 18 months. If a woman is pregnant, she stops lactating before the normal weaning time out of fear "to poison" the baby.

At the age of 5-6 months, the Ntomba complement lactation with a porridge of cassava paste and sugar (fufu) containing more than 50% water and starch. At 10-12 months of age, the infant changes to the adult diet. The median duration of postpartum amenorrhea is 12-13 months; however, within the three months following delivery, 24% of the women are menstruating (first quartile), although nearly all of them are fully nursing. A second peak occurs between 15 and 18 months, when 23% of the mothers resume menstruation. At 18 months, 70% of the mothers have stopped lactating and 78% have resumed menstruation.

Tembo. The median lactation period is 22 months. The custom

Table 1

Proportion of Women with Postpartum Amenorrhea, Lactating,
and Full Nursing by Month Since Live Birth
Equatorial Forest Areas

Months since Previous Live Birth	Ntomba ($l_0 = 285$)			Tembo ($l_0 = 148$)		
	In Postpartum Amenorrhea	Still Lactating	Full Nursing	In Postpartum Amenorrhea	Still Lactating	Full Nursing
0	1.00	1.00	1.00	1.00	1.00	1.00
1	.93	1.00	.94	.96	1.00	.76
3	.76	1.00	.91	.91	.98	.31
6	.70	.98	.12	.76	.96	(.02)*
9	.65	.96		.68	.94	
12	.53	.94		.43	.81	
15	.45	.83		.32	.79	
18	.22	.29		.21	.60	
21	.14	(.02)*		(.16)*	.52	
24	(.06)*	-		(.05)	.40	
27					.21	

* ( ) based on less than 25 women.

is to breastfeed up to the next pregnancy, which explains the
length of the weaning ages. The first quartile is 16 months
long and the third one, 26 months (Table 1).

In the first weeks after birth, the child is fed a pre-chewed
porridge of banana flour and water. At an age of 2 months most of
the mothers introduce a supplement to breast milk. At 5 months,
50% of the children eat cassava paste and fish. At 9 months, 80%
of them share meals with the adults. The median duration of postpartum amenorrhea stands between 11-12 months. The first quartile
is reached at 6 months. Fifteen percent of the women are menstruating between 3 and 6 months when most of them adopt a mixed nursing. After 21 months, 50% of the mothers are still lactating
while amenorrhea persists in only 16% of them.

Highlands

In the Havu, the median duration of lactation is 22 months
(Table 2). After 12 months, only 8% of women have weaned their

Table 2

Proportion of Women with Postpartum Amenorrhea, Lactating,
and Full Nursing, by Month Since Previous Live Birth
Highland Area

	Havu (l_o = 316)		
Months since Previous Live Birth	In Postpartum Amenorrhea	Still Lactating	Full Nursing
0	1.00	1.00	1.00
1	.98	1.00	.66
3	.95	1.00	.51
6	.89	.98	.19
9	.78	.95	(.05)*
12	.67	.92	
15	.60	.87	
18	.49	.74	
21	.36	.57	
24	.14	.38	
27	.09	.21	

* ( ) based on less than 25 women.

child. The first quartile is reached at 18 months, the third at
26 months.

Artificial nursing begins very early: from the first months,
mothers feed their infants supplementary pre-chewed banana porridges.
The median duration of postpartum amenorrhea is 18 months. The
first quartile stands at 9-10 months, the third at 22-23 months.
Normally, according to the custom, the mother breastfeeds her child
up to a new pregnancy, but this social norm is followed by 65% of
the women only. The first postpartum amenorrhea menstruation has
a special name, different from monthly menstruation: "okubonera
omwana", i.e., "menstruation to see the child." This local name
signifies the long expectation of fertility.

FACTORS INFLUENCING THE AMENORRHEA DURATION

Duration of Lactation

The duration of lactation prolongs postpartum amenorrhea in

the three populations (Table 3). In the Tembo of the Tropical
forest, though lactation is protracted beyond two years, postpartum
amenorrhea is only extended a total of 12-13 months. Apparently
postpartum amenorrhea is not extended much longer than one year
with an extension of lactation. In Highlands, on the contrary,
the correlation between the durations of lactation and postpartum
amenorrhea is high (r = 0.7). It has to be noted, however, that
the lactating period is very often determined by the resumption of
menstruation since this generally induces weaning.

Nature of the Nursing

The effect of partial weaning on the mean duration of postpartum amenorrhea is analyzed in Table 4. There is an effect;
earlier partial weaning results in a difference of 2 or 3 months
in the duration of postpartum amenorrhea. It cannot be excluded,
however, that lactating mothers, except for primipara, consider the
anticipated date of menstruation resumption as the time to start
weaning.

Age and Parity

Although there was a slight increase in the duration of amenorrhea with age and parity, the increases were not significant.

Urbanization

The effects of urbanization on the durations of breastfeeding
and postpartum amenorrhea in rural populations are complex: they
cover the life style as well as the social behavior and also the
dietary customs. We were given the opportunity to study the impact
of urbanization on the Ntomba and the Havu. The native cities of
Mbandaka (108,000 inhabitants) (Ntomba) and Bukavu (135,000
inhabitants) (Havu), are not real urban centers from the historical
point of view. These townsmen are mainly rural people who have
been urbanized but still live in close relationship with their
native village.

Table 5 compares the data on lactation and amenorrhea in
urban women obtained from other sources (51) with our findings in
the rural areas. In the Tropical forest (Ntomba), no significant
difference between rural and urban areas is observed in the durations of breastfeeding and postpartum amenorrhea. On the other
hand, in Highlands (Havu) the duration of lactation is 7 months
shorter in the urban area. Neither the type nor the method of
breastfeeding in the urban areas seems likely to account for the

Table 3

Mean Months* of Postpartum Amenorrhea by Duration of Nursing
for Women in Equatorial Forest Area and Highland Area

Equatorial Forest Area				Highland Area	
Ntomba (n = 120)		Tembo (n = 92)		Havu (n = 168)	
Duration of Nursing	Mean Duration of p.p. Amenorrhea	Duration of Nursing	Mean Duration of p.p. Amenorrhea	Duration of Nursing	Mean Duration of p.p. Amenorrhea
12-14	7.8	9-14	6.8	12-15	10.7
15-18	9.5	15-20	8.7	16-21	15.7
18-21	11.9	21-26	12.3	22-27	20.1
				28-36	24.6
Mean 16.9	10.7	18.7	10.4	22.0	18.7

*Means are calculated on absolutely retrospective segments.

Table 4

Mean Duration of Postpartum Amenorrhea Among Women
Who Initiate Partial Nursing Early and Late*
in the Equatorial Forest and Highland Areas

Time of Partial Nursing	Mean Duration of Postpartum Amenorrhea	
	Equatorial Forest	Highland
	Tembo (n = 76)	Havu (n = 193)
Before 3 months	9.1	16.9
After 3 months	11.8	19.6

* The cases where partial nursing follows the beginning of
  menstruation are excluded.

9 month difference in the length of postpartum amenorrhea. Indeed,
in Bukavu, duration of breastfeeding remains dependent on menstruation resumption according to custom, and the introduction of dietary
supplements to breast milk usually takes place at 4-5 months of
age, i.e., one month later than in rural areas.

Table 5

Mean Month of Breastfeeding and of Postpartum Amenorrhea
Among Rural and Urban* Women in the Equatorial
Forest and Highland Areas

	Equatorial Forest (NTOMBA)		Highlands (HAVU)	
	Rural (n=120)	Urban (n=500)	Rural (n=166)	Urban (n=311)
Duration of Breastfeeding	16.9	17.3	21.9	14.9
Duration of Postpartum Amenorrhea	10.7	9.3	18.7	9.6

* Source: A. Devreese, 1960 (51).

In the Highlands, the nutritional differences between urban
and rural areas are quite noticeable. In Bukavu, in the native
city, the supply of calories is adequate according to a nutritional
survey (50). Needs in proteins are also met and the supply of
lipids represents 20-30% of the caloric supplies, i.e., 5 or 6
times more than in rural areas.

The shortening of the duration of postpartum amenorrhea in
urban Havu could, therefore, possibly be related to the improvement
of the supply of proteins and lipids.

Birth Intervals

If the time added by intrauterine mortality is estimated 2-3
months, and with the help of our observations on conception delays,
it is possible to set up the birth intervals for each population,
according to the analytic model by Perrin and Sheps (44). This
analysis is given in Table 6. In Ntomba, the unusual length of
the mean conception delay is partly explained by the influence of
taboos on postpartum intercourse: 18-24 months for a first child,
3-6 months for the others. The other two populations are not
subject to postpartum intercourse taboos. The birth intervals are
obviously strongly influenced by the duration of postpartum amenorrhea. In absence of any clear modification in the methods of
protracted lactation, a 9-10 months difference between birth intervals can be related to the different eco-systems.

Table 6

Estimated Duration of Birth Interval Components for
Populations in the Equatorial Forest and Highland Areas

Population	Gesta-tion	Post-Partum Amen-orrhea	Menstru-ating Interval	Time Added by Pregnancy Wastage	Total Birth Interval Inferred From Components
Equatorial Forest					
Ntomba	9	10.7	12	2-3	34-35
Tembo	9	10.4	7	2-3	29-30
Highlands					
Havu (urban)	9	9.3	7	2-3	28-29
Havu (rural)	9	18.7	8	2-3	38-39

DISCUSSION

Postpartum amenorrhea is obviously prolonged by lactation in
both the investigated ecologic areas. Despite different lactation
lengths due to differences in customs, Ntomba and Tembo populations
from the Equatorial forest display rather equal durations of postpartum amenorrhea. Our observations suggest that this situation
is induced by similar nutritional patterns.

Populations living in the Equatorial forest and Highlands
present clearly different durations of postpartum amenorrhea.
According to our observations, a likely factor to explain this is
the difference between the nutritional patterns and especially
between intakes of lipid and protein from animal origin.

This hypothesis may be supported when we consider the specific
influence of the factor "urbanization" on both the ecological
environments. In the Equatorial forest area (Mbandaka), urbanization does not result in important modifications in the rural nutritional pattern (51). By contrast, among the Havu living on
Highlands, the dropping of the postpartum amenorrhea duration and
correlatively of lactation may be interpreted as a result of the
transition from the dietary intake with seasonal protein and lipid
deficiencies in rural areas, to a relatively balanced diet in
urban areas (Bukavu). In line with this hypothesis, it is interest-

ing that as soon as deficiencies in protein and lipid are corrected, the postpartum amenorrhea duration in the Highlands becomes comparable to that observed in the Tropical forest.

Our observations suggest that, in a homogenous rural environment, a moderate chronic malnutrition, characterized by unbalanced supplies in protein and lipid, induces a 7-9 months prolongation of postpartum amenorrhea in lactating women. The imprecise and fragmentary character of our demographic data due to its retrospective and cross-sectional character, and the absence of individual nutritional criteria, leave us unable to fully explain the relations between malnutrition and postpartum amenorrhea.

In the absence of any postpartum sexual taboo, the birth intervals in rural population living on the Highlands are longer than in the Equatorial forest because of the duration of postpartum amenorrhea. This demographic data led us to consider the importance of a possible self-regulating fertility mechanism through chronic malnutrition which could reduce the fertility long before the advent of overt famine or severe nutritional deficiency with its devastating effects (52). If validated, this assumption of self-regulation would highly modify our conception of the population evolution and of the demographic transition. It would also plead in favor of the indispensable integration of any program aiming at the improvement of the nutritional status of a given population with a family planning program.

                                    APPENDIX

Our conclusions concerning the possible effect of deficiency in lipid and protein supplies as the factor responsible for prolonged duration of postpartum amenorrhea and the observations by R. Frisch (37) on the role of body fatness as necessary determinant for regular menstrual cycles in women led us to measure individual weight for height in lactating amenorrheic and in menstruating women in the Havu (and in the Shi) living in poor rural areas.

In a sample of 549 lactating women, 79 were withdrawn in whom menstruation resumption occurred more than two months before the interview. The sample presents slight irregularities. The results, shown in Table A, lead to two conclusions:

1. All the lactating women in amenorrhea stand above the critical weight for height relation which determines the maintenance of the menstrual cycle in women, according to Frisch and MacArthur (53).

2. The observation of a 3 to 4 kg difference in weight for

equivalent height during the first year of lactation (from 3 to 12 months) favors R. Frisch's hypothesis that the weight for height has a direct or indirect role to play on menstruation resumption; however, the absence of such a difference during the second year of lactation suggests that other factors, most probably of hormone origin, play a role in very prolonged amenorrhea.

ACKNOWLEDGMENTS

This survey has been supported in part by The Pathfinder Fund (Boston).

The author warmly thanks Dr. H. L. Vis for suggesting this study and Dr. W. Wils for his helpful remarks.

Appendix Table A

Mean Weights and Heights of Amenorrheic Lactating and Menstruating Lactating Women by Duration Since Last Live Birth

Postpartum Months	n	Weight (kg) $\pm$ SD*	Height (cm) $\pm$ SD
Amenorrheic Lactating Women			
0- 2	78	53.6 $\pm$ 7.6	153.1 $\pm$ 6.9
3- 5	99	52.1 $\pm$ 6.0	154.6 $\pm$ 6.4
6-11	96	51.2 $\pm$ 5.6	153.5 $\pm$ 6.2
12-24	58	51.3 $\pm$ 6.9	154.3 $\pm$ 6.4
Menstruating Lactating Women			
0- 2	20	56.2 $\pm$ 6.1	154.9 $\pm$ 4.8
3- 5	54	56.5 $\pm$ 8.7	152 $\pm$ 6.5
6-11	34	55.9 $\pm$ 5.9	153.5 $\pm$ 6.9
12-24	31	52.5 $\pm$ 5.4	153.8 $\pm$ 4.9

* SD: Standard Deviation

References

1. Henry, L. La fécondité naturelle: Observations. Théorie. Résultats. Population 16: 631, 1961.

2. Potter, R., Wyon, J., New, M. and Gordon, J. Applications of Field Studies to Research of the Physiology of Human Reproduction (Lactation and Its Effects upon Birth Intervals in Eleven Punjab Villages). J. Chronic Diseases, XVIII: 1125, 1963.

3. Potter, R. G. Birth Intervals: Structure and Change. Population Studies 1125, 1963.

4. Leridon, H. Aspects biometriques de la fecondite. I.N.E.D. cahier nº 65, 184 p., Paris 1973.

5. Rao, M. N. and Mathew, K. K. Rural Field Study in Population Control, Singur 1956-69. All India Inst. of Hygiene, 1970.

6. Kang, K. W., Hong, J. W., and Cho, K. S. A Study on the Inter-relationships Between Lactation and Postpartum Amenorrhea. Korean Inst. for Family Planning, 1973.

7. Chen, L. C., Ahmed, S., Geshe, M. and Mosley, W. H. A Prospective Study of Birth Interval Dynamics in Rural Bangladesh. Population Studies 28: 277, 1974.

8. Caraël, M. Postpartum Amenorrhea Associated with Malnutrition in Central Africa. In press.

9. Bourgeois-Pichat, J. Les facteurs de la fécondite non dirigée. Population 20: 384, 1965.

10. Tietze, C. The Effect of Breastfeeding on the Rate of Conception. Proc. of the Intern. Pop. Conf. vol. 2, I.U.S.S.P. Liege, p. 129, 1961.

11. Van Ginneken, J. K. Prolonged Breastfeeding as a Birth Spacing Method. Studies in Family Planning 5: 201, 1974.

12. Jain, A., Hsu, T. C., Freedman, R., and Chang, M. C. Demographic Aspects of Lactation and Postpartum Amenorrhea. Demography 7: 255, 1970.

13. Mondot, J., Ferry, B., et Cantrelle, P. Durée d'allaitement et d'aménorrhée post partum en France vers 1900. In: Les relations en Afrique entre la fécondité, la mortalité aux jeunes ages et la nutrition. Mondot-Bernard, J. Centre de dévelopement, OCDE, 101 p., Paris: 1970.

14. Perez, A., Vela, P., Potter, R., et Masnick, G. Timing and Sequence of Resuming Ovulation and Menstruation after Child-birth. Population Studies 25: 3, 1971.

15. Delvoye, P., Delogne-Desnoeck, J., and Robyn, C. Serum-Prolactin in Long Lasting Lactation Amenorrhea. The Lancet II, 288, 1976.

16. Hinshaw, R., Pyeatt, P., and Habicht, J.P. Environmental Effects on Child-spacing and Population Increase in Highland Guatemala. Current Anthropology 13: 216, 1972.

17. Rajalakshmi, R. Reproduction Performance of Poor Indian Women on a Low Plane of Nutrition. Trop. Geogr. Med. 23: 238, 1971.

18. Malkani, P. K. and Mirchandini, J. J. Menstruation during Lactation: A Clinical Study. J. Ob. Gyn. India 11: 11, 1960.

19. Cantrelle, P. and Leridon, H. Breast-feeding, Mortality in Childhood and Fertility in a Rural Zone of Senegal. Population Studies 25: 505, 1971.

20. Jelliffe, D. B. Appréciation de l'état nutritionnel des populations. O.M.S. monographie n°53, I vol de 253 p., Geneve, 1958.

21. Antonov, A. Children Born During the Siege of Leningrad in 1942. J. of Pediatrics 30: 250, 1947.

22. Smith, C. A. The Effects of Wartime Starvation in Holland upon Pregnancy. American J. Obstet. Gynec. 53: 599, 1947.

23. Bergues, H. Répercussions des calamités de guerre sur la premiere enfance. Population 3: 502, 1948.

24. Stein, Z. and Susser, M. Fertility, Fecundity, Famine. Human Biology 47: 131, 1975.

25. Sweeney, J. S. et al. An Observation on Menstural Misbehaviour. J. Clin. Endocrinol. 7: 659, 1947.

26. Janz, G. J., Demayer, E. M. and Close, J. Nutrition et Lactation. Ann. Nutr. (Paris) II, 33, 1957.

27. Hitchcock, N. E. and English, R. M. Nutrient Intake During Lactation in Australian Women. Brit. J. Nutr. 20: 599, 1966.

28. World Health Organization. Nutrition in Pregnancy and Lactation. Technical Reports No. 302, 1965.

29. Jelliffe, D. B. and Maddocks, I. Ecologic Malnutrition in the New Guinea Highlands. Clin. Pediat. 3: 432, 1965.

30. Gopalan, C. Studies on Lactation in Poor Indian Communities. J. Trop. Ped. 4: 87, 1958.

31. Venkatachalam, P.S.A. Study of the Diet, Nutrition and Health of the People of the Chimbu Area, New Guinea Highlands. Territory of Papua and New Guinea, Department of Public Health (Monograph No. 42).

32. Rajalakshmi, R. Reproduction Performance of Poor Indian Women on a Low Plane of Nutrition. Trop. Geogr. Med. 23: 238, 1971.

33. Thomson, A. M., Billewicz, W. Z., Thompson, B., and McGregor, I. A. Body Weight Changes during Pregnancy and Lactation in Rural African (Gambian) Women. J. Obstet. Gynec. Brit. Cwlth. 73: 724, 1966.

34. Beaton, G. H., Arroyave, G. and Flores, M. Alterations in Serum Proteins during Pregnancy and Lactation in Urban and Rural Populations in Guatemala. Am. J. Clin. Nutr. 14: 269, 1964.

35. Jacob, M., Hunt, H. I., Dirige, O., Swendseit, M. E. Biochemical Assessment of the Nutritional Status of Low Income Pregnant Women of Mexican Descent. Am. J. Clin. Nutr. 29: 650, 1976.

36. Thomson, A. M., Hytten, F. E. and Billewicz, W. Z. The Efficiency of Human Milk Production. Brit. J. Nutr. 24: 565, 1970.

37. Frisch, R. E. Demographic Implications of the Biological Determinants of Female Fecundity. Social Biology 22: 17, 1975.

38. Platt, B. S. and Mayer, J. Report of Joint FAO/WHO Mission to Ghana. FAO/59/5/3880, 1958.

39. Miller, D. S. and Rivers, J. Seasonal Variations in Food Intake in Two Ethiopian Villages. Proc. Nutr. Soc. 31: 1, 1972.

40. Vis, H. L., Yourassowsky, C. and Van der Borght, H. A Nutritional Survey in the Republic of Rwanda. Musée Royal de l'Afrique Centrale. Sc. Humaines No. 87, Tervuren (Belgique) 1975.

41. Le Roy Ladurie, E. L'aménorrhée de famine. In: Le territoire de l'historien. Ed. Gallimard. 1 vol. de 542 p., Paris: 1973.

42. Vis, H. L. Epidémiologie de la famine. In: Epidémiologie
    des desastres Ann. de Med. Trop. 1 vol., 1976.

43. Warren, M. P., Jelewicz, R., Dyrenfurth, I., Ans, R., Khalaf, S.
    and Vandewiele, R. L. The Significance of Weight Loss in the
    Evaluation of Pituary Response to LH-RH in Women with Secondary
    Amenorrhea. J. Clin. Endocrin. Metab. 40: 601, 1975.

44. Perrin, E. B. and Sheps, M. C. Human Reproduction: A Stochastic
    Process. Biometrics 20: 28, 1964.

45. Vis, H. L., Pourbaix, Ph., Thilly, C., and Van der Borght, H.
    Analyse de la situation nutritionnelle de sociétés tradition-
    nelles de la région du lac Kivu: les Shi et les Havu. Ann. de
    Méd. Trop. 49: 353, 1969.

46. Vis, H. L. et Pagezy, H. 1976. Communication personnelle.

47. Roels, O. A., Leurquin, P. and Marian Trout.   Serum Poly-
    unsaturated Fatty Acids in Groups of Africans with Low and High
    Fat Intakes. J. Nutrition 69: 2, 195, 1959.

48. FAO-WHO. Energy Requirements and Protein Requirements. World
    Health Organization Technical Report Series No. 522, 1973.

49. Ermans, A. M., Thilly, C., Vis, H. L. and Delange, F. In:
    Endemic Goiter, Stanbury, J. B. (ed.), Pan Amer. Health Org.,
    Scientific Publication 193: 101, 1969.

50. Rapport sur l'enquete des budgets familiaux en milieu Africain
    ville de Bukavu. Inst. Nat. de la Stat. Kinshasa, 1 vol. de
    232 p., 1973.

51. Devreese, P. Communication personnelle.

52. Wils, W., Caraël, M. and Tondeur, G. Le Kivu montagneux:
    surpopulation, sous-nutrition et érosion du sol. To be
    published in 1977.

53. Frisch, R. E. and McArthur, J. W. Menstural Cycles: Fatness as
    a Determinant of Minimum Weight for Height Necessary for Their
    Maintenance or Onset. Science 185: 949, 1974.

NUTRITION AND BIRTH INTERVAL COMPONENTS:

THE GUATEMALAN EXPERIENCES

Hernán Delgado, Aaron Lechtig, Elena Brineman,
Reynaldo Martorell, Charles Yarbrough, Robert E. Klein

Institute of Nutrition of Central America and Panama
(INCAP), Guatemala City, Guatemala

INTRODUCTION

A birth interval is defined as the period between one live
birth and the next (1). Beginning with a live birth, it can be
divided into several components: the period of postpartum amenorrhea, the menstruating interval, and the next period of gestation
(2,3). Lactation, initiation of menstruation and ovulation after
delivery, conception and intrauterine development of the fetus each
place a large demand on the nutritional status of women; thus,
malnutrition may lower the biological capacity to conceive, bear,
and deliver a live child (4).

Evidence that these intermediate fertility variables are partially dependent upon nutrition is diverse, and often indirect,
but not unconvincing. Several authors have suggested that the
nutritional status of the mother affects the duration of postpartum amenorrhea in lactating women (5,6,7,8,9). Furthermore,
the duration of postpartum amenorrhea is apparently associated with
per capita income; mothers from high socioeconomic groups (5,7,10)
are amenorrheic for less time than mothers from low socioeconomic
groups (11,12,13). Aside from the implication of a nutritional
impact suggested by socioeconomic comparisons, the possibility that
nutrition may be related to the duration of postpartum amenorrhea
is given additional support by the increased prevalence of amenorrhea reported during times of severe food shortage and famine (14,
15).

Some experimental evidence to date also supports the plausibility of the above hypothesis. Chavez and Martinez (16) compared the

postpartum amenorrhea of a small group of lactating women receiving
food supplementation through pregnancy and lactation to a control
group of lactating women receiving no supplementation. Their
results suggest that one of the effects of supplementing the diet
is to significantly reduce the duration of postpartum amenorrhea.
They reported that postpartum amenorrhea lasted 7.5 months in the
supplemented group and 14.0 months in the control group, although
retrospective information on prior pregnancies showed that both
groups had similar lengths of postpartum amenorrhea before food
supplementation.

LONGITUDINAL STUDIES IN GUATEMALA

Over the past seven years the Division of Human Development
at the Institute of Nutrition of Central America and Panama (INCAP)
has been carrying out longitudinal research in four communities of
eastern Guatemala (17,18). This study examined the major hypothesis
that mild to moderate protein-calorie malnutrition adversely affects
the physical growth and mental development of infants and preschool
children. The longitudinal study is a multidisciplinary project
involving in depth analyses of the sociocultural, psychological,
physical and nutritional condition of the children in these communities.

The study of nutrition, physical growth and mental development
began in January 1969. Since its initiation, basic demographic
data have been collected in the form of a bi-annual census. Moreover, bi-weekly home visits have collected data on the timing and
incidence of various reproduction related events such as births,
conceptions, menstruation, migration and changes in family composition. A core working group of demographers, epidemiologists, and
other related professionals have recently begun to analyze these
data and to extend research efforts in the demographic area.

Population

The population under study live in four Spanish speaking,
subsistence agricultural villages in the department of El Progreso,
Guatemala. The villages were originally chosen on the basis of
their relative isolation, and homogeneity with respect to language,
culture, size and general economic and social structure.

The ethnic background of the population is Ladino, or mixed
Indian and Spanish. The main crops of these agricultural communities are corn and beans, most of which is consumed in the same
village. The median annual income is approximately $200.00 per
family, with most expenditures allocated for food and clothing.
Although schools exist in all of the communities, the average

adult schooling is about 1.5 years and functional literacy is low.
Modern contraception is uncommon. There is little permanent migration, and contact with the outside world is generally limited to
trips to nearby markets. Seasonal migration occurs once a year
when some of the men harvest cash crops in the coastal zones.

The entire population of the four villages was 3359 in the
1975 census. In the period 70-74 the crude birth and death rates
were respectively 42.5 and 6.9 per 1,000. Total fertility rate
was 7.1. The percentage of females age 15 to 45 living in consensual or formal marriages was 68% (average of the 1969 and 1975
censuses). Largely as a result of the free basic medical care and
food supplementation, the infant mortality dropped from between
150 and 200 in the 1960's to about 50 per 1,000 in the early 1970's.

Study Design

To test the basic hypothesis of the longitudinal study, a
quasi-experimental design was employed. Experimental treatment
consisted of food supplementation in the four villages. In two of
the villages, a high protein calorie drink was made available daily
in a central dispensary. This beverage is similar to a popular
local gruel, atole. In the other two villages, a non-protein, low
calorie drink, similar to a local cold drink known as fresco was
provided daily. The nutrient content of both supplements is shown
in Table 1.

The low calorie supplement, or fresco, contained no protein
and provided only one-third of the calories contained in an equal
volume of atole. Both supplements contained the vitamins and
minerals which were limited in the normal diet. Atole and fresco
were carefully measured daily and recorded to the centiliter at
the distribution center in each village. Since consumption of the
supplements was free and voluntary, a wide range of supplement
intake was observed in mothers and infants. In addition, in all
four villages, free outpatient preventive and curative medical
services were provided. These services also provided nutritional
rehabilitation when prescribed.

Methods

The analyses presented here included as subjects all pregnant
and lactating women with infants less than two years of age in the
four villages. The principal data gathered during the prenatal and
postnatal period are presented in Table 2.

The use of the terms dependent and independent variables in
Table 2 is an attempt to describe the hypothetical causes and

Table 1

Nutrient Content of Dietary Supplements
(per 180 ml)

Nutrients	Atole[1]	Fresco[2]
Total calories (KCal)	163	59
Protein (g)	11	--
Fats (g)	0.7	--
Carbohydrates (g)	27	15.3
Ascorbic Acid (mg)	4.0	4.0
Calcium (g)	0.4	--
Phosphorus (g)	0.3	--
Thiamine (mg)	1.1	1.1
Riboflavin (mg)	1.5	1.5
Niacin (mg)	18.5	18.5
Vitamin A (mg)	1.2	1.2
Iron (mg)	5.4	5.0
Fluoride (mg)	0.2	0.2

[1]The local name of a gruel commonly made with corn.
[2]Spanish for refreshing, cool drink.

effects of the interrelationships discussed later. A brief
description of the dependent and independent variables considered
in the present analyses follows.

Dependent Variables. The duration of postpartum amenorrhea
and of lactation was obtained prospectively by monitoring menstruation and lactation every 14 days in all women in the study population. The duration of postpartum amenorrhea was defined as the
interval, in months, between a birth date and the first incidence
of two menses occurring within a three-month period. The duration
of lactation was defined as the interval, in months, between a
birthdate and weaning.

Independent Variables. Because the measurement of nutritional
status is difficult and critical to our analyses, we utilized
several different proxies of this variable:

a) The assessment of supplement intake was expressed in terms
of calories because the normal dietary intake appeared to be more
limited in calories than in proteins. We have previously found
that this food supplementation program increases variability in

Table 2

Relevant Data Collected in INCAP's Longitudinal Study.
Maternal and Child Information

---

1. Independent Variables:

   - Measurement of subject's attendance at supplementation center and quantity of supplement ingested
   - Dietary survey: 24-hour recall
   - Anthropometry

2. Dependent Variables:

   - Birth interval components

3. Additional Variables:

   - Obstetrical history
   - Information on delivery
   - Morbidity survey
   - Clinical examination
   - Socioeconomic survey of the family

---

nutrient intake and represents a true supplement to the habitual diets.

b) Information on home diet was obtained through a 24-hour recall done once during each trimester of pregnancy. For the present analyses, this information was summarized for the last two trimesters of pregnancy and was expressed as the mean home caloric intake.

c) Finally, we used a summation of both home dietary intake and supplement consumption as an estimation of total nutrient intake.

In summary, food supplementation during pregnancy is the main experimental treatment and groups of mothers were categorized by: a) the amounts of supplemental calories and proteins they ingested during pregnancy, b) their home diet, and c) their total calorie-protein intake. While nutrient intake measures are reflective of current nutritional status, anthropometric variables are utilized not only as current but also as long-term indicators of maternal status.

Sample Size

The total sample for analysis was made up of all mothers in the four communities who had a delivery between January 1, 1969 and February 28, 1973, and who had been followed up to January 1975. Because reliable information on menstruation and lactation was not collected prospectively until the end of 1970, we have prospective information for only 438 intervals. It is important to point out that in this sample a woman may contribute more than one interval to the total sample.

RESULTS

Potter, et al. (3) distinguished two types of prospective intervals. If the start and end of an interval fell within the prospective period of data gathering, the interval was called "entirely prospective." The "truncated prospective" intervals started in the prospective period but were truncated by outmigration or termination of the study. Following Potter's approach, we will present our results in two sections: a) results based on entirely prospective intervals, biased toward interval brevity; and b) life table results, which combine entirely prospective and truncated prospective intervals. Furthermore, attention will be confined to the duration of postpartum amenorrhea, because this period has the largest possible variability of any of the components of the birth interval in a non-contracepting population (3). In all of the following analyses we excluded stillbirths and infant deaths.

Entirely Prospective Information. The mean duration of lactation in the study communities is 18 months; the mean duration for postpartum amenorrhea is 14 months. The two variables are highly associated, the correlation coefficient being .62 (377 cases, $p < .01$). The median duration of postpartum amenorrhea in nursing women in our study is comparable to those reported in other rural populations. Potter et al. (3) in a prospective study in India found a median of 11 months. A study of Eskimo women (19) showed a median of 10 months, and Chen, et al. (20), in Bangladesh, reported a median of 18 months.

As shown in Table 3, data from the longitudinal study reveal a negative association between the duration of postpartum amenorrhea and anthropometric measures of the mother taken 3 months after delivery, such as height, head circumference, weight, skinfolds, arm circumference, weight for height and arm circumference for height. Although none of these associations were statistically significant, there was a consistent negative trend. Recently we constructed an index of women's nutritional status by combining standardized measures of weight, arm circumference and triceps

Table 3

Relationship Between Length of Postpartum Amenorrhea
and Anthropometric Measures of the Mother

Variable	Correlation Coefficient	Number of Cases
Height	-.10	395
Head Circumference	-.09	298
Weight	-.14	160
Skinfolds: biceps	-.07	160
triceps	-.08	160
subscapular	-.07	160
mid axillary	-.05	160
Arm circumference	-.13	160
Weight/height	-.12	160
Arm circumference/height	-.07	160

skinfold. We found that this index of nutritional status showed a statistically significant negative association with the duration of postpartum amenorrhea ($p < .05$) (4).

Negative associations were found between the length of postpartum amenorrhea and both home caloric intake and caloric supplementation ingested during pregnancy. As shown in Table 4, we also found a negative association between total caloric intake during pregnancy (sum of home caloric intake and caloric supplementation) and the duration of postpartum amenorrhea in both atole and fresco villages. However, in atole villages this correlation was significant, whereas in fresco villages it was not. The reduction in the duration of postpartum amenorrhea for the same number of supplemented calories, or slope value, was not significantly different between fresco (b = -.0005 months/Calorie) and atole (b = -.0027 months/ Calorie) villages.

Another way of looking at these data consists of comparing the durations of postpartum amenorrhea in three groups (terciles) categorized by increasing total caloric intake within atole and fresco villages. As shown in Table 5, there is a consistent trend towards shorter postpartum amenorrhea in atole communities, but not in fresco communities, within categories of total nutrient intake. Although these results suggest an added effect of protein calorie supplementation over caloric supplementation, these differences were not statistically significant.

All these data suggest that better nutritional status during

Table 4

Relationship Between Length of Postpartum Amenorrhea
and Maternal Nutrient Intake During Pregnancy

Variable	Correlation Coefficient	Standard Regression Coefficient	Number of Cases
Caloric supplementation	-.0694	-.0665	398
Home dietary intake	-.0982	-.0934	339
Total caloric intake (TCI)	-.1163*	-.1151	339
TCI (Fresco villages)	-.0362	-.0345	153
TCI (Atole villages)	-.1780*	-.1756	186

* p < .05

pregnancy results in somewhat shorter lengths of postpartum amenorrhea.

Further indications can be obtained by comparing the duration of postpartum amenorrhea in these groups (terciles) with increasing total caloric intake within several comparable categories of duration of lactation. Table 6 shows clearly the strong association between duration of lactation and length of postpartum amenorrhea. Within all lactation categories, the length of postpartum amenorrhea was shorter in the groups with high calorie intake than in the group with low calorie intake.

Some of the indicators of nutritional status of the infant have also been found to be associated with the duration of postpartum amenorrhea. Weight gain of the infant during the first 9 months after birth was positively related to the duration of postpartum amenorrhea (r = .15, n = 301) and caloric supplementation ingested by the lactating infant during the first nine months was negatively related to the length of postpartum amenorrhea (r = -.14, n = 401). These results could be interpreted in two different ways:

a) If a mother starts supplementing the breastfed infant, the frequency of suckling will decrease. It is known that frequency of suckling is an important determinant of the duration of postpartum amenorrhea (10,21).

b) If a mother starts supplementing the breastfed infant, the nutritional demand of lactation will decrease, improving the nutritional status of the mother. It has been suggested that improved nutritional status of the mother would reduce the duration of postpartum amenorrhea (6). As we discuss later, the lack of specific

Table 5

Mean Durations of Postpartum Amenorrhea in Three Different
Total Caloric Intake Groups Within Atole and Fresco Villages

Total Caloric Intake[1]	Atole	Fresco	Total
	Months	Months	Months
Low	14.33 (64)[2]	14.38 (50)	14.35 (114)
Middle	13.60 (70)	14.04 (48)	13.78 (118)
High	12.29 (66)	14.21 (42)	13.04 (108)

[1]Total caloric intake = sum of home caloric intake and caloric
supplementation during pregnancy·

Low = ≤ 1,308 Cal/day; Middle = 1,309-1630 Cal/day; High = ≥ 1,631
Cal/day.

[2]Numbers in parentheses are number of cases.

information does not permit us to differentiate between these two
alternative explanations.

Finally, other variables such as parity, length of previous
birth interval and age of the mother were found to be positively
and significantly correlated with the duration of postpartum amenorrhea. The last two associations have been previously reported in
the literature (7,22). Salber et al. (22) found no significant
association between parity and duration of postpartum amenorrhea.
In our study, the association may be explained by the high association between parity and age in these mothers.

Life Table Analysis

In order to correct for the bias toward interval brevity
expected in the entirely prospective intervals, we applied a life
table technique so that we could use the truncated prospective
intervals. By this technique we compute the monthly probabilities
of resuming menstruation in two groups of mothers: a group who
ingested less than 10,000 calories during pregnancy and those who
consumed equal to or more than 20,000 calories during pregnancy.

As shown in Table 7, there is a consistent trend towards a
higher monthly probability of remaining amenorrheic in the poorly
supplemented group than in the highly supplemented group. It should
be noted that the approximately one month reduction in the median

Table 6

Mean Duration of Postpartum Amenorrhea in Three Different Total
Caloric Intake Groups Within Categories of Duration of Lactation

	Categories of Lactation (Months)				
Total Caloric Intake[1]	0 - 6	7 - 12	13 - 18	19 - 24	25 & more
	Months	Months	Months	Months	Months
Low	-	6.54 (13)[2]	12.03 (35)	16.44 (45)	19.93 (14)
Middle	-	6.31 (13)	11.64 (33)	15.47 (57)	18.90 (10)
High	-	5.47 (14)	11.13 (30)	14.60 (47)	19.64 (11)

[1]Total caloric intake = sum of home caloric intake and caloric
supplementation during pregnancy.

[2]Numbers in parentheses are number of cases.

length of amenorrhea in the highly supplemented group cannot be
attributed to a reduction in the duration of lactation between the
two groups. As shown in Table 7, high and low supplemented groups
exhibited virtually identical lactation intervals. The differences
found in these comparisons are not statistically significant, but,
as before, give support to the hypothesis that nutrition can have
an effect on the duration of postpartum amenorrhea.

DISCUSSION

In combination, the data presented here support the hypothesis
that improved maternal nutrition is associated with a decrease
in the duration of postpartum amenorrhea. This can result in a
shorter birth interval. This decrease in birth interval appears to
be occurring in our populations. Analyses of the entirely prospective birth intervals (not presented here) showed a 3.1 month reduction in the duration of the birth interval in the highly supplemented
group ($\geq$ 20,000 calories during pregnancy) as compared to the poorly
supplemented group (< 10,000 calories during pregnancy).

Although our results showed an association between maternal
nutritional status and duration of postpartum amenorrhea, some
weaknesses should be mentioned:

1. One of the major difficulties in inferring causality in
the association between nutrition and postpartum amenorrhea from

Table 7

Life Table of Postpartum Amenorrhea and Lactation in Two Groups
of Caloric Supplementation During Pregnancy[1]

Months of Exposure	Number of Cases Exposed	Probability of Remaining Amenorrheic X months P_A (X)	Standard Error of P_A (X)	Probability of Remaining Lactating X Months P_L (X)	Critical Ratio: Difference Between P_A (X) Low and P_A (X) High
		Low Supplemented Group (< 10,000 Cal/pregnancy)			
1	192	0.99478	0.00519	0.99582	
3	186	0.98421	0.00904	0.99582	
6	173	0.91011	0.02098	0.98723	
9	158	0.83248	0.02540	0.96117	
12	130	0.71121	0.03270	0.89454	
15	88	0.49014	0.03768	0.77202	
18	60	0.29409	0.03509	0.54266	
		High Supplemented Group (≥ 20,000 Cal/pregnancy)			
1	169	1.00000	0.00000	1.00000	-1.00261
3	165	0.95815	0.01548	1.00000	1.45309
6	151	0.88613	0.02459	1.00000	0.74184
9	132	0.78295	0.02738	0.97734	1.32624
12	115	0.65550	0.03425	0.91483	1.17650
15	84	0.43093	0.03746	0.78848	1.11462
18	50	0.24278	0.03299	0.54902	1.06519

[1] Based on "entirely prospective" and "truncated prospective"
intervals. It excludes all stillbirths and infant deaths.

these data derives from the fact that the allocation of subjects
in the different categories of caloric supplementation depends upon
the level of their cooperation with the intervention program.
Thus, there has been no means of controlling for possible factors
which might predispose a woman to choose to take both high levels
of supplementation and to have short periods of postpartum amenorrhea.

2. Since the longitudinal study was not originally designed to investigate the relationship between nutrition and the birth interval, another difficulty arises from our lack of data on confounding factors which might cause a spurious association between them. For example, it has been postulated that prolactin, secreted by the anterior pituitary as a response to suckling (23-32) may be the mechanism by which lactation inhibits ovulation. If that is the case, supplemental feeding of the infant, by reducing the frequency of suckling, may affect the duration of postpartum amenorrhea. In our study, we do not have information regarding home dietary intake of the infant, frequency of breastfeeding, or suckling frequency, duration and intensity; all important potentially confounding factors in the association between nutrition and duration of postpartum amenorrhea.

3. Another lack of data is apparent when we try to define the nutritional status of lactating mothers. Our analyses could only explore the effect of nutrition during pregnancy on the duration of postpartum amenorrhea because, in the longitudinal study, home dietary intake, an important parameter of nutritional status, was not collected during lactation nor during the rest of the birth interval.

4. Available evidence indicates that the longer the duration of lactation, the longer the period of postpartum amenorrhea. Our previous data (33) suggested that better nutrition was associated with a longer period of lactation, and therefore, through this mechanism, would prolong the duration of postpartum amenorrhea. These results were not replicated in a larger sample. There could be several reasons for this, one being a change in breastfeeding patterns for social reasons. It is important not to regard the length of lactation as an isolated variable, since it may be partially determined by some of the same behavioral and environmental factors which affect the desired number and spacing of births. If that is the case, it is imperative to study in depth the attitudes and behavior related to fertility and family size in the same population in which the biological aspects of fertility are being studied. The longitudinal study is missing information on these types of variables.

5. Finally, we are concerned with the relative importance of proteins and calories on fertility. Although some of our results indicate a higher impact of a combination of proteins and calories than calories alone, the experimental design and the study sample size do not permit us to differentiate the effect of proteins as compared to calories on the duration of postpartum amenorrhea.

FINAL COMMENTS

In this paper we presented data which indicate that maternal nutrition is associated with the duration of postpartum amenorrhea and, consequently, on birthspacing. We discussed in some detail the weaknesses of our results and believe that more investigation is needed before we can clearly understand the impact of nutrition on fecundity and fertility. We consider a longitudinal study with nutritional interventions and adequate controls for biological, attitudinal and behavioral variables the only way to test the hypotheses that our work and the work of others have generated.

This research was supported by Contract No. NO1-HD-5-0640 from the National Institute of Child Health and Human Development, National Institutes of Health, Bethesda, Maryland, and by Population Council grant No. D75. 49C.

References

1. Potter, R. G. Birth Intervals: Structure and Changes. Population Studies 17: 155-166, 1963.

2. Henry, L. Some Data on Natural Fertility. Eugenics Quarterly 8: 81-91, 1961.

3. Potter, R. G., New, M., Wyon, J., and Gordon, J. Applications of Field Studies to Research on the Physiology of Human Reproduction. J. Chron. Dis. 18: 1125-1140, 1965.

4. Bongaarts, J. and Delgado, H. Effects of Nutrition on Fertility. Unpublished manuscript, 1976.

5. Malkani, P. K. and Mirchardini, J. J. Menstruation During Lactation: A Clinical Study. J. Obstet. Gynecol. India 11: 11-22, 1960.

6. González, N. S. de. Lactation and Pregnancy: A Hypothesis. Amer. Anthrop. 68: 873-878, 1964.

7. Salber, E. J., Feinleib, M., and Macmahon, B. The Duration of Postpartum Amenorrhea. Am. J. Epidemiol. 82: 347-358, 1966.

8. Gopalan, C. and Naidu, A. N. Nutrition and Fertility. Lancet 2: 1077-1079, 1972.

9. Frisch, R. E. Demographic Imiplications of the Biological Determinants of Female Fecundity. Paper presented at the Population Association of America Annual Meeting, April 1974, New York.

10. McKeown, T. and Gibson, J. R. A Note on Menstruation and Con-
    ception During Lactation. J. Obstet. Gynecol. Brit. Emp. 61:
    824-826, 1954.

11. Baxi, P. A Natural History of Childbearing in the Hospital
    Class on Women in Bombay. J. Obstet. Gynecol. India 8: 26-51,
    1957.

12. Bonte, M. and Van Balen, H. Prolonged Lactation and Family
    Spacing in Rwanda. J. Biosoc. Sci. 1: 97-100, 1969.

13. Kamal, L., Hefnawi, F., Ghoneim, M., Tallat, M., Younis, H.,
    Taqui, A., and Abdalla, M. Clinical, Biochemical and Experi-
    mental Studies on Lactation. Am. J. Obstet. Gynecol. 105:
    314-323, 1969.

14. Antonov, A. N. Children Born During the Siege of Leningrad in
    1942. J. Pediat. 30: 250-259, 1947.

15. Smith, C. Effects of Maternal Undernutrition upon Newborn
    Infants in Holland, 1944-1945. J. Pediat. 30: 229-243, 1947.

16. Chávez, A. and Martínez, C. Nutrition and Development of
    Infants from Poor Rural Areas. III. Maternal Nutrition and its
    Consequences on Fertility. Nutr. Rep. Int. 7: 1-8, 1973.

17. Klein, R. E., Habicht, J-P., and Yarbrough, C. Some Methodo-
    logical Problems in Field Studies of Nutrition and Intelligence.
    In: D. J. Kallen (ed.), Nutrition, Development and Social
    Behavior. Washington, D.C.: U.S. Government Printing Office,
    DHEW Publication No. (NIH) 73-242, 61-75, 1973.

18. DDH/INCAP. Nutrición, crecimiento y desarrollo. Boletín de
    la Oficina Sanitaria Panamericana 78: 38-51, 1975.

19. Berman, M. I., Hanson, K., and Hellman, I. Effect of Breast-
    feeding on Postpartum Menstruation, Ovulation and Pregnancy
    in Alaskan Eskimos. Am. J. Obstet. Gynecol. 114: 524-534, 1972.

20. Chen, L. C., Ahmed, S., Gesche, M., and Mosley, W. H. A
    Prospective Study of Birth Dynamics in Rural Bangladesh.
    Population Studies 28: (2) 277-297, 1974.

21. Pérez, A., Vela, P., Masnick, G. S., and Potter, R. G. First
    Ovulation after Childbirth: The Effect of Breastfeeding.
    Am. J. Obstet. Gynecol. 114: 1041-1047, 1972.

22. Salber, E. J., Feldman, J. J., and Hannigan, M. Duration of
    Postpartum Amenorrhea in Successive Pregnancies. Am. J. Obstet.

Gynecol. 100: 24-29, 1968.

23. Meiter, J. and Clemens, J. A. Hypothalamic Control of Pro-
    lactin Secretion. Vit. and Hormones 30: 165-221, 1972.

24. Franz, A. G., Kleinberg, D. L. and Noel, G. I. Studies of
    Prolactin in Man. Recent Progress in Hormone Research 28:
    527-590, 1972.

25. Villa, J. G. and Salto, L. Prolactina y galactorrea. Rev.
    Clin. Esp. 128: 183-194, 1972.

26. Robyn, C., Delboye, P., Nokin, J., Vekemans, M., Bodaw, M.,
    Pérez-López, F. R., and L'Hermite, M. Prolactin and Human
    Reproduction. In: Human Prolactin. Proceedings of the Inter-
    national Symposium on Human Prolactin, Brussels, June 12-14,
    1973, Excerpta Medica Amsterdam, 1973.

27. Friesen, H. G. and Hwang, P. Human Prolactin. Ann. Review of
    Medicine 24: 251-270, 1973.

28. McNelly, A. S. Prolactin and Human Reproduction. Brit. J.
    Hosp. Med. 12: (1) 57-62, 1974.

29. Friesen, H. G., Fournier, P., and Desjardins, P. Pituitary
    Prolactin in Pregnancy and Normal and Abnormal Lactation.
    Clin. Obstet. Gynecol. 16: 25-45, 1973.

30. Jacobs, L. S. and Daughaday, W. H. Physiologic Regulation of
    Prolactin Secretion in Man. In: J. B. Josimovich, M. Reynolds,
    and E. Cobo (eds.), Lactogenic Hormones, Fetal Nutrition and
    Lactation. New York: John Wiley & Sons, Chapter 17, 351-377,
    1974.

31. Tyson, J. E., Friesen, H. G., and Anderson, M. S. Human Lacta-
    tional and Ovarian Response to Endogenous Prolactin Release.
    Science 177: 897-900, 1972.

32. Tyson, J. E. and Friesen, H. G. Factors Influencing the
    Secretion of Human Prolactin and Growth Hormone in Menstrual
    and Gestational Women. Am. J. Obstet. Gynec. 116: 377-387,
    1973.

33. Delgado, H., Habicht, J-P., Lechtig, A., Klein, R. E.,
    Yarbrough, C., and Martorell, R. Prenatal Nutrition. Paper
    presented at the Symposium on Current Concepts in Nutrition:
    Nutrition in the Life Cycle, University of Southern California,
    Los Angeles, September 1973.

EFFECT OF MATERNAL NUTRITION ON FERTILITY IN RURAL BANGLADESH

A. K. M. Alauddin Chowdhury

Cholera Research Laboratory

Dacca, Bangladesh

INTRODUCTION

The Cholera Research Laboratory (CRL) has maintained demographic surveillance of a rural population of approximately 260,000
persons in Matlab Thana and adjacent areas in Comilla District,
Bangladesh, since 1966. During this period of time, the year 1974
was marked by severe economic hardship in Bangladesh. In Matlab
Thana, rice prices increased early in 1974 and remained high until
late 1975. Many people in the area could not afford to buy a
minimally adequate amount of food, and famine conditions prevailed
(1).

The CRL found in this population between 1973 and 1974 that
the crude death rate climbed from 14 to 21 per 1000; in 1975, the
rate fell somewhat to 18 per 1000. The infant mortality rate followed a similar pattern; 125 per 1000 in 1973, 175 per 1000 in
1974, and 152 per 1000 in 1975. During this period, the decline
in fertility was even more dramatic. For these three successive
years the crude birth rate fell from 47.8 to 40.1 to 27.6, a drop
of nearly 45% from 1973 to 1975. These fluctuations in fertility
and mortality reduced the rate of natural increase to 0.9% in 1975
compared with 3% per year between 1966 and 1970.

A reported contraceptive use rate in October 1975 of only
2.4% for married women aged 15-44 suggests that modern contraceptives could not play a major role in the fertility decline. The
famine conditions can be related to the drastic decline in fertility,
although the variables involved have only been partially explored

401

(1,2). It is known that the food shortage beginning in 1974 caused
a threefold increase in net out-migration from the area. The shortage was also probably linked to the decline in marriages and
increase in divorces and separations observed in 1974, and these
undoubtedly affected the fertility rates in 1975. Biologically,
the food shortage probably decreased the nutritional status of
women, a decrease which may have reduced fecundity, lengthened the
period of temporary infertility and increased fetal deaths.

This paper will present a preliminary analysis of maternal
nutrition and its relationship to two components of fertility: 1)
length of postpartum amenorrhea (amenorrhea segment), and 2) length
of time to conception after resumption of menses (menstruating
segment). Information was collected in the Matlab area over a 12
month period beginning in November, 1975.

THE STUDY AREA

Matlab Thana is an administrative unit in Comilla District,
Bangladesh. Like much of the nation, Matlab is situated on a flat
deltaic plain intersected by numerous rivers and canals. The
region has no roads. Internal communication is accomplished by
foot or country boat. The climate is subtropical with three
seasons. Most of the average annual rainfall of 85 inches falls
during the monsoon which extends from June till September. During
this season, it rains almost daily, and most of the low-lying
fields are flooded. The monsoon is followed by the cool-dry season
which lasts until February. The hot-dry season begins in March and
ends with the beginning of the monsoon. Agriculture is the dominant economic activity, with rice as the major staple and jute the
main cash crop. Fishing is the second most common occupation.
The remainder of the labor force is involved in service-related or
labor-intensive activities. There are three harvests annually;
the aman crop, a flood crop, which yields over half of the annual
rice production, is harvested in November. Smaller rice crops are
harvested at the end of the boro season (February) and the aus
season (June).

The people are nearly all indigenous Bengalis; over 85 percent
are Muslim and most of the remainder are Hindu. The population
density exceeds 2,000 persons per square mile, making Matlab one
of the most densely settled rural regions in the world. Villages
have an average population of 1,000 persons. Each village is
divided into many baris, each consisting of two or more patriline-
ally-related families. A family averages approximately six
persons and usually has its own one-or two-room house with a mud
floor, jute stick walls, and a thatched grass or galvanized iron
roof. The houses of a bari are arranged around a central courtyard

and bari members function as an economic and a domestic unit.

METHODS

The study began in November 1975 and will continue through October, 1978. Twelve villages within a five-mile radius of the CRL Matlab Treatment Center were selected for study. These villages contained approximately 2,200 married women aged 15-49 years. An initial interview and existing CRL records provided basic information about the women including age, parity, number of living children, education, religion, husband's occupation and date of last pregnancy termination. Follow-up information is collected by trained female workers who visit each woman once a month to inquire about pregnancy, pregnancy termination, menstrual status, breast-feeding practices, family planning practice, child mortality, and morbidity, and the absence of either the woman or her husband. The height of each woman was measured once and weight and arm circumference are measured each month. Every two months, fingertip blood samples are collected for hematocrit determinations.

DEFINITIONS

The length of postpartum amenorrhea is defined as the number of full calendar months from the date of a pregnancy termination to the date of onset of the first menses. The waiting time for conception (menstruating segment) is defined as the number of full calendar months from the first postpartum menses to the month of conception.

For the purpose of analysis, amenorrhea and menstruating segments were divided into closed-interval and open-interval segments based on cut-off or termination during this period. A closed amenorrhea segment is one which started with pregnancy termination and ended with the onset of menses during the period of the study. An open amenorrhea segment also started with pregnancy termination but continued to the cut-off date without the onset of menses. A closed menstruating segment is one which started with the onset of menses and ended at conception occurring during the study period. An open menstruating segment continued until cut-off date without conception. Any of these segments may have started either before or during the study period. If a woman had more than one amenorrhea or menstruating segment during the year, only the most recent of each kind was included.

This paper covers only the first 12 months of observation and includes only closed intervals, that is, only those amenorrhea and menstruating segments which terminated in the study period. The

nutritional status of the woman is based on the measurements taken
in the month the interval is closed, i.e., in the month of first
menstruation for the amenorrhea segment, and in the month of conception for the menstruating segment. It is recognized that this
analysis will be biased because of a selection for short intervals;
however, this bias should not substantially affect comparisons of
interval lengths by age, nutritional status, or other variables.

RESULTS

Two thousand two hundred eighteen women were studied. Table 1
compares the age distribution of the study population with the
total Matlab population. Forty-one of these women were menopausal
and 204 had no previous pregnancy termination; 1,395 women had
menstruating segments terminating or cut off during the study
period. One hundred forty seven of these had been menstruating
for at least 60 months without pregnancy occurring and were assumed
to be sterile. Of the remainder, 483 had closed menstruating segments and 766 had open menstruating segments; 643 women had closed
amenorrhea segments and 562 had open amenorrhea segments.

Table 2(a) shows the length of postpartum amenorrhea and waiting time for conception by age of the women studied. Age is
positively related to length of both the amenorrhea and menstruating
segments. The mean length of amenorrhea for women of less than 25
years of age was 13.7 months compared to 19.3 months for the age
group 25-34, and 20.6 months for the age group 35 and over. The
differences in mean waiting time for conception by age are not
great - 12.2 months in age group below 25 versus 14.0 in age group
35 and over.

Table 2(b) shows the length of amenorrhea and menstruating
segment by parity. The pattern closely parallels that by age and
is probably due to the age/parity correlation (see below).

Table 2(c) provides the segment lengths by education of the
women. Education shows a negative relationship with length of
postpartum amenorrhea. No evidence exists of any association
between education and waiting time for conception. Again, because
of education and age relationships, any interpretation of this
table may be difficult.

Table 2(d) shows the waiting time for conception by period of
absence of the husbands. As expected, the absence of husbands is
directly related to the duration of the menstruating segments.

Table 2(e) shows the length of postpartum amenorrhea and waiting time for conception as related to the death of children. The

Table 1

Comparison of Study Population with Matlab
Population in 1974 by Age Group

Age Group	Study Women	Married Women in Matlab
10-14	1.7	1.8
15-19	16.4	17.0
20-24	17.6	17.8
25-29	15.2	15.4
30-34	18.7	18.0
35-39	14.0	12.9
40-44	11.0	10.8
45-49	5.4	6.3
	100.0	100.0

average length of postpartum amenorrhea is shorter by at least six months for mothers experiencing child death during the segment. This, of course, reflects the earlier interruption of breastfeeding. The waiting time for conception was found higher among mothers who had a child death since her last pregnancy; however, this cannot be interpreted because of small numbers and no adjustment for age in this tabulation.

The length of amenorrhea and length of menstruating interval by height of the women is presented in Table 3(a). Height showed no effect on the menstruating segment or on amenorrhea segment.

Table 3(b) presents the length of amenorrhea and length of menstruating intervals by weight of the mother. Weight showed only a slight negative relationship both to waiting time for conception and to the length of postpartum amenorrhea. The arm circumference, another index of nutritional status, also failed to show any consistent relationship with the fertility variables (Table 3(c). Hematocrit level showed some positive correlation with fecundity, but none with postpartum amenorrhea (Table 3(d).

Because of interrelationships between variables in the previous tables, a correlation matrix is presented in Table 4 which shows the extent of interrelationship between nutritional, demographic, and socioeconomic factors affecting fertility. In the table, age-parity correlation was found to be 0.84, age-education correlation was -0.16. Age-weight correlation was found -.12, height-weight correlation was 0.42, and weight-arm circumference was 0.73.

Table 2

Mean Duration of Postpartum Amenorrhea and of Menstruating
Interval by Mother's Age, Parity and Education,
Husband's Absence, and Infant Death
Matlab 1975-1976

		Postpartum Amenorrhea		Menstruating Interval	
		No.	Mean Months	No.	Mean Months
(a)	All	643	17.9	482	10.9
	Age				
	< 25	189	13.7	173	12.2
	25-34	304	19.3	226	8.8
	35 +	150	20.6	83	14.0
(b)	Parity				
	1-3	266	16.5	249	12.2
	4-6	197	20.6	151	8.5
	7 +	155	19.0	77	11.8
(c)	Education (Yrs.)				
	None	467	18.6	385	11.1
	1-4	62	17.1	44	8.9
	5 +	74	14.1	53	11.4
(d)	Husband's Absence (Mo.)				
	< 1	-	-	347	8.6
	1-4	-	-	71	11.8
	5 +	-	-	20	15.3
(e)	Infant Death				
	No	600	18.2	430	10.6
	Yes	49	12.9	46	13.6

Multiple regression analyses were done, considering separately
as the dependent variable: 1) the closed interval of postpartum
amenorrhea, and 2) the closed interval of waiting time to conception
to assess the effects of each of the independent variables.

Table 3

Mean Duration of Postpartum Amenorrhea and the Menstruating
Interval by Maternal Height, Weight, Arm
Circumference, and Hematocrit
Matlab 1975-1976

		Postpartum Amenorrhea		Menstruating Interval	
		No.	Mean Months	No.	Mean Months
(a)	Height (cm)				
	< 145	169	18.2	110	10.9
	145-149	255	17.5	206	11.4
	150 +	210	18.5	160	10.5
(b)	Weight (Kg)				
	< 38.5	137	17.9	120	11.3
	38.5-42.4	191	17.5	138	10.7
	42.5 +	174	16.8	161	10.0
(c)	Arm Circumference (cm)				
	< 21	153	18.7	115	10.7
	21-22	302	17.8	219	9.9
	23 +	160	17.6	130	12.1
(d)	Hematocrit (%)				
	< 34	161	17.3	134	9.3
	35-39	222	19.9	185	11.9
	40 +	44	18.6	28	12.7

   Table 5 presents the regression analysis where the independent
variables are age, parity, weight, arm circumference, height and
hematocrit, and the dependent variable is the length of postpartum
amenorrhea. Here, after controlling other factors, only age, parity, and the hematocrit are significantly related to the duration
of postpartum amenorrhea. The relationships are in the expected
directions: increasing age is associated with longer amenorrhea;
higher parity is associated with shorter amenorrhea, possibly
because short birth intervals are required to reach higher parity;
similarly, a higher hematocrit is logically associated with longer
amenorrhea since the hematocrit was measured at the end of the
period of amenorrhea and higher levels must be related to the

Table 4

Correlation Matrix

Variables		Variable Number							
		(1)	(2)	(3)	(4)	(5)	(6)	(7)	(8)
Age	(1)	1.00							
Parity	(2)	0.84	1.00						
Education	(3)	-0.16	-0.14	1.00					
Height	(4)	-0.04	-0.08	0.05	1.00				
Arm Cir.	(5)	-0.01	-0.01	-0.02	0.16	1.00			
Weight	(6)	-0.12	-0.15	-0.02	0.42	0.73	1.00		
Hematocrit	(7)	-0.11	-0.08	0.05	0.08	-0.07	-0.08	1.00	
Husband Absence	(8)	0.06	0.08	0.02	-0.01	-0.01	0.00	0.00	1.00

Sample size 568

sparing of blood loss. The nutrition variables, height, weight, and arm circumference, were not significantly associated with the length of amenorrhea.

Table 6 presents the second regression analysis, putting the menstruating segment as the dependent variable, and age, parity, weight, height, arm circumference, length of husband's absence, and hematocrit level as the independent variables. Not surprisingly, age and husband's absence were positively associated with the menstruating interval, and higher parity was associated with shorter intervals. Again, there were no significant relationships with the nutrition variables.

CONCLUSIONS

A preliminary analysis of the birth interval components, based on prospective observations in rural Bangladesh leads to the following conclusions:

1. Age of women is positively related to both the length of postpartum amenorrhea and waiting time for conception.

2. After eliminating the age effect, parity is negatively related to the length of both the amenorrhea and the menstruating intervals.

Table 5

Relationship of Length of Postpartum Amenorrhea to
Age, Parity and Nutrition Variables
Simple and Partial Correlation Coefficients

Independent Variable	Simple Correlation	Partial	
		R	F
Age	0.283	0.234	36.93*
Hematocrit	0.113	0.119	9.18*
Parity	0.190	-0.097	5.98*
Arm Circumference	-0.043	-0.029	0.53
Height	-0.003	0.016	0.16
Weight	-0.049	0.005	0.02

Multiple R^2 = 0.104
F = 12.28*
N = 641 women

* $p < 0.05$

Table 6

Relationship of Menstruating Interval to Age, Parity,
Husband's Absence, and Nutrition Variables
Simple and Partial Correlation Coefficients

Independent Variable	Simple Correlation	Partial	
		R	F
Age	0.076	0.205	21.67*
Parity	-0.057	-0.183	17.04*
Husband's Absence	0.117	0.120	7.17*
Weight	0.070	0.074	2.75
Hematocrit	0.068	0.074	2.73
Height	0.002	-0.034	0.58
Arm Circumference	0.021	-0.028	0.38

Multiple R^2 = 0.067
F = 5.03*
N = 512 women

* $p < 0.05$

3. The nutritional indicators - height, weight, and arm
    circumference - were not significantly associated with
    either the length of postpartum amenorrhea or the waiting
    time to conception.

4. Longer amenorrhea is associated with a higher hematocrit,
    probably due to sparing of blood loss.

5. Husband's absences are associated with conception delays.

It should be noted that though this longitudinal study was
carried out over the year of a famine and falling fertility, the
data presented here does not begin to explain the fertility decline.
This is in part because this analysis deals only with closed intervals, that is, intervals which terminate in the observation period.
While this may not be a serious problem with reference to postpartum amenorrhea, it may be presenting a bias in measuring fecundability. Specifically, women who cannot conceive, that is, who
have long conception times did not appear in the study group.

There is some evidence that this may be a factor. Preliminary
analysis indicates that among women in the lowest weight group
(less than 38.5 kg) 17.6% had not conceived in five years, as
compared to only 6.7% and 8.4% in the higher weight groups.
Further analysis, adjusting for age for example, is required before
any definitive conclusions can be reached in this area.

References

1. Chowdhury, A.K.M.A. and Chen, L. C. The Dynamics of Contemp-
    orary Famine (mimeo). The Ford Foundation, Dacca, Bangladesh,
    1977.

2. Chen, L. C., Huffman, S. L. and Satterthwaite, P. Recent
    Fertility Trends in Bangladesh: Speculation on the Role of
    Biological Factors and Socioeconomic Change (mimeo). The
    Ford Foundation, Dacca, Bangladesh, 1976.

VARIATIONS IN FERTILITY WITH BREAST-FEEDING PRACTICE AND
CONTRACEPTION IN URBAN FILIPINO WOMEN: IMPLICATIONS FOR A
NUTRITION PROGRAM

Trinidad S. Osteria

University of the Philippines

Manila, Philippines

INTRODUCTION

An important aspect of the present rapid growth in population
in developing countries is the decline in breastfeeding practice.
There is a dearth of literature on trends in breastfeeding practices
in the Philippines although separate studies point toward the reduction. In 1959, a survey of 1000 infants in various hospitals and
health centers in the City of Manila revealed that 64.2% were
breastfed, 23% were artificially fed, and 12% were sustained by
mixed feeding (1). About a decade later in 1970, a nationwide
survey of 1000 Filipino infants indicated that 43.8% were breastfed,
32.1% bottle fed, and 24.1% had mixed feeding (2). Strict compara-
bility could not be warranted due to difference in locale (the first
study was urban, while the latter included urban and rural population). The findings, nevertheless, indicate a shift to bottlefeeding (Table 1). A more recent study based on a food consumption
survey by the Food and Nutrition Research Institute in urban and
rural areas in Luzon indicated a further reduction in the percentage breastfeeding in urban centers. In this study of children aged
0-3 years, it was shown that 26.5% were breastfed, 44.1% had mixed
feeding, and 29.4% bottle fed (3).

This reduction in proportion breastfeeding was attributed to
changing roles and modes of life of urban mothers and their exposure to highly commercialized milk substitutes. Improved technology
in food and dairy industry has made available a wide variety of
milk based infant foods. High pressure advertising and sales promotion gimmicks employed by most manufacturers of these human milk
substitutes has been one of the causes of decline in breastfeeding
and early weaning.

Table 1

Changes in Infant Feeding Patterns in the Philippines
Based on Surveys in 1958, 1968, and 1974

Type of Feeding	1958[1] Urban %	1968[2] Urban & Rural %	1974[3] Urban %	Rural %
Breast	64.2	43.8	26.5	66.1
Mixed	12.7	24.1	44.1	27.5
Bottle	23.1	32.1	29.4	6.4
	100.0	100.0	100.0	100.0

Source: [1]del Mundo, reference (1).

[2]Dulay, reference (2).

[3]Intengan, reference (3).

The relationship between lactation and birth intervals which
operates through the postpartum amenorrhea has been adequately
documented. It has been postulated that with the decline in
breastfeeding practice and the traditional pattern of late weaning,
a corresponding increase in fertility of the women could be experienced. This shortening of birth intervals could be compensated by
the institution of contraceptive programs, a natural link in the
transitional process. The extent to which contraceptive use has
enhanced or competed with the effects of breastfeeding in the
developing nations is a subject worthy of attention (5).

THE PHILIPPINE POPULATION PROGRAM

The family planning program in the country has been operating
on an organized basis in 1970. Between 1970 and 1974, the number
of acceptors rose from 191,700 to 749,900. While a slight shift
toward condom and conventional (foam, diaphragm, and rhythm) acceptance has been noted, oral contraceptives have remained the pre-
dominant method of choice, accounting for almost half of the
acceptances (Table 2). It would be interesting to determine the
extent to which contraceptive use, particularly the pills, could
have compensated for the lack of breastfeeding.

Table 2

Distribution of Contraceptive Acceptors by Method and
Year of Acceptance, Philippines, 1970-74

Year	Total (000's)	IUD	Oral Contraceptives	Others	Total
1976	191.7	21.6	53.2	25.2	100.0
1971	408.8	19.7	60.1	20.2	100.0
1972	621.9	14.1	57.3	28.6	100.0
1973	737.9	10.9	46.6	42.5	100.0
1974	749.9	9.8	49.8	40.5	100.0

Source: Philippine Population Program (Mimeographed)

THE STUDY DESIGN

In this study, attempts were made to answer several questions concerning the relationship of lactation, amenorrhea, contraception, and birth intervals in a group of urban Filipino women. These are:

1. How do socioeconomic and demographic factors relate to breastfeeding practices?

2. How does the duration and type of lactation affect the period of amenorrhea?

3. What is the duration of the menstruating interval, and does this vary by age and between women who do not lactate as compared to those who do?

4. Is there a correlation between contraceptive usage and breastfeeding practices?

5. How does contraceptive use overlap with postpartum amenorrhea where lactation is prevalent? Does such overlap affect the demographic impact of contraception?

Methods

This report describes the results of a prospective, truncated study among 794 married women, residents of the City of Manila, who delivered at J. Fabella Maternity Hospital in June and July, 1973, and were followed up on a monthly basis for 24 months. On

each visit there was a detailed inquiry regarding breastfeeding
and infant supplenentation practices, amenorrhea, contraceptive
usage, and eventual pregnancy. Information was also obtained on
socioeconomic and demographic status, fertility history, interval
between delivery and resumption of sexual relations and infant
survival.

Definitions

1. Lactation was classified into two categories: When a
nursing mother reported giving no food supplement solid or liquid,
full breastfeeding was recorded. If any supplementary food was
given to the infant, breastfeeding was classified as partial.

2. The length of postpartum amenorrhea is taken as the number
of full calendar months from the date of delivery to the date of
the onset of first menses. If the woman became pregnant prior to
menstruation, the date of conception (and thus the duration of
postpartum amenorrhea) was calculated retrospectively after following the mother till the termination of pregnancy.

3. Conception date is computed as the fourteenth date after
the first day of the last menses, or if conception occurred during
amenorrhea, the pregnancy was followed up and the length of gestation ascertained based on the outcome and thereafter the conception
data estimated in retrospect.

4. The menstruating interval is the number of full calendar
months from the first menstruation to conception.

Limitations of the Study

Certain biases are recognized which might restrict generalizations from the findings:

1. All intervals in this study begin with a live birth;
women with fetal wastages and stillbirths are excluded. Further,
since the study group consists of a sample of livebirths delivered
at the same time in the same year, it will be biased toward more
fecund women, and not representative of all married childbearing
women.

2. The 24-month period of the study results in a truncation
bias since a substantial portion of the women had not conceived
during the period and a small number were still lactating at the
end of the study. (There were 31 women who withdrew from the study
in the course of 24 months. However, they terminated lactation
and resumed menses prior to withdrawal.) This potential bias is

minimized by the use of the life table analysis technique.

3. In the course of the twenty-four months, 565 (71.2%) of the wives used some form of contraception. Nineteen pill acceptors began pills before the resumption of menses and were therefore excluded from the estimation of the length postpartum amenorrhea since menstrual cycles resume with pill use. The menstruating interval for non-contraceptors might be biased by the self selection of acceptors. However, since the potential fertility of the two groups is unknown, the possibility of such bias cannot be estimated.

4. The end of postpartum amenorrhea is demarcated by the onset of first menses. This period roughly coincides with the period of infertility but not exactly, since most women who are breastfeeding will have an ovulatory first cycle; that is, they will ovulate two weeks prior to the onset of the first menses.

5. An underlying assumption in the determination of menstruating interval is that it begins the fecundable period. However, some women may not be fecund in the first few cycles.

6. Finally, there is the problem of identifying conception. Obviously, this is observed only with the clinical evidence of the next pregnancy. There always remains the possibility of some conceptions being missed because there were very early fetal wastages.

All of these problems notwithstanding the interpregnancy interval will be divided into its two subintervals in order to better define the sources of variability in interpregnancy intervals for different groups of women.

General Framework

The interpregnancy interval has been defined as the period between the termination of a pregnancy or delivery and the onset of the subsequent pregnancy. It is the difference between the date of delivery and the date of subsequent conception. This can be divided into two additive components: the period of postpartum amenorrhea which is the interval between delivery and resumption of menses and the menstruating interval - the period from the resumption of menses and the start of conception. The length of postpartum amenorrhea is largely affected by the duration of lactation while practice of contraception affects the menstruating interval.

For menstruating interval there will be two groups of women, those who do not choose to practice contraception, the "non-contraceptors", and those who do choose to practice contraception, the "contraceptors." For the non-contraceptors, it can be noted that there are several factors that affect their fecundity. First is age; it is clearly established that fecundity declines with age. Second, there is some variability in the first few menstrual cycles according to whether or not the women ever initiated breastfeeding. For non-breastfeeding women, the early menstrual cycles are not ovulatory, most likely because of residual hormonal activity from the recent pregnancy. Further, even where they are ovulatory the women may appear to be subfecund, that is, not have a detectable conception or pregnancy because of incomplete restoration of normal function of the reproductive organs.

For the contraceptors, the major source of variability will relate to the specific contraceptive chosen and the women's motivation to use the method, particularly if it is a technique such as the pill which requires continuous motivation as compared to the intrauterine device.

RESULTS

Characteristics of the Women

Table 3 gives the distribution of the women by age and parity. Almost half (46%) of the wives were less than 25 years of age and 3.5% beyond 40 years. About a third (33.4%) had one child and a fifth (19.9%) had two children. The average age was 26 years and the average parity 3. The completion of childbearing is approached at the 35-39 group with 6 births. Most of the women were of low socioeconomic status. Although most of the wives had acquired some high school education, more than three-fourths (79.3%) were not working. Employment was mainly limited to around the house, like dressmaking and store tending. Eighty percent of the husbands were blue collar workers - laborers, jeepney drivers, carpenters, street sweepers, and factory workers.

Interpregnancy Interval

Figure 1 depicts the cumulative proportions of pregnancies occurring during the course of the prospective study for all women and for two age groups - less than 30 years and 30 and over. At the end of 3 months, 15.1% became pregnant. After 6 months, the proportion rose to 22.9% and after one year, 32.5% or close to a third conceived. After 18 months, 37.4% became pregnant and after 2 years the percentage rose to 39.7%. Differentials in probabilities of conception were noted between the younger wives (less than 30) and their older counterparts, with the probability being much

Table 3

Distribution of the Study Population by
Age and Parity, Manila, 1973

Age	Parity							Total	%	Average Parity
	1	2	3	4	5	6	7+			
15-19	81	27	5	0	0	0	0	113	14.3	1.3
20-24	117	70	47	14	3	1	0	252	31.7	1.9
25-29	47	52	38	32	20	14	3	206	25.9	2.9
30-34	14	6	15	18	15	16	28	112	14.1	4.6
35-39	4	4	6	7	11	6	45	83	10.5	5.6
40-44	1	0	4	0	1	1	21	28	3.5	6.1
Total	264	159	115	71	50	38	97	794	100.0	3.0
(Percent)	(33.2)	(10.0)	(14.5)	(8.9)	(6.3)	(4.9)	(12.2)	(100.0)		

higher for the younger women.

This interpregnancy interval will be dissected into two major
components - the period of postpartum infertility and the menstruating interval. Each of these components will be analyzed for the
relevant variables that influence these intervals.

Postpartum Amenorrhea

<u>Breastfeeding Practices</u>. Since breastfeeding has been
recognized as a major factor affecting postpartum amenorrhea,
Table 4 presents the breastfeeding practices by age, education,
and employment status. Overall, 76% of the women breastfed their
infants for some time period. Variations in the percentage breastfeeding are insignificant but the median period of lactation for

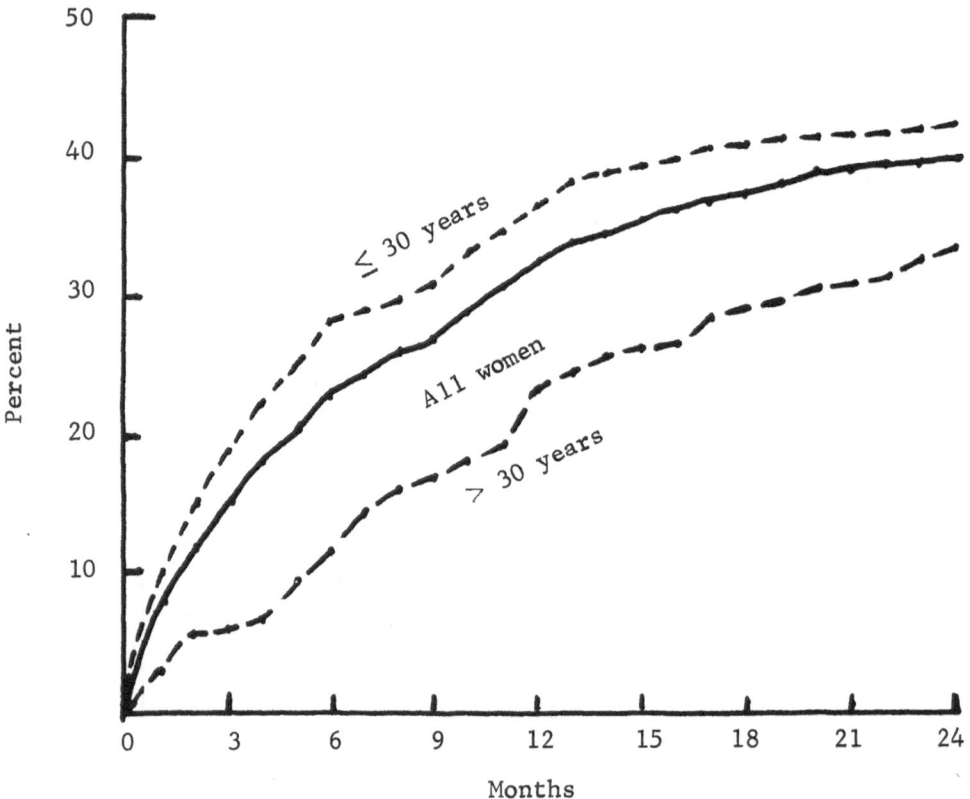

Figure 1. Cumulative percent of women pregnant by month since last
live birth.

Table 4

Distribution of Women by Breastfeeding Status
and Selected Characteristics, Manila, 1973

	Total	Breastfeeding Number	%	Median Length of Breastfeeding
AGE				
<25	365	281	77.0	8.7 ⎫ 9.1
25-29	206	158	76.7	9.7 ⎭
30-34	112	83	74.1	13.6 ⎫
35-39	83	64	77.1	12.0 ⎬ 12.8
40 +	28	18	64.3	12.0 ⎭
Total	794	604	76.1	10.3
EDUCATION OF WIFE				
Elementary or less	337	267	79.2	12.3
High School	314	241	76.8	8.1
College	143	96	67.1	4.3
Total	794	604	76.1	10.3
WIFE's EMPLOYMENT				
Full Time	87	56	64.4 ⎫ 68.2	1.7 ⎫ 3.3
Part Time	77	56	72.7 ⎭	5.0 ⎭
None	630	492	78.1	11.4 ⎭
Total	794	604	76.1	10.3

women below 30 years was 9.1 months while for those over 30 years
it was 12.8 months - a difference of 3.7 months.

With respect to socioeconomic status there is a decline in
the proportion of breastfeeding women with improvement in education.
Whereas 79.2% of the wives who had 6 years of education or less
breastfed, the proportion breastfeeding among those who acquired
some college education was 67.1%. There was a greater difference
in the median duration of lactation. Wives with lower education
breastfed approximately 12 months as opposed to 4 months for their
better educated counterparts. When wife's employment is considered,
a somewhat higher proportion of women who did not work breastfed -
a difference of about 10%. There were great differences in the
duration of breastfeeding - fulltime workers breastfed for less
than 2 months as compared to almost 1 year for non-workers. Thus,
small variations are observed in the proportion breastfeeding for
each category of age and socioeconomic status; the major differences

Table 5

Breastfeeding Status by Socioeconomic Status and Age

| | <30 | | | 30+ | | |
Status	Total	Breastfed	Median Duration of BF	Total	Breastfed	Median Duration of BF
		%			%	
EMPLOYMENT STATUS						
Employed	104	69.2	3.33	60	66.7	4.0
Unemployed	467	78.6	10.35	163	76.7	15.5
EDUCATION						
Elementary or less	203	81.8	6.22	134	75.4	16.6
High School	251	78.1	8.33	63	71.4	6.5
College	117	65.8	2.88	26	73.1	7.5

are in the durations of lactation.

The differences in breastfeeding practices were analyzed in more detail through cross tabulations by age and employment status and by age and education status in Table 5. While very slight variations are noted in the proportion breastfeeding, the median duration of breastfeeding varied significantly by socioeconomic class. Overall, the median duration of breastfeeding is longer for those beyond 30 years of age but within each age category the socio-economic differentiation prevails. Among those employed and less than 30 years of age, the median length of breastfeeding was 3.3 months. For the unemployed, it was 10.4 months. For those beyond 30 years, the median length of lactation for the employed was 4 months and for the non-working mothers, 15.5 months. By education, those who acquired a high school or college education breastfed for much shorter intervals than those with elementary education. There were variations by age group within an education category. Younger women in the highest and lowest education groups breastfed for only one-third as long as their older counterparts. Age had no effect on the duration of breastfeeding among women with a high school education.

A tabulation of breastfeeding practice by nutritional status of the mother using Jellife's nutritional standard (4) failed to show a marked difference in either the proportion or the duration of breastfeeding (Table 6).

Table 6

Breastfeeding Patterns by Nutritional Status of the Mother

Nutritional Status of Mother	Total No.	Breastfed		Median Duration of BF (mos.)
		No.	%	
Nourished	522	410	78.5	11.78
Malnourished	272	194	71.3	10.83
Total	794	604		

Lactation and Amenorrhea. A positive relationship between lactation and amenorrhea has been amply documented. To demonstrate this effect in this study, a life table analysis was undertaken to determine the probability of resuming menstruation by months following delivery for those who breastfed and those who did not. Three life tables were constructed to compare the effect of full and partial breastfeeding as well as non-lactation on the probability of resuming menstruation.

Table 7 indicates that almost half (47.8%) of those who do not lactate resume their menses within the first month after delivery. By the third month, 86% have resumed their menses. Among the women who partially breastfeed, 24% resume their menses in the first month, close to half (49.2%) by the third month, and at the end of one year 87% have resumed menstruating. For those fully breastfeeding, only 12% resume their menses in the first month, 25% by the third month, and 68% by the end of the year.

Contraception

Contraceptive Acceptance. That urban wives tend to accept family planning was borne out by the fact that by the end of the observation period, 565 wives had enrolled at the clinics. The method most commonly used was the IUD since J. Fabella Hospital where the women delivered has a program of postpartum IUD insertion. Differentials in contraceptive status by age and education of the wives are shown in Table 8. Pill acceptors on the average were somewhat younger than acceptors of IUD and conventional contraceptives; 67% of pill acceptors were less than 25 years of age whereas only 44% of IUD acceptors and 35% of conventional acceptors were under this age. Non-acceptors tended to be somewhat less educated than the family planning clients.

Table 7

Cumulative Probability of Resuming Menstruation by
Lactation Status by Month Since Delivery

Months since Delivery	Non-lactating	Breastfeeding	
		Partial	Full
0	.000	.000	.000
1	.478	.241	.115
3	.859	.492	.251
6	.989	.695	.351
9	.995	.792	.477
12	.995	.869	.682
15	1.000	.930	.830
18	1.000	.973	.902

Interval Between Delivery and Acceptance. Table 9 shows the
relationship of contraceptive acceptance, by method to time interval since birth. The majority of the IUD acceptors accepted in
the first month after delivery through a hospital based postpartum
program. For the IUD, the mean and median interval between delivery and acceptance were 1.3 and 0.5 months, respectively. For
pills, they were 5.6 and 5 months and for conventionals, 5.8 and
3.4 months, respectively.

Overlap Between Contraceptive Use and Amenorrhea. An important issue in determining the impact of a family planning program
is the extent to which contraceptive use overlaps with the period
of postpartum amenorrhea - the portion of time when the woman is
ordinarily not at risk of becoming pregnant due to anovulation.
This period of overlap negates any potential demographic impact
of contraceptive use. Since the pills induce menstruation, the
length of overlap could only be measured for the acceptors of IUD
and those of other methods. Table 10 shows that the mean period
between IUD acceptance and first menstruation is 4.3 months, and
for the other methods 2.1 months.

Contraceptive Continuation. Differentials in continuation
rates were likewise observed for the different methods (Table 11).
Among the pill acceptors, 35% have dropped out at the end of 3
months, and 58% terminated use after 6 months. IUD acceptors have
better continuation; after one year, only 21% have stopped using
the IUD. Acceptors of other methods also dropped out at a lower
pace - after 3 months, the percentage was 6.5%; this rose to 21.8%
after one year. The point of overlap noted above is relevant to
these continuation rates, since contraceptives do not exert their

Table 8

Pattern of Contraceptive Use by Age and Education

Age Group	Non-acceptors		Pills		IUD		Conventionals		Total	
	No.	%	No.	%	No.	%	No.	%	No.	%
< 25	118	32.3	49	13.4	129	35.4	69	18.9	365	100.0
25-34	84	26.4	23	7.2	124	39.0	87	27.4	318	100.0
35 +	27	24.4	1	0.9	42	37.8	41	36.9	111	100.0
Total	229	28.8	73	9.2	295	37.2	197	24.8	794	100.0
Mean Age	26.9		24.8		27.7		28.8			
EDUCATION										
Elem. or less	113	33.5	23	6.9	121	35.9	80	23.7	337	100.0
High School	77	24.5	35	11.2	127	40.5	75	23.8	314	100.0
College	39	27.3	15	10.4	47	32.9	42	29.4	143	100.0
Total	229	28.8	73	9.2	295	37.2	197	24.8	794	100.0

Table 9

Interval Between Delivery and Contraceptive Acceptance

| Months since Delivery | Number of Acceptors | | |
	Pill	IUD	Conventionals
1	11	280	28
2	9	3	16
3	5	2	45
4	7	2	22
5	4	2	8
6	6	0	17
7	6	2	6
8	13		3
9	5		14
10	0		4
11	3		8
12+	4	4	26
Total	73	295	197
Mean	5.6	1.3	5.8
Median	5.0	0.5	3.4

effect on the birth interval during the period of overlap, but only by extending the duration of menstruating interval.

Pregnancies Following Termination of Contraceptive Use. Figure 2 presents the probability of pregnancy after termination of use by method accepted. Pregnancies occurred rapidly for all women; from 30% to 40% were pregnant by the third month following discontinuation of use. Pill acceptors did show some initial delay in conceptions as compared to previous users of IUDs and conventionals, but ultimately they had the highest cumulative fertility, probably reflecting their younger age.

Menstruating Interval

The menstruating interval has been defined as the period between the resumption of menses and the start of conception. A life table technique has been used to determine the monthly and cumulative probability of pregnancy by months since resumption of menses.

Table 12 is the life table of the menstruating interval for all women. At the end of three months, since resumption of menses, 14.6% of the wives have become pregnant. After 6 months, 23.1% have conceived, and after a year more than a third of the wives (34.70%) have become pregnant. The median interval between resumption of menses and conception is more than 24 months.

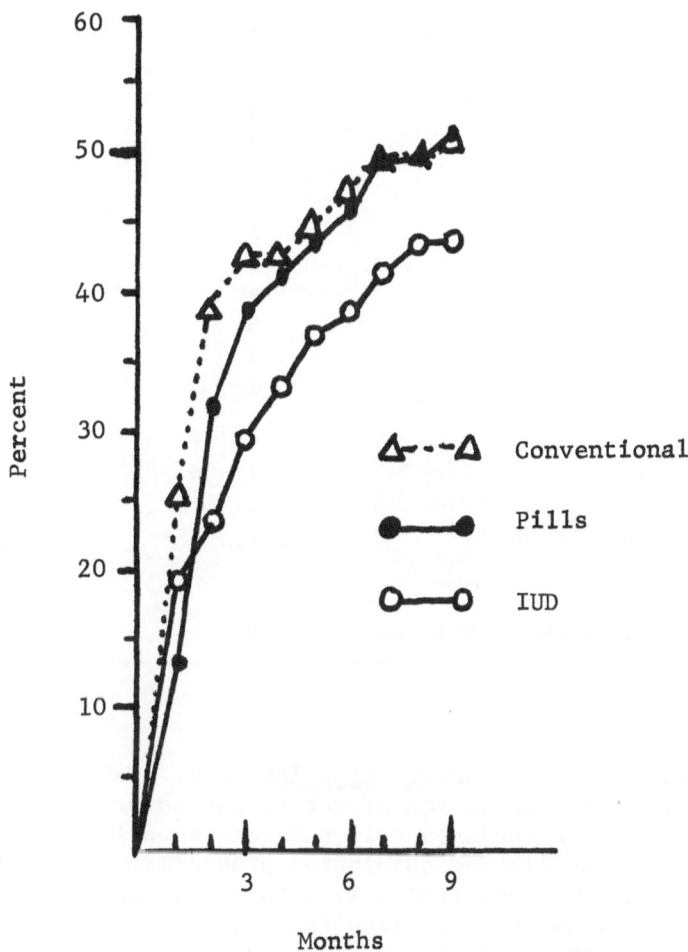

Figure 2. Cumulative percent conceptions by month after discontinuing IUD, pill, or conventional contraceptives.

Table 10

Months Between Contraceptive Acceptance and Resumption
of First Postpartum Menstruation

Months to First Menstruation	Number of Acceptors	
	IUD	Others
0	78	129
1	59	10
2	26	9
3	21	7
4	16	4
5	8	5
6	10	5
7	7	3
8	11	2
9	6	4
10	7	1
11	2	2
12	9	3
13	8	3
14	6	5
15	4	2
16	3	
17	5	1
18	1	
19	1	
20	2	
21	1	
22	1	
26	1	
No menstruation (pregnant)	2	2
Total	295	197
Mean Months with Amenorrhea	4.29	2.14

Factors Affecting Menstruating Interval. Table 13 gives a
more detailed analysis of the effect of age on menstruating interval. This analysis includes only non-contracepting women. At all
intervals, the monthly and cumulative probability of pregnancy is
higher for younger wives (those less than 30) compared to older
women. Among wives who were less than 30 years, 6.8% conceived
before the resumption of menses, 23.0% by the end of 3 months,
36.0% after 6 months. Among older wives, the proportions were
3.3%, 12.0%, and 18.9%, respectively.

Table 11

Cumulative Contraceptive Termination Rates by Method

Months Since Use	Method		
	Pills	IUD	Others
0	.000	.000	.000
1	.216	.038	.016
3	.352	.068	.065
6	.582	.106	.132
9	.634	.164	.180
12	.666	.208	.218
	(n=73)	(n=295)	(n=197)

Menstruating Interval of Contraceptive Acceptors

In order to segregate the impact of contraceptive acceptance, a multiple decrement life table was utilized where adjustment was made by removing women from the risk of conception when they accepted contraception. A basic general methodological point should be made here. First is the definition of an acceptor and a non-contraceptor. All women are initially classified as non-contraceptors. When a woman accepts some method of contraception, she then permanently is classified as an acceptor for the rest of the period of observation, whether or not she uses or discontinues the use of the method. The assumption is that acceptors are women who have been identified as making the behavioral choice to try to delay or prevent the next pregnancy. Once they are identified as acceptors, the question is: How successful are they in preventing the next conception as compared to those who never accept contraception?

Table 14 is a detailed analysis of the menstruating interval of acceptors showing the cumulative probability of pregnancy for acceptors of the various contraceptive techniques. There is a clear difference in conception rates between conventional and pill versus IUD acceptors. At the end of 3 (menstrual) months, 4.5% of the IUD acceptors became pregnant as opposed to 17.8% for conventionals and 19.9% for pill acceptors. After 6 months, the percentage of IUD acceptors pregnant was 7.6% as against 27.1% for conventionals and 33.4% for pill acceptors. After a year, close to half of pill acceptors (46.8%) and conventionals (45.1%) became pregnant compared to only 14.8% for IUD. Figure 3 illustrates

Table 12

Monthly and Cumulative Probability of Pregnancy Since Resumption
of Menses, All Women (Contraceptors and Non-acceptors)

Months Since Resumption	Probability	
	Monthly	Cumulative
**	.0605	.0000
0	.0309	.0605
1	.0305	.0895
2	.0330	.1173
3	.0478	.1464
4	.0284	.1872
5	.0261	.2103
6	.0252	.2309
7	.0331	.2545
8	.0238	.2792
9	.0322	.2964
10	.0222	.3191
11	.0193	.3342
12	.0202	.3470
13	.0212	.3602
14	.0124	.3738
15	.0254	.3816
16	.0053	.3973
17	.0165	.4005
18	.0087	.4104
19	.0032	.4155
20	.0069	.4174
21	.0082	.4214

** Pregnancy before resumption of first menses

that the pill and conventional acceptors got pregnant at about the
same rate as young non-acceptors.

It seems that the IUD is the only method that accounts for a
real reduction in fertility among acceptors. The programmatic
implications of pills and conventionals are minimal. The high
rate of pregnancy for pill acceptors can be accounted for largely
by their poor continuation rates. It could also be possible that
pill acceptors are more fecund, although differential fecundability
after termination of use was not borne out by the data in Figure 2.

Table 13

Menstruating Interval
Monthly and Cumulative Probability of Pregnancy
by Age, Non-acceptors only

Months Since Resumption of Menses	Age < 30		Age 30 +	
	Monthly	Cumulative	Monthly	Cumulative
**	.0683	.0000	.0329	.0000
0	.0504	.0683	.0417	.0329
1	.0537	.1153	.0161	.0732
2	.0809	.1628	.0354	.0881
3	.0893	.2305	.0583	.1204
4	.0480	.2992	.0211	.1717
5	.0631	.3328	-	.1892
6	.0402	.3596	.0460	.1892
7	.0535	.3749	.0482	.2271
8	.0347	.3939	.0267	.2644
9	.0119	.4149	.0278	.2840
10	.0256	.4219	.0615	.3039
11	.0130	.4367	-	.3467
12	.0263	.4440	.0323	.3467

** Pregnancy before first menses

DISCUSSION

The study of birth intervals is useful for understanding the dynamics of changes and trends in marital fertility among child-bearing women. This is particularly true in societies such as the Philippines which are going from traditional to modern contraceptive practices. In such circumstances, there is a very dynamic situation with discontinuance of lactation which would shorten birth intervals and initiation of contraception which would prolong birth intervals. The net effect of combining the two may or may not make much difference in the birth interval. It is likely, however, that if the woman is shortening lactation and initiating contraception in order to enter the labor market, less attention is given to the child with obvious detrimental effects.

Table 14

Menstruating Interval

Monthly and Cumulative Probability of Pregnancy Among
Contraception Acceptors by Type of Contraceptive Accepted

Months Since Resumption of Menses	Pills		IUD		Others	
	Monthly	Cumulative	Monthly	Cumulative	Monthly	Cumulative
**	.0869	.0000	.0209	.0000	.0522	.0000
0	.0755	.0369	-	.0209	.0550	.0522
1	.0282	.1559	.0070	.0209	.0586	.1043
2	.0230	.1797	.0105	.0279	.0253	.1568
3	.0632	.1986	.0247	.0453	.0458	.1781
4	.0594	.2492	.0036	.0689	.0315	.2157
5	.0561	.2938	.0037	.0723	.0405	.2404
6	.0187	.3335	.0221	.0757	.0165	.2712
7	.0566	.3459	.0152	.0961	.0422	.2832
8	.0588	.3829	.0077	.1098	.0362	.3134
9	.0204	.4192	.0157	.1167	.0976	.3383
10	.0211	.4311	.0121	.1306	.0335	.4029
11	.0444	.4431	.0082	.1411	.0488	.4229
12	.0500	.4678	.0084	.1481	.0276	.4511

** Pregnant before resumption of menses

The approach to the study of interpregnancy intervals is by breaking it into its two components: the postpartum amenorrhea and menstruating interval. These two components have very different behavioral and biological elements and are examined separately. Further, there may or may not be linkages between behavioral patterns related to the two components; that is, women who are choosing to abbreviate breastfeeding may or may not choose to accept some form of contraception in order to compensate. The study of the postpartum period confirmed previous observations about the importance of duration and type of breastfeeding in prolonging this interval.

A study of monthly conception rates by method accepted indicated that the pill and conventional contraceptive acceptors were not much better off than non-acceptors in terms of pregnancy

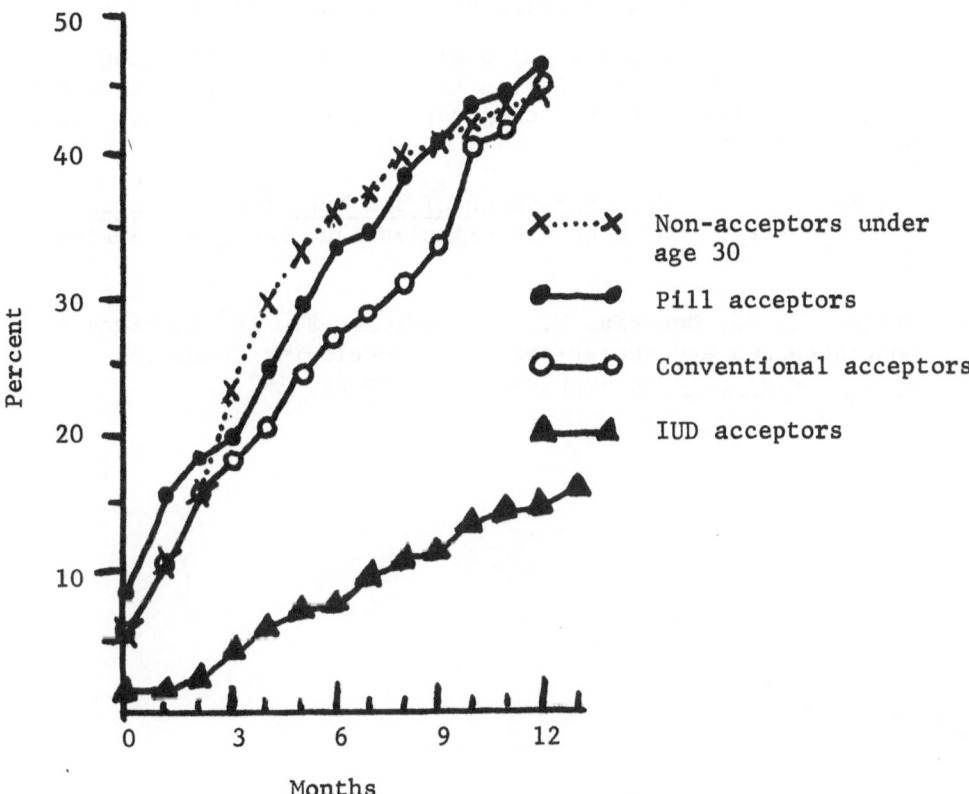

Figure 3. Cumulative percent pregnant by month from first menstruation for contraceptive acceptors, by method, and non-acceptors under age 30.

prevention. In an area where most of the acceptors take to the pills, it would be questionable if contraceptive acceptance could substitute for the shortening of lactation length. With industrialization and urbanization, or with a nutritional supplementation program, a reduction in breastfeeding can be expected. As the study indicates, the demographic impact of these changes may or may not be compensated by contraceptive technology. Experience in the urban areas indicates that introduction of contraception, particularly the pill, may not be contributing to the prolongation of birth intervals.

References

1. Del Mundo, P. Present Trends in the Feeding of Filipino Infants. P. J. of Pediatrics 8: 229-237, 1959.

2. Dulay, L. G. Current Feeding Patterns as Observed Among 1000 Filipino Infants. P. J. of Pediatrics 19: 95-103, 1970.

3. Intengan, C. L. Nutritional Evaluation of Breastfeeding Practices in Some Countries in the Far East. Paper presented at the 10th International Congress of Nutrition, Kyoto, Japan, August 3-9, 1975.

4. Jelliffe, D. B. The Assessment of the Nutritional Status of the Community. World Health Organization, Monograph Series No. 53.

5. Mosley, W. H., Osteria, T., and Huffman, S. Interactions of Contraception and Breastfeeding in Developing Countries. J. Biosocial Science Supplement, in press, 1977.

A STUDY OF BIRTH INTERVAL DYNAMICS IN RURAL JAVA

Valerie J. Hull

Gadjah Mada University, Yogyakarta, Indonesia, and
Australian National University, Canberra,
Australia

INTRODUCTION: JAVANESE FERTILITY

Recent demographic studies have shown that Java, the most populous and densely settled island of Indonesia, has the lowest recorded fertility of the country's major regions (1,2). Within Java, fertility is lower among the ethnic Javanese of the provinces of East and Central Java than among the smaller group of Sundanese in West Java. Furthermore, there is evidence that among the rural Javanese, differences also exist in fertility according to socioeconomic status; that is, fertility is lower among poor villagers than among relatively better-off rural dwellers (3,4,5,6). (See Chart 1).

These fertility patterns are of considerable interest from both a theoretical and policy viewpoint. Several researchers have suggested possible reasons why the Javanese, and particularly poor Jananese peasants, have lower fertility. It has been hypothesized that there is voluntary restriction of fertility in response to the extreme population density and adverse economic conditions which characterize rural Java (1). The author's previous sociodemographic research* has indicated that involuntary as well as voluntary

---

* Reported in Hull (5,7). These data are based on year-long intensive research carried out by T.& V. Hull, during which time the researchers were resident in the study community of Maguwoharjo. In addition to a detailed marriage and pregnancy history of just under 2000 women, this study also collected interval data retrospectively for 325 women for whom dates of live births were fully

Chart 1: Total Fertility Rates among Regions and Groups
          in Indonesia ca 1965-70.

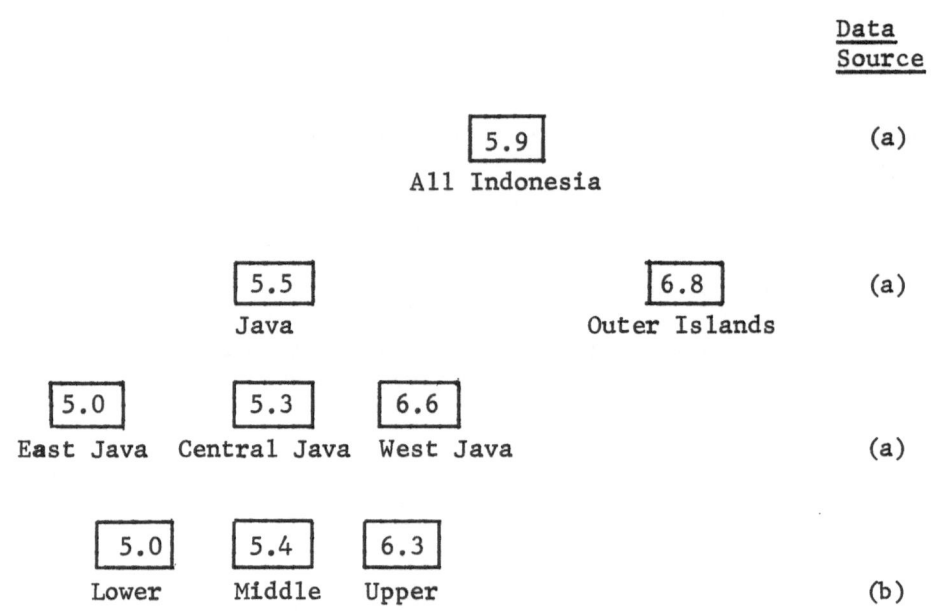

Source: (a) McDonald, Yasin and Jones (2), p. 50. See references
             for the exact geographical areas represented by these
             figures.

         (b) Hull (7), p. 331, based on data collected in the
             villages of Maguwoharjo, Yogyakarta, central Java.

---

mechanisms act to restrain fertility; these include factors such
as marital disruption and apparent secondary sterility. However,
it is also clear that even among fecund, currently married women
fertility is not unrestricted; birth intervals are long - averaging three years - despite very low rates of usage of modern
contraceptives. Long durations of lactation, postpartum amenorrhea,
and abstinence have been recorded (3,5). Furthermore, there is
evidence of differential child spacing patterns, with intervals
tending to be longer among ethnic Javanese and among those in the

---

documented by birth certificates.

lower socioeconomic status groups.*

THE PROSPECTIVE STUDY IN RURAL JAVA

Background

Research into all factors which might account for the observed fertility patterns and differences is limited. In the case of birth spacing patterns, for example, the only available information is from studies which did not focus on birth intervals specifically; often the interval lengths presented have not been analyzed according to maternal age, birth order, or pregnancy outcome. Perhaps most important, birth interval data in the past has been based only on retrospective studies which, although they can adequately distinguish broad patterns of postpartum behavior, cannot provide us with the reliable information needed for a thorough examination of the subject.

The need for better information on this important topic prompted the research now in progress. The study was originally envisaged as an attempt to investigate prospectively, and in detail, factors which determine the long average birth intervals recorded among rural Javanese. Though its main emphasis was demographic, a secondary goal was to collect more information on the sociocultural context influencing postpartum behavior. Finally, the opportunity to collaborate with the Faculty of Medicine, Gadjah Mada University, allowed for the addition of a nutrition and health component to the study.

Although the main focus of the initial two-year study is on breastfeeding, amenorrhea, and abstinence patterns, attention will also be given to the influence on birth spacing of other factors such as infant mortality and marital disruption. Also important will be the analysis of more general information on pregnancy and childbirth practices, some retrospective analysis of birth intervals, and basic fertility data collected for a large base population. The final research design was funded early in 1976** and collection of baseline data began in May 1976.

---

* More detailed data on the findings of past studies into birth interval dynamics can be found in an earlier version of this conference paper, available from the author.

**The research is being funded by a Rockefeller Ford Population and Development Policy Research grant.

The Study Area

The project is located in two villages (<u>kelurahan</u>) in the sub-district of Ngaglik, about 15 kilometers north of the city of Yogyakarta in central Java. Both villages include areas of well irrigated rice land, as well as poorer quality land suitable only for dry-cropping. Most adults are engaged in agriculture; however, there are also fairly large numbers of traders, craftsmen, and some civil servants who commute daily into the city of Yogyakarta. Although the majority of the population are nominal Muslims, only a small proportion strictly adhere to Islamic teachings.

A community health center combined with a Maternal Child Health Center is located on the main road to the study villages, and serves a population of about 40,000 people. It is staffed by paramedical personnel supported by weekly visits from a doctor. Although charges are inexpensive and those unable to pay are supposedly given free services, the center is not frequently used by people in the study community. In part this may be due to feelings of embarrassment related to the status differential between clinic personnel and the villagers, but people also complain that they cannot afford the basic transport cost (5 to 10 cents) for a ride in a cart or bus to reach the clinic. An obstetrics clinic is located near the health center, staffed by a midwife and visited twice weekly by a doctor. Costs for delivery and postnatal care are high by local standards (Rp.5000, or about U.S. $12), and the clinic is used virtually exclusively by members of the village elite.

Stages of the Study

In May-June 1976 a complete census of the two villages was carried out to collect information on the age, sex, marital status, educational attainment, and economic activities of each household member. The base population recorded was over 15,000 people in nearly 3500 households. In the same interview, a detailed household economic survey was completed, collecting data on land ownership and control, housing conditions and household consumption patterns, and an overall estimate of total household income. In the second round of interviewing, a fertility survey was administered to all ever-married women aged 15-49 (a total of over 2500), in order to estimate the fertility levels and patterns in the community. During this survey stage, field assistants also determined the date of most recent pregnancy termination (live birth, still-birth, or abortion). All women found to have delivered since January 1, 1976 were eligible for the third and prospective phase of the study, which began with a complete marital and pregnancy history, followed by regular monthly interviews for a period of

two years (see below). The Stage II fertility survey also identified women who were currently pregnant and they too, became eligible
for the prospective phase. Thus, eligible women for the two-year
prospective interviews were those who had already experienced, or
would experience, a terminated pregnancy in the calendar year 1976,
plus a small number of women in the early stages of pregnancy whose
estimated delivery date was early in 1977. The total prospective
sample numbers just under 500 women.

The reasons for the selection of the sample in this manner
relate primarily to considerations of maximizing sample size* in
the face of budgetary and time constraints. With a time limit of
only one and a half years from the start of prospective interviewing to final report, we wanted to maximize the number of postpartum
women from whom we could collect accurate prospective and partially
retrospective information on pregnancy, delivery, lactation, amenorrhea, and abstinence. The inclusion of recently delivered women
was predicated on the assumption that we could still determine
dates of their pregnancy termination accurately.** We found that
the vast majority were still breastfeeding, were amenorrheic, and
had not yet resumed intercourse at the time of the first visit.***

---

*This was felt to be especially important for later analysis, in
order to be able to divide respondents into age and parity groups
as well as nutritional level or socioeconomic status.

**Javanese society is highly numerate, and a great deal of emphasis
is placed on important dates. Periodic rituals are held at specified times after an event (for example, at 5 days, 35 days, 105
days, and 7 Javanese months after birth, in the 5th and 7th month
of pregnancy; on the 3rd, 7th, 40th, 100th, yearly, and 1000th day
after death). As such, recent birth dates, and even dates of pregnancy wastage, can usually be determined with high accuracy.
Furthermore, even instances of recent resumption of menses or
intercourse can frequently be determined with precision, for women
often remember the Javanese month and the particular hari dan
pasaran (a combination of the Javanese day and international calendar day, which occurs in 35-day cycles and which is the basis of
important calculations). This can then be converted using a
special almanac (T. Hull (11)).

***First visits to 256 women with a living child showed that 98%
were still breastfeeding; 95% still amenorrheic; and 96% had not
resumed intercourse. For the postpartum sample as a whole (that
is, including those experiencing infant death, abortion, or stillbirth, N=284) the proportion still amenorrheic was 90% and 95%
were still abstaining from sexual intercourse.

In selecting currently pregnant women, all birth interval segments
will be prospective, but the total months of followup time will be
shorter, and for these women in particular we might expect a large
proportion of truncated intervals at the end of the two years.

PRELIMINARY FINDINGS

Characteristics of Respondents

Respondents selected for the prospective survey are, as would
be expected, concentrated in the peak childbearing years, with 50%
being between the ages of 20-29 and a further 35% aged 30-39. Census data showed that nearly a third (31%) had no schooling, and
29% have had only a few years of primary school. Average monthly
household income for respondents were estimated at just below Rp
10,000, or about U.S. $24, and about half of all households did
not own any irrigated rice land, an important indicator of economic
status. At the time of the census, the majority of women (84%)
were reported as engaging in economic activities during 1976.
These were evenly divided among household enterprises (such as
farming on one's own land, cottage industries) and non-household
enterprises (the most common being a hired farm laborer).*

Preliminary tabulations of average cumulative fertility
(children ever born), surviving children, and survivorship ratios
according to income group (Table 1) confirm the pattern observed
in other studies; upper income women in each age group have had
more live births, and their children have a higher rate of survival
than is found among the lowest income group. This pattern is also
found in tabulations according to other indicators of socioeconomic
status, including amount of land owned, education, and a composite
economic index based on ownership of a variety of consumer items.
The positive relation between economic status and fertility also
holds for the larger population of all ever-married women aged 15-
49 according to the stage II fertility survey.**

---

* Detailed information on economic activities of respondents is
collected each month during the prospective phase.
** Overall, women eligible for the prospective phase have higher
fertility than for the community as a whole, since the group consists of only currently married, fecund women. Average completed
fertility for ever-married women in the stage II fertility survey
was 5.0, similar to overall levels recorded in other studies in
the region. There is thus the need to analyze determinants of the
fertility patterns of all women, looking at such factors as marital
disruption and secondary sterility, which have been shown to be
important in previous research on Javanese fertility (5,7).

Table 1

Average Number of Children Ever Born, Children
Still Living, and Survivorship Ratios. All
Women Eligible for Prospective Phase
According to Income Group and Current
Age. Ngaglik Study 1976

| | Income Group | | | |
Age Group	Lower	Middle	Upper	Total
	Children Ever Born (CEB)			
15-19	0.75	0.44	1.00	0.68
20-24	1.46	1.40	1.64	1.49
25-29	1.98	2.21	2.87	2.33
30-34	3.39	4.11	4.74	4.04
35-39	4.92	5.45	5.90	5.31
40-44	6.82	7.58	(8.62)	7.45
45-49	-	(6.00)	(7.00)	(6.50)
	Children Still Living (CSL)			
15-19	0.75	0.44	1.00	0.68
20-24	1.27	1.27	1.43	1.32
25-29	1.71	1.97	2.74	2.11
30-34	2.76	3.43	4.23	3.43
35-39	3.72	4.22	5.09	4.17
40-44	4.76	5.91	(7.00)	5.62
45-49	-	(6.00)	(6.00)	(6.00)
	Survivorship Ratios (CSL + CEB)			
15-19	1.00	1.00	1.00	1.00
20-24	0.87	0.91	0.87	0.89
25-29	0.86	0.89	0.95	0.91
30-34	0.81	0.83	0.89	0.85
35-39	0.76	0.77	0.86	0.79
40-44	0.70	0.78	(0.81)	0.75
45-49	-	(1.00)	(1.86)	(0.92)

Note: : Figures in parentheses indicate N < 10.
Source: Preliminary tabulations, Ngaglik Study.

Table 2

Reported Behavior Patterns During Month Preceding Interview, December 1976
All Post Partum Respondents According to Month Post Partum

Behavior	Month Post Partum											Total
N =	$\frac{1}{28}$	$\frac{2}{32}$	$\frac{3}{40}$	$\frac{4}{31}$	$\frac{5}{37}$	$\frac{6}{46}$	$\frac{7}{39}$	$\frac{8}{46}$	$\frac{9}{34}$	$\frac{10}{24}$	$\frac{11}{31}$	$\frac{}{388}$
1. Pregnancy Outcome (%)												
Child still living	100	91	88	90	84	91	100	87	91	88	84	91
Child died during month	0	0	0	0	0	0	0	2	0	8	0	1
Abortion, stillbirth, child died previous month	0	9	13	10	16	9	0	11	9	4	16	9
2. Breastfeeding (%)	100	100	100	100	100	100	100	93	100	95	92	98
3. Supplementary food (%)	96	93	91	93	90	98	85	100	97	95	81	93
4. Menstruation (%)	0	6	18	10	14	15	5	13	15	17	32	13
5. Possible pregnancy (No.)	0	0	0	0	1	0	0	0	0	0	0	1
6. Abstinence (%)	100	97	90	94	95	89	92	80	79	83	87	89
7. Contracepting (No.)	0	1	2	1	2	3	2	2	1	1	1	16
8. Economic activities % Participating	14	19	50	35	49	52	33	57	44	46	39	41

Source: Preliminary tabulations, Ngaglik Study.

Table 3

Timing of Initiation of Breastfeeding Following
Birth According to Place of Delivery[1]

| Initiation of Breastfeeding | Place of Delivery | | | | | |
| | At Home | | Clinic/Hosp. | | Total | |
	No.	%	No.	%	No.	%
Within first 12 hours	68	18	1	5	69	17
13-24 hours	101	27	3	14	104	26
25-48 hours	101	27	5	24	106	27
49-72 hours	71	19	6	29	77	19
73 hours +	20	5	6	29	26	7
Not yet begun at time of interview[2]	8	2	-	-	8	2
Did not breastfeed[3]	6	2	-	-	6	2
Total	375	100	21	101	396	100

[1] N = all post partum respondents with a live birth as of 1 January 1977.

[2] These are cases in which the respondent was visited within the first 1-2 days postpartum.

[3] Includes 4 cases in which the infant died before breastfeeding was initiated. Two respondents still have living children who were not breastfed.

Source: Preliminary tabulations, Ngaglik Study.

Prospective Findings

By December 1976, four months of the prospective phase had been completed, and some interesting information had already begun to emerge. A general summary of some postpartum patterns is presented in Table 2 which shows behavior during the month preceding the December 1976 round of interviews. All of this is based on preliminary hand-tabulations. Planning for life table analysis of interval segments is still in preliminary stages. Nevertheless, it is useful to review the data being generated at present to see why and how particular questions are being asked and to examine the patterns we are finding.

Lactation

Breastfeeding behavior was one of the main initial areas of research. Previous Javanese studies have indicated durations of breastfeeding ranging from one to two years, with the reported averages being shorter in West Java (9,12) than in Central Java (13,14) and East Java (15,16). The Maguwoharjo study cited earlier (7) recorded a slight tendency for younger women to breastfeed for shorter durations, and recent research in an urban elite group* showed an average duration of lactation of only 7.6 months. These studies collected almost no information, however, on aspects of breastfeeding such as timing and frequency of feeding. Early findings from the Ngaglik study show some interesting patterns.

Initiation of Breastfeeding Following Birth. All women who experienced a live birth were asked how much time elapsed before the newborn infant was given the breast for the first time. "Common knowledge" among medical personnel was that rural mothers began breastfeeding immediately, but data show that among all women, even older non-educated women, breastfeeding frequently does not begin until after two or three days. Some women claimed to wait until the infant began to cry as a sign that it was hungry; it received nothing to eat until that time. Most women who delay two days or longer, however, said they were reluctant to feed colostrum to the infant. The colostrum was expressed and carefully discarded, for the mothers believe that misfortune can result if the discarded colostrum is eaten by insects or foraging animals. The infant is given the breast only when "true milk" appears. During this time, infants are usually fed small amounts of either honey, lime juice, or young coconut water.

Table 3 compares the initiation of breastfeeding among women who gave birth at home with those delivering in a clinic or hospital. Although the total numbers in the latter group are small, it is clear that breastfeeding is postponed for longer periods among these women, reflecting the common hospital practice of separating mother and infant, with the baby receiving bottle feedings.

Frequency and Duration of Suckling. Survey data on frequency of breastfeeding indicate modal replies of five times during the day and three times at night, when the babies generally sleep with their mothers. Breastfeeding sessions were reported to last on average 7-8 minutes. Although survey data can provide us with a fairly good estimate of the range of response, we plan to supplement these with the results of direct observation of a subsample of

---

* See Hull et al. (10). The study interviewed women in the Gadjah Mada University community, including 52 female lecturers and 333 wives of male lecturers.

women in an attempt to obtain data of greater accuracy.

Sucking Substitutes. In the four interview months to December 1976, between one-quarter and one-third of the mothers surveyed were giving some type of sucking substitute to their infants. Substitutes included bottles, pacifiers, both bottle and pacifier, and, in a few cases, sucking at a grandmother's breast. Substitutes were used primarily when mothers went out to work, when they were doing time consuming household tasks, and in some cases if the child cried after being breastfed. In each of the first four months of interviewing, working mothers (those with economic activities other than domestic duties) were more likely to give a sucking substitute to the infant than were non-working mothers.*

Working Mothers and Breastfeeding. Working mothers were asked how they arranged breastfeeding. We were particularly interested in women who worked away from home, usually in the market place or rice fields. Because working hours are often short and flexible, most women reported that they were able to breastfeed just before leaving and upon returning home from work.** The planned direct observation of breastfeeding patterns will select both working and non-working mothers.

Supplementary Foods. Unlike many other societies, the Javanese begin supplementary feeding very early in an infant's life (12,16). Even among infants aged one month, fewer than one in ten received the breast exclusively. Retrospective data was collected at the time of first visit for infants who had already begun receiving supplementary food. The most common first food was mashed banana, given in the first week postpartum in 37% of cases and within the first month by 80% of respondents. Common supplementary foods mentioned during the first four months of interviewing were banana, rice flour porridge, and soft cooked rice. By December, the majority (66%) of infants were receiving rice at least once or twice a

---

* Depending on the interview month, percentages giving sucking substitutes ranged between 28% to 52% among working mothers, and from 23% to 29% among non-working mothers. There is a tendency for the proportion giving sucking substitutes to decline in later interview months, perhaps as the proportion of older infants in the sample increases. Later analysis will be carried out according to age of child.

** Only a few carried their babies with them. One woman reported that if her baby at home cried while she was in the fields, she would be summoned home to breastfeed by the beating of a kentongan, a hollow wooden instrument which hangs outside many homes and is commonly used as a signal.

day, usually mixed with coconut sugar or the cooking water from vegetables. In December 1976, 14% of breastfed infants were receiving milk or prepared formula*, most of these through daily bottle feedings. The most commonly reported pattern of feeding was for a mother to breastfeed upon arising in the morning, then for breastfeeding to follow the one or two supplementary feedings during the day (usually mid-morning and early evening), with additional breastfeeding sessions on demand. When we select a subsample for more detailed study of these aspects, we will try to measure the actual quantity of the additional foods being given to infants.

Changes in Mother's Diet/Consumption of Herbs. Previous surveys in Java (12,16) have reported various food taboos associated with lactation. Rather than asking about general beliefs, the present study asked women specifically whether they a) avoided or b) reduced the quantity of foods they would normally eat, because they were lactating. About one-third of the women interviewed each month claim to have made such changes in their diet. Particular foods mentioned most frequently are those which have a "fishy" taste, sour fruits, chilis, and cold drinks, among others. The deleterious effects which such foods are believed to have (such as diarrhea, colds, eye disease, vomiting in the child, but also such effects as bringing on menstruation too quickly in the mother) were also recorded. Women were also asked about additions or increases in certain foods, and nearly half reported increasing consumption of particular foods such as green vegetables (spinach, papaya leaves, watercress, and other) in order to improve the quality and/or quantity of the breastmilk. Virtually all women (96 to 98%, depending on the month of interview) drink herbal mixtures as an aid to breastfeeding.

Weaning. Up to December 1976, there were only 3 cases of infants weaned during the study's prospective phase, at months 6, 7,8 postpartum. The reasons for weaning were: one infant "didn't want to suckle" any longer; one infant had diarrhea and its mother was advised by a doctor to change to prepared formula; and one woman reported that she resumed menstruation, which ruined the milk and caused the child to lose weight. In all those cases, the mothers began bottle feeding the child with formula. Similar data is being collected for all subsequent cases of weaning. Once an infant has been weaned, a new questionnaire is administered monthly which asks about the infant's diet (according to food groups); food taboos for the infant; whether the infant still sucked at the breast; who has major responsibility for selecting, preparing, and giving food to the child.

---

* Of these 47 infants, 7 were given powdered skim milk, and the remainder prepared formula manufactured in Indonesia.

   <u>Other Topics for Research Related to Breastfeeding.</u> Important
subjects which will be investigated through supplementary surveys
include support and advice concerning breastfeeding given to the
new mother from other family members, the traditional or trained
midwife, or from women of her peer group; attitudes and practices
concerning breastfeeding in public; and socioeconomic and age
differentials in these factors.

                    Amenorrhea and Menstruation

   Retrospective studies of durations of amenorrhea have reported
averages ranging from only 3.5 months among the urban elite population cited above (10) to 18.7 months in the poor village south of
Yogyakarta studied by Singarimbun (3). In the relatively prosper-
ous village of Maguwoharjo (7) the recorded average was 12.9
months, with slightly longer durations associated with increasing
birth orders and age of mother. In this latter study population,
the average reported duration of postpartum amenorrhea following
abortion was 4.1 months, while after stillbirths it was 4.6 months.

   Women in the present study are asked on each monthly visit
whether they menstruated since the previous visit and, if so, when
and for how many days.* In December 1976, 13% (52 out of 388 postpartum women) had experienced menstruation during the month preceding the interview. For women who have already entered the
menstruating interval we will be able to analyze the length of
menstrual cycles, as well as identify cases of subsequent pregnancy.** Each month a woman who has not experienced menstruation
(whether she has already menstruated since delivery, or whether
she is still amenorrheic) is asked whether it is possible that she
is pregnant. The Javanese recognize and have a specific word for
pregnancy which occurs without resumption of menstruation postpartum
(mbumbung). In the early stages of the survey, the majority of
amenorrheic women - and amenorrheic women still made up the vast

---

* It should be pointed out that the date of interview is determined
by the date of parturition. Thus, a woman giving birth on the 12th
day of June, for example, would be visited each month on the 12th
(or at the most within 2 days thereafter); thus interviews are
conducted at each exact completed month postpartum. Dates of menstruation can be fixed with a high degree of accuracy.

** By December, there were 5 instances of women who had become
pregnant again in the course of the study. These included two
cases of women who had had spontaneous abortions and both became
pregnant again in the eighth month postpartum; and three cases of
early infant death, where the women became pregnant again in month
5, 6, and 8 postpartum.

majority of the total sample as of December 1976 - report that they
are not at risk of pregnancy because they are still abstaining from
sexual relations.

Factors Influencing Postpartum Abstinence and Coitus

Data from rural studies have recorded instances of postpartum
abstinence lasting more than two and one half years (3) with
average durations of between one and two years (3,7,8). Reported
abstinence in West Java appears to be shorter, ranging from the
minimum of 40 days, in accordance with the Islamic proscription,
to about six months (9). The average duration of postpartum
abstinance for the elite sample in Yogyakarta City was 3.0 months.
In the villages studied by Singarimbun (3) and Hull (7), it was
found that the majority of women, but not all, disapprove of sex
before menstruation resumed or during breastfeeding, and the
claimed behavior of these women conformed to these attitudes.
There were, however, substantial differences between the two areas.
In the poor village studied by Singarimbun, resumption of intercourse before menstruation occurred in only 12% of recorded cases,
and intercourse prior to weaning in 38%. Corresponding figures
for Maguwoharjo were 43% and 51%, respectively. Thus, while many
women do in fact abstain during amenorrhea and lactation, the
practice is by no means universal. The Maguwoharjo study indicated
differences in these patterns according to current age and economic
class, with young educated women in particular being less likely
to observe the taboos.

It is difficult to ascertain precise motives for abstinence
practices. There is a belief that pregnancy while breastfeeding
(called kesundhulan in Javanese) is a cause for disgrace, but even
this is not a universal notion. In some cases, too, women believe
that intercourse during breastfeeding ruins the milk, particularly
during the first 12 months of lactation when the infant is still
very vulnerable. For many women, abstinence during lactation was
not associated with any specific belief or taboo, but was con-
sciously practiced in order to space pregnancies. The practice of
abstinence is facilitated in the society by a fairly strong position of women within the family (7,17), which allows them to refuse
their husbands, and by the fact that men who find it too difficult
to abstain may seek out prostitutes during this time (3,18), sometimes with the tacit approval of their wives. However, the factor
which is perhaps most important in supporting the practice of
abstinence is the high value Javanese culture and religion place
on all forms of abstaining and self-control, which is said to
increase a person's spiritual strength (3,19). While this belief
supports long postpartum abstinence, it can also be seen as possibly leading to inflated reports of durations of abstinence,

particularly in retrospective studies. Although even a prospective
study cannot completely eliminate the possibility of misreporting,
it is hoped that the data obtained nevertheless have greater validity than the information presently available.

Preliminary analysis of Ngaglik data indicates that in December
89% of all women reported that they had abstained from intercourse
during the preceding month,* with the figure being 95% among women
who were less than six full months postpartum and 85% among those
in months 6 to 11. Reasons given for abstaining conform to what
has been gathered in the retrospective studies described above (see
Table 4). In later months, the question on reasons for abstinence
may reveal more instances of involuntary abstinence, for example,
abstinence due to fairly prolonged separation of husband and wife,
illness of either spouse, or possibly abstinence for religious
reasons, which have not been systematically researched in Java.

Husband-wife separations for short periods, or occasional
taboos on sexual intercourse, may also be important factors determining coital frequency among women who report sexual relations during
the reference month. Results of interviews carried out thus far
among the small number who have resumed sexual relations postpartum**
indicate average monthly coital frequency of around three times,
though there was fairly wide variation. During the first months of
interviews, anywhere from 10 to 19% of respondents had been separated from their husbands for more than a 24 hour period, and about
one-third to one-half of respondents reported that they observed
certain occasions when intercourse was taboo.***

_____

* An important distinction must be made here between a woman's
behavior in a particular reference month, as opposed to her postpartum status. For example, a woman may resume sexual relations
after childbirth for the first time at 8 months postpartum; her
postpartum status would thus no longer be "abstaining" but "resumed
intercourse postpartum." She may for various reasons, however, not
have sexual relations during month 10 postpartum. For that month's
interview, (i.e., month 10) her behavior is coded as "abstained
during reference month;" however, her status remains "resumed intercourse postpartum." As pointed out above, this is also true for
menstruation, for a woman can resume menses postpartum but not menstruate during a particular month. Both types of information are
recorded and will be used in analysis.

** It should be noted that the women who had already resumed intercourse during the first months of the study are biased toward those
who experienced a pregnancy loss or infant death; there is reason
to believe that their behavior will not be representative of the
group of postpartum women as a whole, as the study progresses.

*** Most commonly during menstruation, and on certain days of

Table 4

Reasons Given for Abstaining from Sexual Intercourse
December 1976

| | Month Postpartum | | | | | |
| | 1-5 | | 6-11 | | Total | |
Reasons	f	%	f	%	f	%
Breastfeeding taboo[1]	47	30	64	34	111	32
Postpone pregnancy[2]	40	25	61	33	101	29
No desire/interest[3]	43	27	35	19	78	23
Not yet healed from childbirth[4]	14	9	0	0	14	4
Husband wife separated[5]	5	3	10	5	15	4
Other[6]	10	6	17	9	27	8
Total	159	100	187	100	346	100

Types of responses included:

[1]Milk would become "fishy"/stale and child would become sick/weak/
have eye disease; disgrace to get pregnant while breastfeeding;
cannot have intercourse until child is weaned.

[2]Afraid of becoming pregnant again too quickly; too soon to have
another child because present child still needs attention/ would
be too difficult to manage/ cannot afford it.

[3]No interest in sex; no desire; husband and wife do not want sex
yet; R is working hard so has no interest in sex.

[4]Just gave birth recently and not yet healed/recovered.

[5]Husband working in capital city/outer islands; temporary separation due to marital difficulties; husband staying with second wife.

[6]Still grieving over death of child; do not want to have any more
children at all; custom; no response (3 cases).

Source: Preliminary tabulations, Ngaglik Study.

---

either the Javanese or Gregorian calendar which have particular
meaning or mystical qualities, for example, on a _hari_ _dan_ _pasaran_
combination which marks the day on which they were born or on
which a relative died; dates in the ritual cycles following a
death; and Senin and Kemis (every Monday and Thursday), a frequent
time for abstaining from sex, food, or sleep.

Contraception

Women who have engaged in sexual relations during the month are also asked whether they are at risk of becoming pregnant. Those who claim they are not are asked how they are protected. In the interviews to date, responses have included: the voluntary use of some form of contraception (see below); women who believe they cannot become pregnant while breastfeeding; women who believe praying to God will protect them; and those who simply believe that unless they really want to they will not become pregnant.* In December, 16 out of 43 non-abstaining women were using a form of birth control; six using condoms, four oral contraceptives, four withdrawal, and two rhythm (See Table 2).

The study has also collected data on the past use of various methods of family planning among women in the prospective sample and from the much larger group of women in the Stage II fertility survey. Overall, very few women have ever used modern methods of contraception, with 5% or less having used either the pill, IUD, or condom, and 6% having used rhythm. Only small numbers (1-4%) had ever used withdrawal, massage (retrofexion of the uterus by a midwife), or traditional herbs. In fact, the only methods reported as having been used by a significant proportion (36%) of women were abstinence and breastfeeding, generally used in combination, for a period of one year or longer. There were no substantial differences in these proportions between the prospective sample women and those in the baseline survey; however, there was a tendency for more educated respondents to have higher rates of usage of modern methods and lower rates of traditional methods. For example, condoms had been used by only 1% of those with no schooling, but 14% of secondary school graduates. At the same time, nearly 40% of those with no schooling claimed to have used abstinence, as compared with less than 20% of secondary school graduates. It is interesting to note here that among the elite women studied in urban Yogyakarta, the most popular methods were rhythm, condom, and withdrawal, often used in combination; that usage rates of methods such as the pill and IUD were very low; and that very few women had ever even heard of using prolonged abstinence as a spacing method (10).

---

* This type of response was also encountered in the author's previous village research. Women both wanting and not wanting to get pregnant occasionally reported that unless they were "calm", "settled", and mentally prepared for pregnancy it did not occur. It is interesting that very poor women not infrequently cited worries over their economic situation as an explanation for long durations of time without conceiving.

Nutritional Indicators

The most recent national nutrition survey carried out in Indonesia recorded an average per capita daily caloric intake in Java of 1404 calories, 49% from rice. The total daily average protein consumption was 37.8 g. of which only 4.5 g. was animal protein (20). The same survey estimated that among Javanese children under age one, 24% were suffering from protein calorie malnutrition (PCM), including 12% who were considered to be cases of moderate to severe PCM. Among children aged one year, the respective estimates were 41% and 15%.* Nutrition of pregnant and lactating women has been recently evaluated for a sample in rural East Java (16), indicating that among pregnant women the percentages with moderate and severe malnutrition** in the first, second and third trimester were 39%, 42% and 50% respectively. Average weight gain during pregnancy was estimated at only six kilograms.*** Among lactating women, proportions with moderate to severe malnutrition ranged from 38% to 55%, depending on the geographic area surveyed. In comparison, the figures for non-pregnant, non-lactating women were generally around 30-36%, although in one very poor area, a figure of 60% was obtained.

In the current study, both pregnant and postpartum women are visited once a month by a team which carries out a basic anthropometric examination and obtains data on illnesses (i.e., symptoms, duration, treatment) experienced by both mother and child in the month preceding the interview. Information is also collected on infant tooth formation and on BCG innoculation. The mother is asked about her diet (according to food groups) during the month.**** Anthropometric data includes: height; head circumference (for the mother, this was done for the first three

---

* Prevalence of PCM was estimated using age in months and upper arm circumference for infants less than 1 year; body height and upper arm circumference for children 1-4 years.

** Using 76-80% of standard upper arm circumference (for adult women) as indicating moderate malnutrition, and $\leq$ 75% as indicating severe malnutrition.

*** Another study in West Java indicated a very low average daily caloric intake of 1273 for pregnant women in the third trimester, as compared to 1434 calories for non-pregnant women, using cross-sectional data (21).

**** It will be remembered that information on the infant's diet is collected on a separate monthly form, along with data on breast-feeding for babies not yet weaned, and on a separate questionnaire for weaned infants.

visits, for the baby it is done each month); chest circumference
of the infant; weight; upper arm circumference; and triceps skinfold measurement. Weights of mothers are obtained using a Homs
beam scale. At present infants are also weighed using the Homs
scale, with a pillow placed on it. Triceps skinfold measurement
is taken using Lange skinfold calipers.

These data have not been analyzed in detail, although cross-
sectional tabulations obtained thus far indicate some interesting
general patterns. Mean body weights for babies fairly closely
follow the Harvard standard up to age 5 or 6 months, after which
there is a sharp fall away. Average skinfold measurement and upper
arm circumference show the same pattern. If this is confirmed by
longitudinal data on individual infants, further examination of the
finding would include investigation into the quality and quantity
of supplementary feedings, and also research into illnesses experienced. The monthly interviews tabulated thus far (July to October)
are recording fairly high incidence of illnesses, which, even
though the majority are minor, may affect feeding habits and weight
patterns. Respiratory complaints and fever in particular are
frequently reported, with the former occurring in as many as 51%
of infants during the October interviews. There is a slight
tendency for higher proportions of infants falling ill during that
month, the start of the rainy season, which may reflect the expected seasonal fluctuations in reported illness. If there is indeed
a tendency for sickness to be more prevalent during the rains, we
would expect peaks to occur during the November-February period.

Data collected on birth weights should also prove important
in the analysis of morbidity and mortality of infants. Available
data for 42 babies born during the prospective phase indicates a
total of 8 with birth weights under 2.5 kilograms. Mean birth
weight for these infants was 2.9 kg.

Anthropometric data for mothers is largely unanalyzed at this
stage, except for distributions of upper arm circumference measurement according to pregnancy and lactation status which were prepared in order to compare results with the East Java data cited
above. The findings indicated much lower proportions of Ngaglik
women with measurements below 80% of standard than were found in
East Java. Interestingly, there is a slight increase in the percentage below 80% in the third trimester of pregnancy, and lactating
women have the highest percentage (24%) of women in this group.
Later analysis will be able to focus on actual changes in nutritional indicators longitudinally as a supplement to this cross-sectional
data. Although the nutritional and health data are fairly basic,
they should be able to identify women in poorly nourished and
better nourished categories in order to observe possible differences in postpartum patterns, in particular lactation and
amenorrhea.

Pregnancy Wastage

Pregnancy histories carried out in rural Java have recorded pregnancy wastage rates in the range of 8-10% (3,7), with higher rates among women aged 15-19 and age 35+ at the time of event. The 8-10% figure is most probably an underestimate due not so much to recall error* as to the fact that spontaneous abortions occurring during early pregnancy go undetected.

Data from the 2507 women in the baseline fertility survey in Ngaglik showed pregnancy losses were 9.5% of all completed pregnancies, and the figure from pregnancy histories of the women in the prospective sample was 8.7%. It is hoped that, especially if the present study can continue beyond the initial two years, more reliable data will be able to be collected prospectively on pregnancy wastage. A major difficulty will be the early identification of pregnancy, particularly in a society where irregular menstrual periods may prove to be fairly prevalent.** At present in the study, all those not menstruating after a 30 day period (that is, since the previous visit of the field assistant) are provisionally considered "pregnant" until followup checks can confirm the possibility.***

Infant Mortality

Among the more important data generated by the prospective

---

* Whereas in many societies spontaneous abortions (or even stillbirths) are not considered important and/or are easily forgotten, in Java the fetus is given a ritual burial, sometimes in a grave marked by a tombstone, and occasionally is also given a name. In the pregnancy history of the current study, we encountered a woman who had obtained official birth certificates for two abortions she had experienced.

** It is interesting that one of the most popular herbal mixtures sold in both rural and urban areas is called "the late period mixture," said to be a fairly reliable means of bringing on one's period. As with all the traditional herbs, more research is needed on the extent of use and the composition of these mixtures.

*** Thus far, there have been several cases of women being amenorrheic during the menstruating interval for long durations, followed by resumption of menses. The respondents themselves claim they were not pregnant and had no other symptoms of pregnancy. Further study of the cases will have to be made to try to determine whether these were instances of early spontaneous abortions or irregular menstrual periods.

study will be an estimate of infant mortality. Estimates based on
census statistics have indicated a Javanese infant mortality rate
for 1960-70 of 138 per 1000, although the rate is lower in the
Yogyakarta region (1). As would be expected, there are also sharp
differences in the incidence of infant mortality in different socioeconomic groups. For all of rural Indonesia, for example, infant
mortality is estimated to range from 155 among children born to
mothers with no schooling, to 68 where mothers are secondary school
graduates (4). The role which infant mortality, and particularly
neonatal mortality, plays in shortening birth intervals needs to
be investigated in Java. It is clear that shorter periods of
amenorrhea and postpartum abstinence follow early infant death (3,
7). As was reported above, three out of the five women who have
become pregnant within the prospective phase of the present study
are women whose infants died shortly after birth.

Unfortunately, the Ngaglik study will not be able to carry
out clinical examinations, but it does collect detailed descriptions
of symptoms preceding the death of a child. We will also be able
to examine the health and anthropometric indices of the child
recorded in interviews prior to the death.

Pregnancy and Childbirth: Beliefs and Practices

Although there is considerable ethnographic data on various
beliefs and practices associated with pregnancy and birth, much of
it is based on research carried out decades ago, and also seems to
relate to cultural ideals rather than to what the majority of
village people actually do. We began to collect information on
these aspects during the monthly interviews with women who were
currently pregnant at the beginning of the prospective study. At
parturition, they are asked a series of questions concerning the
delivery and immediate postpartum period.

It seems apparent from data already collected that for the
large majority of women, pregnancy changes little in their basic
daily activities. Cross sectional data collected on time spent in
both household tasks and outside economic activities indicates
almost no change in the former and only a slight decrease in the
proportions working in outside activities in later months of pregnancy. Cumulating data obtained up to December, we find that
nearly half of all cases in the third trimester of pregnancy are
working at these outside activities.* During pregnancy, the

---

* Further analysis will distinguish among women working at economic
activities outside the home, economic activities at home, and domestic tasks only at home. Estimates of total hours spent in each
of these activities have also been collected, as well as the actual

majority (70% to 80%, depending on the interview month) of women
did not have a medical examination. Those who did consult doctors
or trained midwives were concentrated in the third trimester.
There were only two cases of women who were examined by a traditional midwife during their pregnancy, but the vast majority of
respondents did consume herbal mixtures. Each month, less than
10% of currently pregnant women reported that they had avoided or
decreased the amount of certain foods because of pregnancy*. A
slightly larger proportion of women claimed they did change their
diet by eating more of certain types of food, particularly green
vegetables, but this, too, was not very frequently encountered.**
A question on coital frequency asked of pregnant women showed that
abstinence from sexual relations during the reference month increases from 26% to 48% to 78% in the first, second, and third
trimester, respectively.

All women who give birth during the course of the study and
those who were postpartum at the time of first contact are asked
about beliefs and conditions surrounding the birth. It is clear
that we¹l over 90% of births take place at home, assisted by a
traditional midwife. For nearly one third of these cases, however,
the midwives have been to a short government upgrading course and
use the basic set of equipment given to them by the program. The
technique of massage is perhaps the midwife's main skill, used in
manipulating the fetus into correct position for birth, massaging
the abdomen to help expel the placenta, and postpartum massage
of both mother and infant.

A supplementary survey on some of the beliefs and practices of
childbirth was administered to all respondents who were postpartum
in October (n = 314). It revealed that in over 90% of births, the
umbilical cord was cut after the placenta had been expelled (most
respondents estimated from 15 to 20 minutes afterwards, after the
mother had been cleaned and massaged). Although ethnographic

---

type of job held. Preliminary examination of the data indicates
that most women work as petty traders, farmers, or farm laborers,
and that there is fairly wide variation in numbers of hours and
days worked per month. Hours worked will presumably also show
seasonal fluctuations.

* The women who did report such changes in diet mentioned especially chillies, ice, and salty foods.

** Addition of certain foods also includes such things as sour
fruits and "watery"vegetables such as cucumber which, unlike the
added green vegetables, are eaten because of a craving rather than
for health reasons.

studies have stressed the spiritual importance of the placenta as
the "younger sibling" of the newborn infant, most respondents in
Ngaglik perceived it as a "companion" or "helper" to the infant,
or simply as a cushion or resting place in utero. Nevertheless,
virtually all respondents followed the practice of ceremonially
burying the afterbirth. Certain beliefs are also associated with
the stub of the umbilibal cord which falls off some days after
birth. The majority of women reported to have saved this, claiming
it can be used as medicine for the child. It is interesting to
note, however, that in all the cases of child illness and treatment
recorded since the study began, we have not yet encountered this in
actual practice.

As a very simple means of detecting complications of pregnancy
and birth, questions were asked on duration of labor, color and
smell of amniotic fluid, duration of bleeding and discharge after
birth, and a general appraisal by the respondent herself as to
whether the birth was "easy", "average," or "difficult." Preliminary analysis of this material indicates very few cases of apparent difficulty. Duration of labor was obtained by asking the
respondent how long it took from the time she felt pain until the
birth. The very short reported durations probably indicate that
"pain" was not defined until later stages of labor. Overall, over
half (55%) of the women reported durations of less than three
hours, although among first births, only 29% took place within this
short time. Average duration of postpartum discharge was 14 days
although variation was great and this question, too, relied on the
respondent's definition of "How many days before you were clean of
blood and discharge after the birth?" Reports by respondents on
the retrospective questionnaire indicated dark and/or bad smelling
amniotic fluid in 3% of cases.

Most women (59% of all women, 49% of those of parity 1)
reported that they got up and walked around within one hour after
delivery, usually to go to bathe. Resumption of normal household
duties also began without much delay, occurring within the first
three days postpartum in about one-third of the cases, and within
the first week for a further third of the women.

A supplementary survey concerning pregnancy, childbirth, and
related practices is currently being undertaken among the 18
traditional midwives (dukun bayi) in the research area. The interviews, carried out by two highly skilled field assistants, consist
largely of open-ended questions concerning the midwife's experiences,
beliefs and advice given to patients. These sessions with the dukun
bayi may take as long as three hours. Where agreed to by the
respondent, the interviews are being tape recorded and will later
be transcribed and translated.

DISCUSSION

The Ngaglik Study is a two-year research project aimed at gathering prospective data on factors which determine the long average birth intervals found among women in rural Java. This paper describes the types of data being collected by the project, and reviews some preliminary findings drawn from a baseline survey and from the first four months of prospective interviews. On the basis of these early results, there are several areas of interest which will receive more focused attention as the study progresses.

Patterns of long voluntary postpartum abstinence may prove to be one of the most distinctive components of long birth intervals among the Javanese, in contrast to many other societies, including other ethnic groups in Indonesia. Although we cannot yet predict whether durations of abstinence will prove longer than postpartum infecundity, data from retrospective studies suggest this may be the case for a substantial proportion of women with surviving infants. Motives for abstinence are varied, and include belief in a lactation taboo as well as the conscious use of abstaining to space pregnancies. Significantly, however, past research has indicated that the practice of prolonged abstinence is less prevalent among the young and educated. This finding was confirmed in the present study by retrospective data on the use of voluntary abstinence. We will be investigating this pattern prospectively, looking at the extent to which other forms of voluntary fertility control - if any - are being substituted for abstinence by this group of women.

Duration of breastfeeding among women in Ngaglik can influence both abstinence - among women who observe a lactation taboo - and amenorrhea, through nutritional or hormonal effects. As such, attitudes and behavior patterns related to breastfeeding are a crucial topic for study. The generally reported pattern of breastfeeding in rural Java is one of demand feeding, lasting for 1½ to 2 years. Interestingly, however, some of the factors which are thought to interfere with successful and prolonged breastfeeding seem to be present in Ngaglik. The majority of women report delays in initiating breastfeeding following birth, in most cases related to a belief that colostrum is unfit for the child. Very early supplementary feeding - as early as the first month of life - is virtually universal, although more research is needed into the actual quantity, quality, frequency, and timing of these feedings. One indication that supplementary food may be inadequate is the slowing of infant growth at about age six months which is seen in cross-sectional anthropometric data. Sucking substitutes - bottles and pacifiers - are used with some frequency and to a greater extent by mothers involved in extrafamilial economic activities. Overall, fairly high proportions of women work outside the home, particularly in the later postpartum months and among higher parity

women. While these elements could act to inhibit prolonged breastfeeding among women in the study, there are several factors which
facilitate and directly support breastfeeding. Flexible working
hours among most women who work generally allow for breastfeeding
sessions to take place without long interrruptions. There is
almost universal and fairly frequent night feeding, a generally
supportive social milieu (although later research may point up
socioeconomic status differentials in this factor); and perhaps
also important, there is widespread consumption of herbal mixtures
taken to promote lactation.

The relation between lactation and amenorrhea will be examined
by comparing women who have different breastfeeding patterns and
women of different nutritional statuses. As with all factors under
analysis, these differences will in turn be related to contrasts
in age, parity, and socioeconomic status.

In addition to the three main foci of abstinence, breastfeeding, and amenorrhea, the study will yield data on pregnancy
wastage, regularity of menstrual cycles, factors influencing coital
frequency during the non-abstaining interval, infant mortality, and
other information which is of value intrinsically as well as in
terms of its relation to birth intervals.

The study can, in fact, be seen as an exploratory one, for
much of the data being gathered deals with topics on which there
has been little reliable research. It is hoped that the Ngaglik
Study itself will be able to be extended beyond its initial two
years in order to examine in more detail the trends recorded during
this initial phase. It is also hoped that work of this nature will
be carried out in other areas of Java and in the outer islands of
Indonesia, as an important step toward better understanding of the
substantial fertility differentials which exist within the country.

References

1. McNicoll, C. and Si Gde Made Mamas. The Demographic Situation
    in Indonesia, Papers of the East West Population Institute,
    No. 28, Honolulu, 1973.

2. McDonald, P. F., M. Yasin, and G. Jones. Levels and Trends in
    Fertility and Childhood Mortality in Indonesia, Indonesian
    Fertility-Mortality Survey 1973, Monograph 1, Lembaga Demografi,
    FE-UI, Jakarta, 1976.

3. Singarimbun, M. and C. Manning. Fertility and Family Planning
    in Mojolama, Population Institute, Gadjah Mada University,
    Monograph No. 1, Yogyakarta, 1974. See also Singarimbun, M.

and C. Manning, Breastfeeding, Amenorrhea, and Abstinence in a Javanese Village: A Case Study of Mojolama, Studies in Family Planning 7(6): 175-179, 1976.

4. Hull, T. and V. Hull. The Relation of Economic Class and Fertility: An Analysis of Some Indonesian Data. To be published in Population Studies 31(1): 73-87, 1977.

5. Hull, V. The Positive Relation Between Economic Class and Family Size in Java: A Case Study of the Intermediate Variables Determining Fertility. Monograph Series No. 2, Population Institute, Gadjah Mada University, Yogyakarta, 1976.

6. Demographic Institute. Indonesian Fertility-Mortality Survey 1973, Preliminary Reports 1-3: (West Java, Central Java, East Java), Demographic Institute, University of Indonesia, Jakarta, 1974.

7. Hull, V. J. Fertility, Socioeconomic Status and the Position of Women in a Javanese Village. Unpublished Ph.D. thesis, Department of Demography, Australian National University, Canberra, 1975.

8. Gille, H. and R. H. Pardoko. A Family Life Study in East Java: Preliminary Findings, In Berelsen et al. (eds.), Family Planning and Population Programs: A Review of World Developments, 503-521. Chicago University Press, Chicago, 1966.

9. Borkent-Niehof, A. Fertility in Kecamatan Serpong, Family Planning Project Serpong Paper No. 6, Jakarta, 1974.

10. Hull, V., Kodiran, and I. Singarimbun. Family Formation in the University Community: Preliminary Results of a Case Study. Report Series No. 9, Population Institute, Gadjah Mada University, Yogyakarta, 1976.

11. Hull, T. Almanak Penanggalan Jawn-Masehi untuk Penelitian Sosial Ekonomi (Javanese Almanac for Social and Economic Research), Methodology Series No. 2, Population Institute, Gadjah Mada University, Yogyakarta, 1976.

12. Tan, Mely, et al. Social and Cultural Aspects of Food Patterns and Food Habits in Five Rural Areas in Indonesia. National Institute of Economic and Social Research and Directorate of Nutrition, Jakarta, 1970.

13. Bailey, C. V. Rural Nutrition Studies in Indonesia VII: Field Surveys in Javanese Infants, J. Trop. Geogr. Med. 14: 111-120, 1962.

14. Lembaga Penelitian Ilmu-ilmu Sosial (Institute of Social
    Science Research). <u>Base Line Data Usaha Perbaikan Gizi
    Keluarga Propinsi Jawa Tengah</u> (Base Line Data, Applied Nutri-
    tion Program, Central Java), Universitas-IKIP Kristen Satya
    Wacana, Salatiga, 1973.

15. Biro Pengabdian Masyarakat (Bureau of Social Services),
    <u>Laporan Hasil Penelitian Perbaikan Gizi Keluarga Propinsi Jawa
    Timur</u> (Results of a Study of the Applied Nutrition Program,
    East Java), Universitas Gadjah Mada, Yogyakarta, 1973.

16. Kardjati, Sri, et al. Geographical Distribution and Prevalence
    of Nutritional Deficiency Diseases in East Java Indonesia,
    Interim Report 1 (draft). Airlangga University, Surabaya
    Provincial Health Services and Royal Tropical Institute,
    Netherlands, 1976.

17. Geertz, Hildred. <u>The Javanese Family: A Study of Kinship and
    Socialization</u>, 94-98, Glencoe, Illinois: The Free Press of
    Glencoe, Inc., 1961.

18. Jay, R. R. <u>Javanese Villagers: Social Relations in Rural
    Modjokuto</u>, 94-95, The MIT Press, Cambridge, Mass., 1969.

19. Geertz, C. <u>The Religion of Java</u>, 323-325, New York: The Free
    Press, 1960.

20. Sajogyo, Ringkasan Hasil Survey Evaluasi Proyek Usaha
    Perbaikan Gizi Keluarga (Summary of Results of the Evaluation
    Study of the Applied Nutrition Program), Lembaga Penelitian
    Sosiologi Pedesaan, Institut Pertanian Bogor, 1974.

21. Martoatmodjo, S. et al. A Survey among Pregnant and Non-
    Pregnant Women in a Rural District of West Java Indonesia,
    <u>Gizi Indonesia</u> (Journal of The Indonesian Nutrition Association)
    5: 8-13, 1973.

ECONOMIC DETERMINANTS OF BREAST-FEEDING BEHAVIOR:

THE CASE OF RURAL HOUSEHOLDS IN LAGUNA, PHILIPPINES

Barry M. Popkin

University of the Philippines

Manila, Philippines

INTRODUCTION

It is quite common to ascribe the decline in breastfeeding practices to misinformation and commercial malpractice. There is little doubt that commercial milk and baby food interests have made a negative impact on breastfeeding behavior either directly or through an influential medical profession. Moreover, the medical profession and others who are consulted about breastfeeding are often misinformed about the effects of breastfeeding and the ways to encourage it (1). Yet, the decline in breastfeeding has occurred concurrently with vast social and economic changes in the status of women, household size and income, wage rates, food prices, and even the nature of the work undertaken by the women. This does not, however, mean that exogenous forces such as the marketing pressures of baby food companies and the misinformed medical profession are benign factors; rather, all of these forces affect breastfeeding behavior.

This study attempts to examine the determinants of breastfeeding behavior in the light of some socioeconomic and demographic forces. The study differs from previous similar research in that it emphasizes analysis of correlates of actual behavior within a multivariate framework. We do not attempt to explain longitudinal breastfeeding trends, as available Filipino data are inadequate for such an endeavor. Rather, we use cross-sectional data to analyze some of the factors which are associated with breastfeeding behavior. The model pays less attention to exogenous factors but fully concentrates on factors endogenous to the household, i.e., wage rates and income of family members and family composition. Community price changes, the availability of contraceptives and

the influence of commercial milk advertisers are considered
potential factors.

CONCEPTUAL FRAMEWORK

An understanding of the factors affecting the production of
infant nutritional status, the available household resources, and
the money and time inputs of infant dietary intake can be used to
understand the demand for breastfeeding. If the health and other
nonnutritional factors which affect infant nutritional status are
excluded, the dietary intake can be viewed as the chief factor.
Both money and time are required for feeding the infant milk-
formulae, breast-milk or other solid foods. Time is used to purchase and feed the infant milk or formulae, and money is used to
purchase the feeding utensils and milk/formulae. Similarly, much
maternal time is needed to breastfeed the child, and money is
needed to purchase the food consumed to support lactation. An
artificial or shadow price of infant nutritional status can be
developed by placing a value on the time and goods used in breastfeeding, milk-formulae feeding and also the feeding of other solid
foods.

The household has limited time and money resources with which
to obtain the desired level of infant nutritional status and other
desired consumables.* The demand for breastfeeding and other forms
of infant nutrition are derived from this relationship. The demand
for breastfeeding is affected by the relative price of breast milk
and its substitutes (shadow prices), the nature of the production
relationship between breast milk, milk formulae, and infant nutritional status and the household's knowledge about this relationship, the factors such as the health and nutritional status of the
mother which may shift this production relationship, and the available household resources.

Popkin and Gonzalo have attempted to estimate the time and
money price of infant dietary intake for rural households. They
find that breastfeeding requires relatively more of the mother's

---

* If the household decision to breastfeed is based partially either
on the desire to have a healthier child or on the effect of lactation on postpartum amenorrhea, a broader formulation is needed in
which the quality and quantity of children would be considered as
two attributes of the household's utility function. Breastfeeding
would relate to a derived demand for child health (quality) and/or
the number of children. Butz and Habicht (2) present a formulation
which appears to be implicitly based on this type of utility-
maximizing behavior. The formal model is presented in Appendix I.

time and the money price of milk formulae feeding is much greater
than that of the food costs used to support lactation, especially
for poor households which do not consume many extra lactation
calories.*

We are interested in using this formulation to understand the
factors which may affect breastfeeding behavior. We can not
estimate the time and goods prices for breast milk, bottle milk,
and other food which face each household. We can, however, examine
the effect of the factors which affect these prices such as the
value of time and availability of mother surrogates, such as older
children, the price of substitute foods and so forth. We can
include a variety of biological factors which may affect the infant
nutrition production relationship such as the infant's ingestion of
competing foods, the nutritional status of the mother, and the
mother's knowledge about the production process.**

Dependent Variables

From a fertility perspective, the frequency of breastfeeding
or the total sucking time may be most useful. Results of the
frequency and time data analysis are not presented due to reliability problems with the recall of these variables and the availability of more accurate observation data only for a small sample.
The two variables examined here are breastfeeding participation
during the first three months of life and duration of breastfeeding in months.

Independent Factors Endogenous to the Household

It is useful to consider these factors separately as they are
amenable to different types of societal forces and are changed by
policy more indirectly than the community factors.

---

* A brief summary of the money and time price of breast and bottle
milk for rural women is presented in Appendix II.

** For example, Dr. Samuel Wishik pointed out to this author that
the stomach emptying time of the child is a key biological factor.
He felt that the stomach emptying time, which relates to the age
and development of the child and the content of the food consumed,
is faster for breast milk than cow's milk and also faster during
the day. This biological relationship is not considered here.

Child Care Organization: Who Cares for Infants. Child care
norms determine when older siblings of different ages and sexes
and other persons can take care of the infant. A great deal of
variation in the child care patterns exists in this sample population (4). Girls aged 13-15 appear to provide more time to younger
infants and younger girls aged 7-12 are more important for older
infant and preschooler care. Given these child care practices,
the availability of older girls are expected to reduce breastfeeding participation and of younger girls, the duration of breastfeeding.

The allocation of the child care time among household members
relates to the value of time and the roles of the mother and other
members (father, children, others) in this sample. The use of
children for home and market production partially relates to the
economic position of the family and to the mother's role in market
production; thus separate relationships for the children of rich
and poor working and nonworking mothers have been examined. A few
noteworthy relationships include: older poor girls aged 13-15 are
strong mother substitutes whereas the younger (aged 7-12) poor
girls complement the child care time of the mother, especially in
non-working households; the effects of girls in rich households
are less significant; and the addition of other nonnuclear, family
household members (grandparents, unrelated residents, relatives,
servants) are associated with increased child care time. These
conclusions are derived from the effect of older children aged 7-
12 and 13-15 on the child care time provided by the mother, father
and themselves. In cases where the children or others substitute
for the mother's child care time, we expect this to reduce the
mother's breastfeeding participation and duration.

The number of preschool children present in the home affects
the mother's behavior. Additional preschool children should
increase the mother's productivity at home relative to the market
and, consequently, enhance her probability of staying home and
breastfeeding. Of course, the number of preschoolers may be based
on the preference of the mother for shorter spacing or more children, which in turn, may also relate with the desire to breastfeed
the child.

Mother's Value of Time. This is a critical variable for the
time-intensive breastfeeding activity. The extent of increases in
this variable are expected to have a stronger impact on the extent
of breastfeeding. Higher paid women will have more to lose in
terms of a job tenure experience relationship in the sense that
absence from work may interrupt these women's career ladders more.
Once the woman is breastfeeding, a higher wage rate may provide
a level of needed income and allow her to work fewer hours per week
so she can provide more child care and breastfeeding time. The

predicted relationship between increases in the value of the
woman's time and her breastfeeding behavior are not unambiguous
since the price changes of the different foods are not the only
ones experienced by the households. Household income will also
increase and this "income effect" may be expected to be positive
to work more out of economic necessity and income increases will
allow them more time for child care and breastfeeding activities.
For rich women, the decision to work is based more on wage considerations and choice rather than on necessity. Their labor
force activity will also increase as their wage rate increases (5).
Value of time changes do not have to affect breastfeeding behavior
because of the possibilities of changing home production activities
not related to the infant.

The predicted wage of the mother based on estimated wage rates
for working women is used.* This variable is not included in the
regression analysis of the behavior of only nonworking women.

Compatitility of the Mother's Job with Child Care. One of the
more interesting differences between industrialized and less industrialized areas is the greater prevalence of jobs in less industrialized areas, allowing the mother to be more responsive to child
rearing needs. Hours may be less rigid, the job may be located in
the house, or there may be greater possibilities that the child
can accompany the mother to the work site. It may be very possible
that the mother selects market-related jobs which are compatible
with child care (7). Other anthropologists feel that child rearing
practices are adopted to the requirements of market labor (8).
Compatible jobs may allow the rural Filipino mother to supervise
her older children and others who are engaging in child care. For
this reason, we do not necessarily expect that compatible jobs
will increase breastfeeding behavior. For working women, it may
have the opposite effect of allowing them to allocate the time of
others more efficiently, as was found in the analysis of child
care time (9).

This concept was based mainly on a questionnaire given to
each member of the survey field staff to determine the general
compatibility of certain occupations with child care. Some
empirical testing was used to validate the various groupings. For
example, women who washed clothes or engaged in weaving were listed
as working in jobs compatible with child care. School teachers and

---

* For a number of statistical and theoretical reasons, the predicted wage of the mother was estimated from a regression equation
for which the dependent variable was the hourly wage rate of working women and a set of factors affecting the mother's potential
and actual productivity (age, education, wealth status) were the
independent variables (6).

itinerant saleswomen were placed in the incompatible category. It
should be noted that several other indicators of job compatibility
were tested. These include the location of the work in relation
to the home, the time to travel to work, and the cost of traveling
to work.

The Mother's Human Capital. The education level, knowledge
level, and nutritional status of the mother are included in this
set of human capital elements. Knowledge about breast milk is
expected to play a role in determining the breastfeeding activities
of the mother and possibly even the market labor force status of
the mother. Women were asked which form of infant feeding was
best. The answer was coded so that the variable equals one when
the mother felt that breastfeeding was best and 0 when she did not.
Unstudied were preferences which affect the length of breastfeeding. These may be very different from those which affect the
extent to which the mother breastfeeds. For example, one inter-
viewer reported that several sample mothers felt that the taste
of breast milk deteriorated with a prolonged duration of breastfeeding and stunted the child's personality.

The mother's education may be inversely related to the age at
which solid foods are introduced. Better educated mothers may
more efficiently utilize older children to take care of their
infants. Thus, we could expect an inverse education-duration
relationship. On the other hand, better educated mothers may
understand the greater health and psychological benefits to the
child of continued lactation and may breastfeed for a longer time.
Since education may have a major effect on beliefs or preferences,
both variables will not be used together in the regressions.

The effect of the nutritional status and dietary intake of
the mother on the quantity and quality of breast milk is an unsettled issue. Continued breastfeeding, nevertheless, is a severe
drain on women and we expect that healthier women may be able to
breastfeed more. The lactating mother, especially the lower income
ones, may lose weight, get cracked nipples and become anemic. The
less healthy mother may not be able to begin to breastfeed or to
continue to breastfeed as long as the healthier one. Understanding this health relationship is made more difficult by a psycho-
logically related let-down reflex factor and the health advice
given to mothers by misinformed persons. In addition, healthier
mothers will be more productive in both market and home. If the
market productivity of the healthier woman increases relative to
her home productivity, the healthier mother may be more likely to
have a lower probability and length of breastfeeding.

Only indirect health status variables are available. A 0-1
anemia variable based on a 13 grams/100 ml hemoglobin cutoff and a
percentage of weight for height variable are used. The hemoglobin

data were collected by a specialized Department of Health laboratory team with the use of a Sahli's hemoglobinometer. These
nutritional data are available only for a subsample.

Pregnancy Status. Earlier Filipino studies have found that
pregnancy was an important reason given by women for not breastfeeding (10). To analyze this pregnancy effect in a behavioral
analysis, it is necessary to have a prospective study which follows
the mother's behavior from month to month. For example, the pregnancy effect could be studied by infant age groups in a manner
similar to the lifetable study on lactation behavior presented in
this volume by Osteria. One prospective study found that 13 percent of the studied mothers who were in their fourth month of
pregnancy were still breastfeeding (11). We do not have prospective data for an adequate sample to analyze this relationship.

Let-down Reflex of "Milk Ejection Reflex". This is partly
a psychosomatic reflex which affects the production of breast milk
(12). Anxiety, emotional tension, stress and strain can inhibit
this reflex and subsequently dry the breast. Although the woman
is physically able to breastfeed, she is unable to get the milk
from the alveoli to the collecting lacteals in the areoli area (13).
In many societies a doula or female assistant - be she a mother,
traditional midwife, friend or helper - provides psychological
support for the lactating woman (14). In modern societies and in
urban areas, such support may be less available. This may be the
one reason for the unexplained differences in breastfeeding
behavior between urban and rural women in the Philippines found by
Popkin and Solon (15). Also, it may explain why in previous
Filipino breastfeeding studies urban mothers gave "no breast milk"
as a prominent cause for the discontinuance of lactation (16).

No anxiety or psychological data are available and adequate
proxy variables are unknown. It would appear, however, that
absence of the extended family support and urban residence are two
factors which may be associated with a poorer let-down reflex.

Contraceptive Effect. It is often argued that any birth control pill with an estrogen component will interfere with or
suppress lactation in women. This is an unsettled issue. The
estrogen pill may probably suppress the maintenance of lactation,
but it is unlikely to prevent its establishment. If milk production is diminished, the child may have to seek supplemental food
and, in turn, reduce the amount and vigor of his/her sucking time
and the duration of feeding. We do not examine this effect as too
few women used the pill and the sample was felt to be too small.

Age the Child is Fed Supplementary Foods. When the child
receives other foods, his appetite and sucking vigor may be

reduced and, in turn, may lessen the duration of breastfeeding. The normal supplemental rice lugao (porridge), which has a small nutritional effect, can act, however, to diminish the sucking behavior of the infant. This effect, in turn, can affect lactation behavior. The price of these substitute foods, positive breastfeeding beliefs, and other maternal human capital characteristics such as the value of the mother's time may affect the age when supplementary foods are introduced to the child. Thus, we could view the age the child is fed supplementary foods as an endogenous variable jointly determined with the length of breastfeeding. The correlations of these variables with other independent variables will be carefully tested. The actual age of supplementation is unavailable for the entire sample. A variable based on asking the mothers what the best time was to begin feeding the infant other foods is used.

Value of Time of Father. Increases in the value of time of the father will increase breastfeeding behavior if additional income allows the household to undertake desired activities - such as breastfeeding. On the other hand, increases in the value of the father's time will lower breastfeeding if market foods are generally substituted for more time intensive goods or if richer persons look down on breastfeeding as an inferior activity. For the poor, it is expected that increased income will be spent in meeting family subsistence needs and breastfeeding will not decline but increase if it proved to be a desirable practice. For the rich there is a greater likelihood that breastfeeding is an inferior activity and households will respond to time price increases with increased goods purchases and market work (17).

The actual wage of the father and the combined income of other household members, excluding the mother, are used as alternate variables. The wage of the father is examined only for its price effect. The income of other members is split into the income of the rich and the poor. The value of children's time is not estimated, but the demographic parameters indirectly capture the productivity effects of children of different ages and sexes.

Wealth represents a type of return to nonlabor income. Wealth changes do not affect the value of time considerations mentioned earlier. If breastfeeding is a preferred form of infant feeding, then the effects of wealth on breastfeeding behavior will be positive. The present value of all household wealth is used for our wealth parameter.

Stratification

The sample is stratified according to the mother's market labor force participation. The working-nonworking separation

allows a clearer analysis of the job compatibility factor. Moreover, this stratification may separate women with different
attitudes toward child rearing and child welfare. Women may work
because they do not like child care or other household activities
or because their productivity in the home is lower than that in
the market. Clearly, all mothers work and the term "working" is
used only for convenience. Work is defined to include market and
income related activities which include gardening and the tending
of livestock and poultry.

While stratification will allow us to understand certain key
relationships, it may hide the beliefs effect. This is because
women with positive beliefs toward breastfeeding are expected to
be more likely to stay with their infant rather than join the labor
force. That is, if maternal working status is correlated with
independent variables such as breastfeeding preferences, stratification will bias these parameters. For this reason, we present
results for the total and stratified sample.

Independent Factors Exogenous to the Household

These factors may be the most crucial ones as it is often
easier for public policy to change them. At the same time, analysis of such factors requires larger samples so enough variation
in the prices of foodstuff, the type of milk industry effects, and
so forth, are obtained. There are two relevant types of exogenous
factors. One is the impact of community perceptions of important
issues such as the economic value of children, the probability of
each child's survival, and the value of breast milk and bottle
milk. These community attitudes would be based on aggregate
statistics which may be the same as or different from each household's preferences or experiences. Second are community supply,
price and knowledge factors such as the price of milk, infant non-
milk foodstuffs and other items purchased in the market or at local
sarisari shops (very small stores), the local public and private
health workers' knowledge about breastfeeding, the price and supply
of contraceptives, and the practices of the private baby food and
milk companies in the community. Few of these factors could be
examined in this study.

Baby Food - Milk Industry. The following are often labelled
as reasons for the decline in breastfeeding: the promotion of
baby formulas and milk in hospitals, clinics and doctors' offices;
the manipulation of government and private medical personnel with
gifts and samples of baby formulas; the use of paid nurses or other
personnel to pressure mothers to bottle feed; the prejudices of
medical personnel who believe bottle feeding is better or who do not
understand how to encourage breastfeeding; the status symbol of

having firm breasts (breastfeeding is associated by many with sag-
ging breasts); the distribution of free milk powder by international agencies to infants (which encourages a decline in breastfeeding);
and the milk advertisements which promote bottle feeding over breast
feeding (18,19,20,21).

Each of these factors occurs in the Philippines but the major
problems may be the prejudices and misinformation of the health
profession and the advertising for condensed and evaporated milk
(22). Direct advertising for infant formulae is not prevalent.
The health profession is affected in many ways by the infant food
and commercial milk industries. Included are the provision of
research support, office equipment, medical equipment, and travel
and conference money. No efforts, however, have been made to
properly educate this sector on the benefits of breastfeeding and
the methods of encouraging it. It may be that misinformed health
personnel are responsible for many women who feel "the breast is
not best."

An attempt at determining what effect the milk/infant formula
industry may have was made. Information was collected for a subsample on households who were visited in the past by representatives of this industry. Of the 140 mothers with infants, 9 percent
had been visited by milk company representatives. A variable was
constructed to determine the effect of this factor. The influence
of the milk/infant formula industry on the medical clinics and
hospitals was not measured nor were the attitudes of doctors and
nurses with whom the households have had contact. Such data is
being collected in an on-going survey.

Urbanization. Residence in urban areas has been a key factor
used to explain the decline in breastfeeding. In urban areas,
jobs may be less compatible with child care; home production may be
less valuable; the greater presence of milk industry advertising
and other types of social inducements may discourage the continu-
ance of breastfeeding; the psychological stress and strain on the
urban women is greater (let-down reflex effect); and the psychological support (the doula effect) may be minimal. It is unclear
whether or not there is a pure "urban" effect. Most likely,
urbanization is positively correlated with each of these adverse
effects on breastfeeding. Thus, the use of an urbanization parameter without the inclusion of each of the other factors would
significantly bias the urban parameter. Policies should be directed
at certain problems rather than at urban women in general. There
is one possible and important urban effect. It may also be that
more goods which can substitute for breast milk are available only
in the urban areas. Each of the rural barrios studied had at least
one store (sari-sari) which sold canned milk. Hence, this may not
be an issue in the Philippines.

Multivariate analysis allows for the analysis of the job and other socioeconomic and demographic factors separately from the urban effect, but the let-down reflex and milk industry effects cannot be adequately captured.

Price of Market Purchased Goods. The ratio of the price of infant nutrition relative to other items purchased and of the market goods component of breast milk relative to other forms of infant nutrition could be important parameters. First, among the key 0-3 month age group, commercially purchased weaning foods or other solid foods appear to be unimportant. Second, it was not possible to develop a price index facing each household or each barrio with adequate price variation in this cross-sectional analysis. For this reason, these potentially important price factors are not analyzed.

STUDY DESIGN

The data used in this paper comes from a multipurpose multivisit survey of 573 households in 34 barrios in the higher income rural province of Laguna, Philippines, a province which is richer than most other provinces but which provides more variance in the economic and occupational structure. Initially, 573 households were selected at random from household listings in the 34 barrios which are representative of four rural occupational groupings: lowland and upland farming, fishing and semi-urban industrialized barrios. Several of these barrios could only be reached by walking more than a kilometer. Cross-sectional information on economic, demographic and nutritional factors were collected during five visits to each household. A smaller sample of 99 households were revisited successively after four, seven and nine months. During each revisit the activities of each person in the household were observed by interviewers stationed with the mother and individual dietary intake data were obtained by weighing and measuring methods. During the first revisit, the time and dietary data collected on the first day were discarded and the data collected on second day were used (23).

Based on these visits, breastfeeding information was obtained for 314 infants. Recall data on whether or not the child was breast fed and the length of breastfeeding were used for infants mainly under the age of two and none older than three. We expect some error in the recall of the duration data. In most cases, we are able to link the breastfeeding participation and duration answers with concurrent socioeconomic data. The labor force, income, wage and wealth data come from very detailed profiles based on about two hours of interview time. The age composition data will contain some errors, as we found in reinterviews that the mother's recall of ages varied. Hemoglobin data were obtained

during the cross-section survey and weight and height during the
cross-section survey and each revisit. One problem, however, lies
in these nutritional status data: they should be obtained at birth
or soon thereafter as had been done for about a third of the sample.
For another third, the data represent the latter periods of lactation and for the others, the data was obtained before or after
lactation.

Wealth is used to separate the sample into rich and poor
groups, relating not only to the flow of income from land, carabao,
tools and other productive assets, but also representing the clos-
est approximation to class stratification possible with a highly
heterogenous sample. The sample is split into the lower seventy
percent and the upper 30 percent according to this wealth parameter.
For convenience, all households with wealth of less than ₱5000 are
termed the "poor" and the others, the "rich." Descriptions of each
specific variable are presented in Table 1.

RESULTS

Factors Associated with Breastfeeding Participation

Among the 314 sample rural children, 93 percent were breastfed. At the age of 4-6 months, 88 percent were still being breastfed, and by the age of 12 months 77 percent continued to be breastfed. In Table 2 the sample is split into those mothers who did and
did not breastfeed their children. Better educated and lower income
persons were more likely to breastfeed their children. Those income
and educational differences are significant.

The key relationships between the socioeconomic, preference
and demographic parameters and breastfeeding participation are
examined in a multivariate framework. Table 3 presents the regression results* for the stratified and the total samples.

Mother's Characteristics. In the total sample (Table 3,
Column 5), the beliefs relationship is large and significant.
Women who feel breast milk is best are 22 percent more likely to
breastfeed their children than women who feel the opposite. This
effect is strongest for the nonworking mothers and insignificant
for the working mothers. This preference pattern of the mother is
not correlated with her education level. In fact, the Pearson

---

* In this and all subsequent regression tables, ordinary least
squares regression results are presented. A logit or probit model
was also tested, but found to produce similar results.

Table 1

List of Independent Variables

Belief toward breast	Variable = 1 when mother feels breast milk is best (0 = bottle is best)
Wage mother poor (rich)	Predicted wage rate for low (high) wealth mother (Peso/hour)
Income others poor (rich)	Household income of others excluding mother for low (high) wealth households
Wage of father	Peso per hour father earns
Wealth	Gross wealth of the household which includes liabilities since these were mainly for fertilizer and seeds in crops planted ($1000 units)
No anemia	(Variable = 1 if mother has hemoglobin concentration count = 12 mg/100 ml or more) (Variable = 0 if mother has anemia)
% WTHTM	Mother's % of her weight over a weight standard based on her height
Good job	(Variable = 1 if mother's job is compatible with child care, i.e., can take child with her on her job) (= 0 if incompatible)
Kids 1-6	No. of siblings aged 1-6
Boys 7-15	No. of boys age 7-15 living in household during one or more months during previous year
Girls 7-12 poor (rich)	No. of girls age 7-12 in low (high) wealth households
Girls 13-15 poor (rich)	No. of girls age 13-15 in low (high) wealth households
Others	No. of servants, relatives, unrelated residents in the households
Milk company visit	(Variable = 1 if household was visited by a milk company) (variable = 0 otherwise)
Age fed food	Age supplementary food is fed to the child (months)

correlation coefficient between these two variables is .014. There is a small overall correlation between the education levels of the mothers and their breastfeeding participation ($r = .05$) and there is a significant difference in participation between those mothers with very little education and those with at least an intermediate level of education (Table 4).

Table 2

Factors Associated with Breastfeeding Participation of the Mother

	Did not Breast feed	Did Breast- feed	Total	p*
1. Total Household Income	₱9387	₱4351	₱4720	.001
2. Income per capita of other household members (excluding mother's income)	₱1563	₱ 565	₱ 638	.002
3. Weekly value of per capita household expenditures	₱ 28	₱ 19	₱ 20	.000
4. Total household wealth	₱7699	₱6017	₱6140	.558
5. Average imputed weekly wage rate of mother	₱ 29	₱ 21	₱ 22	.123
6. Average household size	5.7	6.4	6.3	.163
7. Education of mother	2.6 yrs.	3.2 yrs.	3.1	.084
8. Percentage of anemic mothers	5.3%	7.1%	6.9%	.768
Number of Cases	23	291	314	

* T-test level of significance; 2-tail probability; pooled variance

Increases in the predicted market wage of the rich mother in the total sample have a significant negative effect on breastfeeding participation. This follows the threshold income hypothesis laid out above. The coefficients for poor women are not significantly different from zero. The compatibility of the mother's job with child care might be expected to be related positively with breastfeeding behavior. In all cases, there is an insignificant association between compatibility of the job and breast-feeding

Table 3(a)

Factors Associated with Breastfeeding Participation
Results of Regression Analysis
Dependent Variable: 0-1 Breastfeeding Participation

	working Mother			
	(1)		(2)	
Constant	1.03		0.97	
Belief breast is best	-0.03	(-0.35)	-0.02	(-0.20)
Wage mother poor	-0.01	(-0.77)	0.002	(0.10)
Wage mother rich	0.001	(0.03)	0.003	(0.13)
No anemia	-		-	
% WTHTMI	-		-	
Good job	-0.04	(-1.09)	-	
Wage father	0.0004	(0.03)	-	
Wealth	0.0001	(0.05)	0.001	(0.27)
Kids 1-6	0.003	(0.19)	0.01	(0.36)
Boys 7-15	0.01	(0.35)	0.01	(0.48)
Girls 7-12 poor	0.01	(0.23)	0.002	(0.06)
Girls 7-12 rich	0.002	(0.07)	0.005	(0.15)
Girls 13-15 poor	-0.21	(-5.66)*	-0.22	(-5.75)*
Girls 13-15 rich	0.01	(0.08)	0.003	(0.04)
Others	0.02	(0.96)	0.02	(0.91)
Income others poor	-		-0.002	(-0.91)
Income others rich	-		-0.0004	(-0.18)
Milk company visit	-		-	
R^2	0.23		0.23	
$\bar{R}$	0.17		0.16	
F	3.29		3.24	
N	158		158	

(t-values are in parenthesis: Level of significance: * = 1%)

behavior (Table 3).

Better nourished mothers have a higher probability of breast-feeding but the relationship in Column 6, Table 3, is insignificant. Lactation may reduce the nutritional status of the mother, thus the fact that some of these women's height, weight and hemoglobin data were collected after the breastfeeding period may bias these nutritional status coefficients in an unknown manner.

Table 3(b)

Factors Associated with Breastfeeding Participation
Results of Regression Analysis
Dependent Variable: 0-1 Breastfeeding Participation

	Non-working Mother			
	(3)		(4)	
Constant	0.47		0.44	
Belief breast is best	0.32	(3.06)*	0.32	(3.15)*
Wage mother poor	-		-	
Wage mother rich	-		-	
No anemia	-		-	
% WTHTMI	-		-	
Good job	-		-	
Wage father	-0.02	(-2.10)**	-	
Wealth	-0.002	(-1.03)	0.0004	(0.24)
Kids 1-6	0.09	(3.09)*	0.08	(2.95)*
Boys 7-15	-0.01	(-0.51)	-0.01	(-0.45)
Girls 7-12 poor	-0.02	(-0.35)	-0.01	(-0.24)
Girls 7-12 rich	0.01	(0.09)	-0.04	(-0.63)
Girls 13-15 poor	0.07	(0.88)	0.07	(0.96)
Girls 13-15 rich	0.05	(0.42)	0.05	(0.46)
Others	0.02	(8.86)	0.04	(1.34)***
Income others poor	-		0.01	(1.42)***
Income others rich	-		-0.01	(-3.41)*
Milk company visit	-		-	
R^2	0.16		0.22	
$\bar{R}^2$	0.10		0.16	
F	2.48		3.31	
N	140		140	

t-values are in parenthesis: Level of significance: * = 1%,
** = 5%, *** = 10%

Other Variables. Increases in the wage of the father were
inversely related to the participation of nonworking women in
breastfeeding. When the combined income of the father and others
are examined (Columns 2, 4 and 5, Table 3), this negative effect
holds true for the rich. These income results were expected. This
may indicate that the income effect for the rich reflect changes in
the value of time to the household and/or preference patterns. For
the nonworking poor, a significant positive relationship with increases in income of others occurred in the nonworking mother's
group.

Table 3(c)

Factors Associated with Breastfeeding Participation
Results of Regression Analysis
Dependent Variable: 0-1 Breastfeeding Participation

| | Total Sample | | | | | |
	(5)		(6)		(7)	
Constant	0.64		0.48		0.91	
Belief breast	0.22	(3.18)*	0.32	(3.48)*	0.10	(0.84)
Wage mother poor	0.06	(0.63)	-0.02	(-0.15)	-0.01	(-0.38)
Wage mother rich	-0.12	(-1.83)**	-0.18	(-2.68)*	-0.06	(-3.65)*
No anemia	-		0.07	(0.96)	-	
% WTHTMI	-		0.001	(0.43)	-	
Good Job	-		-		-0.06	(-0.82)
Wage father	-		0.01	(0.67)	0.004	(0.24)
Wealth	0.001	(0.42)	-0.0004	(-0.27)	0.001	(0.51)
Kids 1-6	0.04	(2.59)*	0.05	(2.20)**	0.01	(0.27)
Boys 7-15	0.01	(1.01)	0.01	(0.74)	-0.01	(-0.27)
Girls 7-12 poor	-0.02	(-0.87)	-0.02	(-0.82)	0.02	(0.41)
Girls 7-12 rich	0.02	(0.52)	0.05	(1.20)	0.06	(1.02)
Girls 13-15 poor	-0.14	(-3.70)*	-0.16	(-3.60)*	0.04	(0.43)
Girls 13-15 rich	0.01	(0.16)	0.02	(0.19)	0.06	(0.53)
Others	(0.02)	(1.34)***	0.02	(0.90)	0.01	(0.27)
Income others poor	-0.002	(-0.80)	-		-	
Income others rich	-0.001	(-0.49)	-		-	
Milk company visit	-		-		0.06	(0.78)
R_2^2	0.14		0.20		0.19	
$\overline{R}$	0.10		0.14		0.10	
F	3.45		3.27		1.92	
N	298		199		130	

(t-values are in parenthesis: Level of significance: * = 1%,
** = 5%, *** = 10%)

Table 4

Relationship Between Breastfeeding Participation
and Education of the Mother

Education Level	Percentage Breastfeeding Child	Number of Cases
1. None or primary undergraduate	82%*	54
2. Intermediate undergraduate	86%	115
3. Intermediate graduate	96%	95
4. Secondary undergraduate or higher education	92%	50
Total	93%	314

* T-test between first and other education groups significant
  at .01 level.

The demographic relationships are clearer. The presence of
additional preschool children should increase the need for and
productivity of the nonworking mother in child care. Thus, it is
not surprising that increases in breastfeeding behavior are significantly associated with additional preschool children in the non-
working mother and total samples. This may mean that mothers are
aware of these joint relationships or even space their children to
allow child care of several children at once.

The addition of girls in the 13-15 age group in rich and poor
working households fits the pattern found in the child care analysis. In poor households, additional girls in this age group are
associated with the reduction of the mother's child care time and
breastfeeding participation while the opposite holds true in rich
households. The addition of girls aged 7-12 has a minimal insignificant impact on breastfeeding behavior which may relate to
their small role in infant child care. The addition of other
household members had a positive effect on breastfeeding participation as it has on child care time.

Exogenous Variables. Visits by milk company representatives
were associated with a small insignificant increase in breastfeeding participation (Column 7, Table 3). This may be because this
analysis controls for many of the preference, and demographic
parameters which cloud this relationship in most other studies.
Of course the relationship may be totally spurious and this analysis
certainly does not measure the total effect of milk companies. For

instance, milk companies may select active breastfeeding households
or rich breastfeeding households.

Factors Associated with Duration of Breastfeeding

The mean length of breastfeeding is 11.4 months with a
standard deviation of 7.3 months. The factors affecting duration
are clearer than those affecting breastfeeding participation. The
economic, belief, and demographic variables are all significant.
The regression results are presented in Table 5 for the stratified
and total samples.

Endogenous Variables. The belief variable is positive and
significant in all the regressions. It is interesting that the
strength of the belief effect on duration of breastfeeding is
quite similar in both the working and nonworking samples which
contrasts with the insignificant effect of positive beliefs on
breastfeeding participation of the working mothers. The mother's
education, on the other hand, has a different effect. In Table 6
women with at least a secondary education breastfeed significantly
fewer months than the others in the sample. This may relate to a
better understanding of the needs of older infants for solid foods
and the resultant decline in breastfeeding behavior. Another personal characteristic is the mother's nutritional status. An
insignificant positive effect is found.

Positive and significant relationships are found for mother's
predicted wage for the poor for whom a positive wage-duration
relationship is expected. For the rich working mother, a significant positive wage rate coefficient was found. Once the rich
working mother decides to breastfeed, the wage increase may affect
her behavior in a manner similar to the poor. For the total sample,
an insignificant negative relationship exists between job compatibility and breastfeeding duration. The reasons are the same as
those discussed earlier.

The other household economic variables show that the length
of breastfeeding is sensitive to price and income effects. A
significant positive wealth effect was found. The wage of the
father is negatively associated with breastfeeding duration (Table
5, Columns 1 and 3), as is the income of others in rich households.
These economic relationships, like those in the participation
section, fit our a priori expectations.

Additional children have a large impact on the duration of
breastfeeding. The addition of children aged 7-12 is significant
because younger children seem to be used in the child care of older
infants. The impact is positive and significant in poor households

with working mothers. The negative insignificant rich girls aged 7-12 effect is not easily explained since the addition of girls of these ages in wealthy households is associated with large and significant child care time increases. The effect of older poor girls is similar to that found in the participation analysis. Boys aged 7-15 have a significant positive impact on the duration of breastfeeding in the total sample, indicating the older boy's role in replacing the mother in market production and the younger boy's participation in home production and child care (24). The ideal age for supplementation was also positively associated with the duration of breastfeeding. Of course, we pointed out that this variable may capture both a biological and a preference relationship.

Exogenous Variables. The milk company effect was found similar to that in the participation analysis. Being visited by a milk company was associated with a significant increase in the duration of breastfeeding (Table 5, Column 7).

DISCUSSION - SIMULATION ANALYSIS

The analysis has shown that the preference, economic and demographic factors have major effects on breastfeeding behavior. In Table 7 the mean value of variables represented in the regressions in Tables 3 and 5 are used to develop predicted breastfeeding values. Simulated changes in the predicted variables are based on the estimated regression coefficients. Working mothers have a lower probability of breastfeeding but breastfeed longer than the nonworking mothers. Table 7 can be used to evaluate the results of this analysis.

First, the value of time of the mother as represented by her wage rate, has a significant though small positive impact on the breastfeeding behavior of rich households. Wage increases are associated with a decline in the extent and an increase in the length of breastfeeding of the rich. This may indicate that large changes in the wage rates of working women in low income countries may be one source of the decline in breastfeeding participation.

Second, variables which can be changed and which have a strong positive impact on breastfeeding behavior include certain characteristics of the mother, especially her belief pattern. The preference pattern analyzed is a very simple one and it will be necessary to conduct more detailed research on this issue before meaningful programs which would attempt to change preferences could be developed. More specifically, the type of knowledge factor which can be changed should be studied. Formal education may not be as important as the many other factors which affect preferences.

Table 5(a)

Factors Associated with the Duration of Breastfeeding
Results of Regression Analysis
Dependent Variable: Months Mother Breastfeeds the Child

	Working Mother			
	(1)		(2)	
Constant	2.13		0.25	
Belief breast is best	5.35	(1.68)**	5.76	(1.81)**
Wage mother poor	0.63	(1.15)	0.99	(1.41)***
Wage mother rich	1.56	(2.49)*	1.96	(2.80)*
No anemia	-		-	
% WTHTMI	-		-	
Good Job	-1.30	(-1.04)	-	
Wage father	-0.09	(-0.30)	-	
Wealth	-0.01	(-0.09)	0.08	(0.69)
Kids 1-6	0.29	(0.53)	0.45	(0.82)
Boys 7-15	0.29	(0.51)	0.22	(0.38)
Girls 7-12 poor	1.88	(2.20)**	1.97	(2.26)**
Girls 7-12 rich	-0.67	(-0.66)	-1.14	(-1.06)
Girls 13-15 poor	-3.17	(-2.45)*	-3.34	(-2.58)*
Girls 13-15 rich	-2.01	(-0.73)	-2.16	(-0.79)
Others	-0.20	(-0.28)	-0.48	(-0.67)
Age fed food	0.31	(1.65)**	0.26	(1.39)***
Income others poor	-		-0.02	(-0.31)
Income others rich	-		-0.11	(-1.40)***
Milk company visit	-		-	
R^2	0.16		0.17	
$\bar{R}^2$	0.09		0.09	
F	2.00		2.08	
N	158		158	

(T-values are in parenthesis: Level of significance: * = 1%,
** = 5%, *** = 10%)

The mother's nutritional status is another variable amenable to
policy change but we have little indication whether or not its
impact is significant.

Third, the results of the analysis of child care are very
useful in understanding the impact of household composition changes
on breastfeeding behavior. Younger girls seldom care for younger
infants and, consequently, have a significant impact only on the

Table 5(b)

Factors Associated with the Duration of Breastfeeding
Results of Regression Analysis
Dependent Variable: Months Mother Breastfeeds the Child

| | Non-working Mother | | | |
	(3)		(4)	
Constant	1.47		1.11	
Belief breast is best	5.64	(2.08)**	5.66	(2.12)**
Wage mother poor	-		-	
Wage mother rich	-		-	
No anemia	-		-	
% WTHTMI	-		-	
Good job	-		-	
Wage father	-0.19	(-0.92)	-	
Wealth	0.09	(2.10)**	0.13	(2.84)*
Kids 1-6	1.94	(2.67)*	1.80	(2.49)*
Boys 7-15	0.50	(0.88)	0.51	(0.91)
Girls 7-12 poor	-0.61	(-0.52)	-0.58	(-0.51)
Girls 7-12 rich	-1.05	(-0.60)	-1.85	(-1.07)
Girls 13-15 poor	0.99	(0.49)	0.99	(0.50)
Girls 13-15 rich	-2.18	(-0.72)	-2.16	(-0.72)
Others	-0.70	(-0.96)	-0.45	(-0.63)
Age fed food	0.21	(1.27)	0.23	(1.36)***
Income others poor	-		0.07	(0.74)
Income others rich	-		-0.10	(-2.33)*
Milk company visit	-		-	
R^2	0.17		0.20	
$\bar{R}^2$	0.11		0.14	
F	2.37		2.71	
N	140		140	

(T-values are in parenthesis: Level of significance: * = 1%,
** = 5%, *** = 10%)

duration of breastfeeding while older girls aged 13-15 have a significant effect on both breastfeeding participation and duration.
In poor working households older girls substitute for the mother
and reduce her breastfeeding participation and do the opposite in
rich households. Other household members are associated with
increased child care time inputs and breastfeeding participation.
The presence of others could allow the nonworking mothers to
reallocate their time toward child care (including breastfeeding).

Table 5(c)

Factors Associated with the Duration of Breastfeeding
Results of Regression Analysis
Dependent Variable: Months Mother Breastfeeds the Child

	Total Sample		
	(5)	(6)	(7)
Constant	1.91	-1.98	1.42
Belief breast is best	5.49 (2.73)*	7.42 (3.26)*	4.02 (1.28)
Wage mother poor	1.36 (0.48)	0.43 (0.16)	1.00 (1.48)*
Wage mother rich	-1.10 (-0.60)	-2.34 (-1.43)***	-0.53 (-1.19)
No anemia	-	1.37 (0.73)	-
% WTHTMI	-	0.01 (0.23)	-
Good job	-	-	2.65 (1.32)
Wage father	-	0.05 (0.17)	0.14 (0.32)
Wealth	0.14 (3.70)*	0.13 (3.28)*	0.11 (2.42)*
Kids 1-6	0.82 (1.91)**	0.57 (1.08)	-0.90 (-1.22)
Boys 7-15	0.90 (2.38)*	1.25 (2.71)*	0.81 (1.23)
Girls 7-12 poor	0.56 (0.78)	1.41 (1.86)**	2.36 (2.29)**
Girls 7-12 rich	-1.15 (-1.24)	0.12 (0.12)	2.32 (1.50)**
Girls 13-15 poor	-1.98 (-1.83)**	-2.50 (-2.26)**	-2.83 (-1.22)
Girls 13-15 rich	-1.47 (-0.77)	-1.23 (-0.48)	-6.00 (-1.85)**
Others	-0.53 (-1.08)	-0.79 (-1.18)	-0.18 (-0.24)
Age fed food	0.23 (1.89)**	0.45 (2.76)*	0.43 (1.98)**
Income others poor	-0.003 (-0.04)	-	-
Income others rich	-0.05 (-0.80)	-	-
Milk company visit	-	-	3.90 (1.71)**
R^2	0.14	0.24	0.24
$\bar{R}^2$	0.10	0.19	0.15
F	3.17	3.93	2.39
N	298	199	130

(T-values are in parenthesis: Level of significance: * = 1%,
** = 5%, *** = 10%)

Table 6

Relationship Between Duration of Breastfeeding
and Education of Mother

Education Level	Months Breastfeed	N
1. None or primary undergraduate	11.4	54
2. Intermediate undergraduate	11.5	115
3. Intermediate graduate	11.2	95
4. Secondary undergraduate or highest education	9.5*	50
Total	11.1	314

*Statistically significant difference between highest
 education and other 3 groups. T-test at .09 level.

It is also possible that the others provide more direct influences
on breastfeeding. They may promote traditional child rearing
practices or provide comfort so that the mother is more confident
about her ability to breastfeed (doula effect).

Also, a job compatible with child care is associated with
increased time inputs of older children in child care and subsequently with reduced breastfeeding participation although the
effect of this variable on breastfeeding is insignificant. In an
earlier work, a significant positive compatible job effect on
breastfeeding participation was found (25). In that case, compatibility could only be defined by physical proximity of the mother's
job to the house.

Fourth, this study was unable to find an important negative
milk company effect and did not produce a meaningful test of the
possibility that milk companies have no effect on breastfeeding
behavior. However, this framework could be used to explore this
milk company relationship if more work is done on the quantifica-
tion of other milk company effects. A key issue here will be an
examination of the attitudes, knowledge and practices of the
medical profession.

Fifth, the income of other household members, the father's
wage rate and household wealth may explain changes in breastfeeding practices but the effect of marginal changes in these
variables appear to be small.

Table 7

The Effects of Simulated Changes in Economic, Demographic
and Other Variables on Predicted Breastfeeding Behavior[1]

| | Breastfeeding Participation | | | Duration of Breastfeeding | | |
	Non-Working	Working	Total Sample	Working	Non-Working	Total Sample
Pre-dicted value	0.89	0.96	0.93	11.78 mo.	11.11 mo.	11.44 mo.
10% increase in mother's wage rate						
poor	-0.001	-	0.002	0.06	-	0.05
rich	0.0001	-	-0.002**	0.16*	-	-0.02
Belief change to breast is not best	+0.03	-0.32*	-0.22*	-5.35**	-5.64**	-5.49*
Add 1 child age 1-6	0.003	0.09*	0.04*	0.29	1.94*	0.82**
Add 1 girl age 7-12						
poor	0.01	-0.02	-0.02	1.88**	-0.61	0.56
rich	0.002	0.01	0.02	-0.67	-1.05	-1.15
Add 1 girl age 13-15						
poor	-0.21*	0.07	-0.14*	-3.17*	0.99	-1.98**
rich	0.01	0.05	0.01	-2.01	-2.18	-1.47
Add 1 other	0.02	0.02	0.02***	-0.20	-0.70	-0.53
Change to com-patible job	-0.04	-	-	-1.30	-	-

[1]Predicted values are based on the coefficients from Table 3 and
 Table 5 for the mean values of each independent variable.
Statistical significance is based on significance of the coeffici-
ent's t-value in Tables 3 and 5   * = 1%, ** = 5%, *** = 10%.

CONCLUSION

This paper has attempted to examine the effects of factors exogenous to the household on breastfeeding behavior. Is the mother's behavior rational in an "economic sense"? Is this approach meaningful? On the one hand, the regression results explain less than 25 percent of the variance in this behavior and we would have to say we cannot explain very much. On the other hand, there are few unexpected results which proved logical in most cases (e.g., the Good Job effect). Moreover, given a more complete set of variables, a larger sample size, a better measurement of certain variables, such as the health and nutritional status of the mother, and a wider variance in the dependent variables, the results may have been much better. Also, these households' breastfeeding responses to economic and demographic changes are similar to their child care responses to the same changes so it is unlikely that the mother views breastfeeding as some type of leisure or other activity which is unrelated to socioeconomic and demographic issues.

It is easier to affirm that this method of analysis can offer insights into breastfeeding behavior than it is to accept these findings as being representative of the rural Philippines. Laguna is a rich rural province not comparable with other provinces in the Philippines. Urban samples must also be examined. It is clear that this approach may offer insights into the type of data which should be collected for future studies and also into the types of programs which may affect breastfeeding behavior. There are a number of other reservations. Cross-sectional analysis entails critical assumptions about the underlying structure of the relationships studied which may change greatly over time. Also, a key component of this analysis - the value of the mother's time - has rarely been explored in low income rural settings. It may very well be that attributes of the mother's job, such as the compatible job variable, are more reasonable approximations of this value of time effect.*

The final issue is the type of future research or policy suggestions that may be developed from this study, tentative as it is. They should include:

1. Determining the main factors to consider in trying to promote breastfeeding behavior. The belief factor is a key variable which should be examined in more depth;

---

* This was the feeling expressed to this author by William Butz (August 1976).

2. Recognizing the promotion of early child supplementation may have adverse breastfeeding effects with subsequent fecundity increases;

3. Understanding that the enhancement of maternal nutritional status as a factor which might enhance breastfeeding behavior should be studied further;

4. Understanding that in this case the promotion of structural changes in the nature of a woman's job may not promote breastfeeding but that increases in female market labor force participation may carry the tradeoff of reducing the extent of breastfeeding.

ACKNOWLEDGEMENTS

The author wishes to give particular thanks to Ms. Susan de Jesus and Susan Ybañez-Gonzalo who have participated with the author in the overall breastfeeding study and to Mr. Angelito Bernado, Ms. Leticia Buela-Dizon and Ms. Anicia Sayos for their superb assistance. Anne Burgess and Monica Yamamoto are thanked for commenting on earlier versions of this paper. This paper utilizes data from the multipurpose Laguna rural households study which has been supported by the Agricultural Development Council, the Population Center Foundation, the Interdisciplinary Communications Program of the Smithsonian Institution and the U.P. School of Economics. During the preparation of this paper, the author was a visiting associate professor, UP School of Economics associated with the Social Science Division of the Rockefeller Foundation.

APPENDIX I. THE INFANT NUTRITION MODEL

Infant nutrition can be viewed as a direct welfare commodity which can be produced by either bottle or breastfeeding of the infant or a combination of both practices. Both time and goods are required for each practice and there are an infinite number of combinations of breast and bottle feeding for a given amount of infant nutrition. At the same time, there is a limited range for household expansion of the production of infant nutrition because of the biological limitations of both the infant's stomach and the mother's breast milk supply and limitations on the mother's time.*

---

* Breast milk banks exist in some countries and a series of these banks may be developed in the U.S. Also, wet nurses are used in some countries to substitute for (or supplement) mother's milk. The latter practice is rare in the Philippines.

There is a basis, however, for developing a production surface for
infant nutrition. A traditional household economics model is then
used to lay out the basic relationship studied here (26,27).

According to this model, households are assumed to maximize
infant nutritional status N and a composite commodity of all other
items desired by the household, Z where

$$U = U (N, Z)** \qquad\qquad [(1)]$$

The household production function of N has the following components:

$$N = f(X_1, X_2, X_3, t_1, t_2, t_3, HKm) \qquad [(2)]$$

where X_1 is the market purchased vector of goods needed for breastfeeding. Included in X_1 are goods required to support the lactation needs of the mother. X_2 is a vector of goods purchased for
bottlefeeding such as cow's milk or infant formulae and the various
utensils required for preparing and feeding this food. t_1 is the
time used for breastfeeding and t_2, the time for bottle feeding.
These time variables include the purchasing, preparation and feeding components. X_3 and t_3 are the goods and time inputs for other
food fed the infant. HKm is a human capital vector which stands
for education, knowledge, and health/nutritional status of the
mother. These factors can shift the actual or perceived production
relationships. Similarly, Z is produced by a combination of goods
and time.

The household desires to maximize its utility (equation 1)
subject to its resource constraints. Thus the shadow prices per
unit of N, π_n, and Z, π_z, multiplied by the amount of each item used
must be less than the full household income laid out in equation
3. These prices, π_n, π_z, reflect both the prices of goods and
time components. We say shadow price since rarely does a household pay for all aspects of infant nutrition. A time and money
price can be attributed to each component. For example, the value
of time utilized to breastfeed the child multiplied by the breastfeeding time is the time price. The cost of each component of
infant nutrition should be reflected in this shadow price of infant
nutrition. The full income of the household similarly values both
the home time and earned income of the household. Equation 3

** Other components of Z or separate elements of the utility function could include the quantity of children and quality of each
child. Clearly, a mother who desired to reduce the number of
children might either breastfeed longer or use other means of
population control. A desire for a healthy child would increase
the demand for breastfeeding.

presents a constraint whereby the units of infant nutrition multiplied by the price of infant nutrition plus the units of other
consumables times the price of these consumables must be less than
or equal to the full household income

$$N \pi_n + Z \pi_z \leq \sum_k \sum_j W_j T_{jk} + A \qquad [(3)]$$

$$\pi_n = \sum_i P_i X_i + \sum_i \sum_j W_{ij} t_{ji} \qquad [(4a)]$$

$$\pi_z = P_z X_z + \sum_j W_{zj} t_{jz} \qquad [(4b)]$$

$$\sum_i t_{ij} = T_j \qquad [(5)]$$

where

A = nonlabor (unearned) household income,

W_j = weighted average value of time for person j
      (j = mother, father, others in the household),

T_{jk} = total productivity time for person j in producing k
      (k = N, Z),

      = shadow price per unit of infant nutrition (N),

      = shadow price per unit of composite commodity Z,

N,Z = number of units of N and Z,

P_i = the price per unit of market good X_i (i = 1,2,3)

t_{ij} = the time per unit of producing and consuming item i by
      person j, and

W_{ij} = the value of time of person j in producing item i.

This full income constraint considers the possible substitution between the time of the mother and other household members
in the production of bottled milk, other infant food and composite
Z commodity. For breastfeeding, only the mother's time is involved.
Both goods and time are limitative in the sense that a minimal
amount of each is necessary to produce N. For example, very little
of the mother's time would be needed to bottle feed if a maid were
employed. Nevertheless, some supervision time would be necessary.
Similarly, a mother may breastfeed without purchasing lactation
food; however, she will deplete her nutritional stores quickly.

If maternal nutrition (M) is part of our Z commodity, we could assume the mother would not deplete her nutritional stores for her to purchase some lactation food ($P_1X_1 > 0$). An empirical estimate of the shadow price of the milk portion is presented in Appendix II.

Changes in the Value of the Mother's Time

A great deal of energy has gone into attempts to measure the value of the mother's time and then to determine how fertility and other decisions are based on it (27,28). The value of the person's time is based on the value of his/her marginal output at home or market activities. Appropriate valuations of household production are unavailable in most cases so the actual or potential market wage rates of each person are used as proxy variables. Putting aside these estimation problems for the moment, consider how changes in the value of the mother's time may affect her breast-feeding behavior.

The mother is the only person who breastfeeds the infants in the areas studied whereas many others bottlefeed the child (Appendix II). As the value of her time in market related production increases, it is more likely that the working mother will substitute the market goods or other person's time for her home production time. This will mean that she may switch from breast to bottle feeding and/or reallocate her purchases of other items (X_z) to spend less time on the nonmarket produced elements of this Z-vector. We assume the mother wishes to minimize the cost of producing N, π_n or at least household money costs and her own costs. When goods or other persons' time are substituted for the mother's time, bottled milk or formulae and/or other foodstuffs will replace the mother's breast milk as sources of infant nutrition.

If we assume no X_3 is consumed by the infant, the maximization (or cost minimization) relationship can be viewed in two dimensions in Figure 1. N is the desired level of child nutriture. There is a high degree of substitutability between X_1 and X_2; however, they are obviously imperfect substitutes. If they were, the isoquant would be a straight line and there would be only corner solutions with no mixed feeding. For many households, clearly a corner solution is the case but not for all households. A corner solution means the household only breastfeeds or bottle feeds the child. AB is the isocost line for a mother with a low value of time and CD is the cost curve for a woman with a high value of time. An isocost curve represents all the combinations of breast milk (X_1) and bottle milk (X_2) which can be purchased for set breast and bottle milk prices and a given resource level. If total resources equal T, point A equals T divided by the full price ($P_1X_1 + tm_1W_{m1}$)

for breast milk. Thus as the cost of X_1 increases, the household obtains less X_1 for the same amount of resources. The equilibrum for mothers with a low value of time is point E where N consists mainly of breast milk. For a high time value of the mother, equilibrum may be at point F.

Knowledge or Preferences

The knowledge level of a mother may affect her perception of the production relationship between X_1 and X_2 which was represented in Figure 1 by N_0. If the true value of the mother's time leads to isocost curve AB and the true production relationship is N_0, the child will be fed both X_1 and X_2. If the perceived production relationship is N_1, then the child would be fed only X_1. By being better informed, the mother will perceive the correct costs and benefits of her actions.

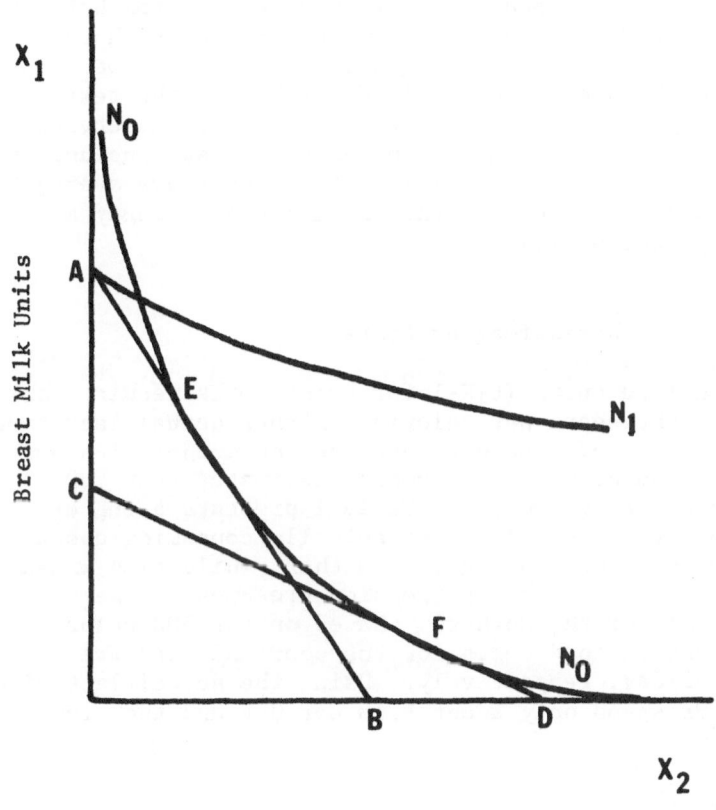

Figure 1. Production of Infant Nutrition

The Breastfeeding Model

These relationships provide the basis for deriving a model which relates breastfeeding behavior to the wage rates of the mother and other household members who bottle feed, the human capital vector which shifts these actual or perceived relationships, and the availability of substitutes. A second shift factor is the ability of the child to breast feed. Children who are sick or who consume other foods will be less able to consume many units of breast milk. In turn, the lowered breastfeeding may make it more difficult for the mother to breastfeed and may raise the fecundity of the mother.

APPENDIX II. COSTS OF BREAST AND BOTTLE FEEDING*

The money or goods and time price per day of breastfeeding and bottle feeding can be derived from the actual behavior of rural Laguna mothers. The results reported here are from both the larger data base of 573 households and a subsample of 99 households for whom direct time and diet data for each person were collected. The Laguna household survey is described in the text. The time and dietary data come from the more accurate observation data, therefore these results can not be used to draw conclusions about the behavior of the larger sample. Also these are average costs which do not reflect the tremendous variance in money and time prices between households.

Breastfeeding Costs

The lactation food costs (P_1X_1) for breast milk require the calorie intake and the costs per calorie. Either actual lactation food or the lactation food needed to provide the mother with her necessary calories can be used.* Thompson estimates that 500 calories are needed for the mother. Table 1 presents a regression where we find poor breastfeeding women actually consuming about 101 calories more than the nonlactating mother, while rich women consume 502 calories more. This regression presumes the same health status for all of the mothers. Based on the 500 calorie approach, the lactation food costs for the poor and rich are ₱0.87/day and ₱0.93/day, respectively. Using the actual lactation food cost, the poor spend only about ₱.18 per day and the rich spend ₱.93 per day.

---

*Calories are selected as our lactation food component as better estimates of the needs of lactating women for calories exist. See Thompson, A. M., F. F. Hytter and W. Z. Billewitz, "The Energy Cost of Human Lactation," British J. of Nutrition 24:565-72, 1970.

Appendix II-Table 1

Regression: Factors Associated with
Caloric Intake of the Mother

Dependent Variable: 1000 Calorie Units

Constant	1.68
Breastfeeding participation of rich mother (Yes = 1; No = 0)	0.502 (1.92)**
Breastfeeding participation of poor mother (Yes = 1; No = 0)	0.101 (.63)
Household income per capita (₱)	0.009 (1.04)
Household wealth (₱)	0.0003 (0)
Mother's education (level)	.14 (1.15)
Household size (Number)	-.054 (-1.69)**
R^2	.10
$\bar{R}^2$	.06
F	1.76
N	98

(T-values in parentheses) **=significant at 5% level.

The poor mother spends 69 minutes per day breastfeeding for a time cost of ₱.54 and the rich mother spends 116 minutes per day for a larger time cost of ₱1.07. The latter may be due to the fact that the rich mother has a higher predicted wage rate. The time data came from the observations on 33 mothers who were breast-feeding. The children had an age range of about 13 months.

Bottle Feeding Costs

The private costs of bottle feeding include the milk and utensils costs and the time costs. It is surprising, but the rich spend much more time than the poor in bottle feeding. The bottle feeding time data came from a smaller sample of 17 children and include only the actual feeding time. The time requirements for actual feeding of 20.0 and 29.1 minutes for the poor and rich households appear low. The time and total costs for the rich are significantly greater than those for the poor. The money costs of ₱0.92 and ₱1.25 for the poor and the rich, respectively, are quite similar, but the time costs of the poor of ₱.42 and the rich of

Appendix II-Table 2

Private Costs per Day for Breastfeeding

	Poor	Rich
1. Costs/500 calories	₱.87	₱.93
2. Actual lactation	101 kcal.	502 kcal.
3. Actual costs per day	₱.18	₱.93
4. Time used to breastfeed minutes/day	68.6	116.3
5. Wage per hour	₱.47	₱.55
6. Time costs per day	₱.54	₱1.07
7. Actual costs	₱.72	₱2.00
8. 500 calories-costs	₱1.41	₱2.00

Appendix II-Table 3

Private Costs per Day for Bottle Feeding

	Poor	Rich
Daily costs of milk	₱.91	₱1.23
Costs of feeding utensils[1]	₱.014	₱.02
Total money costs	₱.924	₱1.25
Bottle feeding time[2]- Minutes per day		
Mother	11.5	13.9
Father	6.2	2.3
Children	4.3	2.6
Other relatives	.0	10.3
Wage rate-Peso per hour		
Mother	₱.52	₱1.80
Father	₱1.98	₱4.08
Children	₱1.64	₱1.73
Other relatives	₱1.38	₱2.54
Total time costs	P .42	₱1.08
Total costs	₱1.23	₱2.31

1/ Based on use for 270 days. Prorated for daily costs.
   Only bottles were purchased.

2/ Total bottle feeding time for the poor and rich are 22 minutes
   and 29.1 minutes, respectively. The 17 families observed fed
   children in all age groups. The actual time holding the child
   is counted.

3/ The sample size was 33 mothers who were observed. The children belonged to all age groups. The actual time in which the
   child is held is counted.

₱1.08 are very different.

Comparison

The actual money or goods costs for breastfeeding are lower than those for bottle feeding, especially for the poor, while the time costs of bottle feeding are less for the poor and similar for the rich. Moreover, the mother has to put much less time into bottle feeding. The poor mother spends almost one hour per day more breastfeeding than bottle feeding, and for the rich the difference is greater. Thus, we conclude breast milk is relatively time-intensive and bottle milk relatively goods-intensive.

References

1. Burgess, A. P. A Study of Attitudes to and Knowledge of Breastfeeding among Health Personnel, School Teachers and Social Workers in Pasay City. Unpublished MPH Thesis, Institute of Public Health, University of the Philippines, March 1976.

2. Butz, W. P. and Habicht, J. The Effects of Nutrition and Health on Fertility: Hypotheses, Evidence, and Interventions. In: Ridker, R., ed., Population and Development, The Search for Selective Interventions, 210-238, Resources for the Future, Washington, D.C. 1976.

3. Popkin, B. Economic Determinants of Breastfeeding Behavior: The Case of Rural Households in Laguna, Philippines. Discussion Paper 76-25, U. P. School of Economics, October 1976.

4. Popkin, B. The Role of the Rural Filipino Mother in the Determination of Child Care and Breastfeeding Behavior. Discussion Paper 76-12, U. P. School of Economics, Aug. 1976.

5. Encarnacion, J. O. Fertility and Labor Force Participation: Philippines, 1968. The Philippine Review of Business and Economics 11: 113-144, December 1974.

6. Popkin, B. op. cit.

7. Brown, J. A Note on the Division of Labor by Sex. Am. Anthropologist 72: 1073-78, 1970.

8. Nerlove, S. B. Women's Workload and Infant Feeding Practices: A Relationship with Demographic Implications. Ethnology 13: 207-214, 1974.

9. Popkin, B. op. cit.

10. Guzman, V. B. and Tantengco, V. Effect of Nutrition and
    Illness on the Growth and Development of Filipino Children
    (0-4 years) in a Rural Setting. J. of the Phil. Med. Asso.
    47, 1971.

11. Osteria, T. Lactation and Childhood Mortality in the Urban
    Area in the Philippines. Unpublished Paper 1976.

12. Jelliffe, D. B. and Jelliffe, E.R.P. Doulas, Confidence and
    the Science of Lactation. J. of Pediatrics 84: 462-64, 1974.

13. Buchanan, R. Breastfeeding: Aid to Infant Health and
    Fertility Control. Pop. Reports, Series J-4: 49-68, July 1975.

14. Jelliffe and Jelliffe, op cit.

15. Popkin, B. M. and Solon, F. S. Income, Time, and the Working
    Mother and Child Nutriture. J. Trop. Ped. and Env. Child
    Health (forthcoming).

16. Del Mundo, F. Present Trends in the Breastfeeding of Filipino
    Infants. Phil. J. of Ped. 8: Oct.-Dec. 1959.

17. Encarnacion, op. cit.

18. Burgess, op. cit.

19. Dwyer, J. T. The Demise of Breastfeeding: Sales, Sloth or
    Society? Priorities in Child Health 2: 1975.

20. Greiner, T. The Promotion of Bottle Feeding by Multinational
    Corporations: How Advertising and the Health Professors have
    Contributed. International Nutrition Monograph Series No. 2,
    1975.

21. Jelliffe, D. B. and Jelliffe, E.F.P. Human Milk, Nutrition
    and the World Resource Crisis. Science 188: 557-561, 9 May
    1975.

22. Burgess, op. cit.

23. Evenson, R. E. and Popkin, B. Notes on the Laguna Household
    Study in the Philippines. Unpublished Paper, Institute of
    Agricultural Development and Administration, Aug. 1976.

24. Boulier, B. The Influence of Children on Household Economic
    Activity in Rural Philippines. Paper presented at the ADC
    Seminar on Household Studies, Singapore, August 1976.

25. Popkin and Solon, op. cit.

26. Becker, Gary. A Theory of the Allocation of Time. Econ. J. 75: 493-517, 1965.

27. Nerlove, Mark. Household and Economy: Toward a New Theory of Population and Economic Growth. J. of Political Economy 82 (Supplement): 200-218, 1974.

28. Gronau, Reuben. The Effect of Children on the Housewife's Value of Time. J. of Political Economy 81 (Supplement), 168-199, 1973.

CONTRIBUTORS

Dr. John Bongaarts, The Population Council, New York, New York.
Dr. Jo Anne Brasel, Associate Professor of Pediatrics,
   Columbia University, New York, New York.
Dr. William Butz, Research Staff, Economics Department,
   The Rand Corporation, Santa Monica, California.
Dr. Pierre Cantrelle, Director de Recherches, Office de la
   Recherche Scientifique et Technique Outre-mer, Paris, France.
Dr. Michel Carael, Centre Scientifique et Medical de l'Universite
   de Bruxelles en Afrique Centrale, Bruxelles, Belgique.
Dr. Kevin Catt, Chief, Section on Hormonal Regulation,
   Reproduction Research Branch, NICHD, NIH, Bethesda, Maryland.
Dr. Lincoln C. Chen, The Population Council, Program Officer,
   Ford Foundation, Dacca, Bangladesh.
Dr. A.K.M.A. Chowdhury, Head, Statistics Branch, Cholera Research
   Laboratory, Dacca, Bangladesh.
Dr. Hernan Delgado, Division of Human Development, Instituto de
   Nutricion de Centro America y Panama, Guatemala City, Guatemala.
Dr. Rose Frisch, Lecturer in Population Sciences, Harvard Center
   for Population Studies, Cambridge, Massachusetts.
*Dr. Jean-Pierre Habicht, National Health Survey Division, Health
   Resources Administration, Rockville, Maryland.
Dr. Valerie J. Hull, Population Institute, Gadjah Mada University,
   Jakarta, Indonesia.
Dr. Aaron Lechtig, Instituto de Nutricion de Centro America y
   Panama, Guatemala, Central America.
Dr. George S. Masnick, Head, Department of Population Sciences,
   Harvard University, Boston, Massachusetts.
Dr. Jane Menken, Research Demographer, Office of Population
   Research, Princeton University, Princeton, New Jersey.
*Dr. W. Henry Mosley, Chairman, Department of Population Dynamics,
   Johns Hopkins School of Hygiene and Public Health, Baltimore,
   Maryland.
Dr. Trinidad S. Osteria, Assistant Professor, Institute of Public
   Health, University of the Philippines, Manila, Philippines.
Dr. Barry M. Popkin, Department of Nutrition, School of Public
   Health, University of North Carolina, Chapel Hill, North Carolina.

*Dr. Robert G. Potter, Department of Sociology, Brown University, Providence, Rhode Island.

Dr. Ananda S. Prasad, Department of Medicine, Wayne State University School of Medicine, Detroit, Michigan.

*Dr. Jeanne Clare Ridley, Center for Population Research, The Joseph and Rose Kennedy Institute, Georgetown University, Washington, D. C.

*Dr. John Stanbury, Massachusetts Institute of Technology, Department of Nutrition and Food Science, Cambridge, Massachusetts.

Dr. Zena Stein, Professor, Division of Public Health, Columbia University, New York, New York.

Dr. John E. Tyson, Associate Professor, The Johns Hopkins University, School of Medicine, Baltimore, Maryland.

Dr. Jeroen K. van Ginneken, Evaluation and Social Sciences Department, International Planned Parenthood Federation, London, England.

Dr. Wilbur Wils, Foundation for Business Administration, Delft, Netherlands.

*Dr. Joe Wray, Acting Head, Department of Population Sciences, Harvard University, Boston, Massachusetts.

* Member, Subcommittee on Nutrition and Fertility, Committee on International Nutrition Programs, National Research Council

PARTICIPANTS

Dr. Barbara Anderson, Sociologist-Assistant Professor, Department of Sociology, Brown University, Providence, Rhode Island.

Dr. Inese Z. Beitins, Assistant Professor, Harvard Medical School, Massachusetts General Hospital, Boston, Massachusetts.

Dr. Daniel Bermeo-Chaparro, Director, University Center for Population Studies, Universidad Del Valle, Cali, Colombia.

Dr. Roy E. Brown, Associate Professor, Department of Community Medicine, Mt. Sinai School of Medicine, New York.

Dr. Richard Cash, Harvard Institute for International Development, Cambridge, Massachusetts.

Dr. O. L. Ekpechi, Professor of Medicine, University of Nigeria, Enugu, Nigeria.

Dr. John Fernstrom, Assistant Professor, Department of Nutrition and Food Science, Massachusetts Institute of Technology, Cambridge, Massachusetts.

Dr. Hector Aliaga Gambino, Medico Nutriologo, Santiago, Chile.

Dr. Martin Forman, Office of Nutrition, Department of State, AID, Washington, D. C.

Dr. Linda Haverberg, Instructor, Human Nutrition and Nutrition Analyst, International Nutrition Planning Program, Massachusetts Institute of Technology, Cambridge, Massachusetts.

Dr. Margot Higgins, Senior Fellow, Washington, D. C.

Dr. Lee M. Howard, Director, Office of Health, Department of State/AID, Washington, D. C.

Dr. Sandra Huffman, The Johns Hopkins University School of Hygiene and Public Health, Baltimore, Maryland.

Dr. Terence H. Hull, Population Institute, Gadjah Mada University, Jakarta, Indonesia.

Dr. Elizabeth Hutchins, Associate Professor, School of Nursing, Virginia Commonwealth University, Richmond, Virginia.

Ms. Cressy Kateregga, East Lansing, Michigan.

Dr. John Knodel, Associate Professor, Population Studies Center, Ann Arbor, Michigan.

Dr. James H. Leathem, Director, Bureau of Biological Research, Rutgers University, New Brunswick, New Jersey.

Dr. James Levinson, Director, Office of Nutrition, Department of State/AID, Washington, D. C.

Dr. Janet W. McArthur, Professor, Harvard Medical School, Massachusetts General Hospital, Boston, Massachusetts.

Dr. James McCabe, Assistant Professor, Economic Growth Center, Yale University, New Haven, Connecticut.

Dr. Charles Nobbe, Special Adviser (Population), Canadian International Development Agency, Ottawa, Canada.

Dr. Clifford Pease, Office of Health, Department of State/AID, Washington, D. C.

Dr. Dana Raphael, Human Lactation Center, Westport, Connecticut.

Dr. Merrill S. Read, Division of Family Health (Nutrition), Pan American Health Organization, Washington, D. C.

Dr. Franz W. Rosa, Director, Medical Operations Branch ACTION, Washington, D. C.

Dr. Allan G. Rosenfield, Director, Center for Population and Family Health, International Institute for the Study of Human Reproduction, Columbia University, New York, New York.

Dr. Pedro Rosso, Assistant Professor of Pediatrics, Institute of Human Nutrition, Columbia University, New York, New York.

Dr. Carolos V. Serrano, Medical Officer-Project Coordinator, Organizacao Pan-Americana Da Saude, Sao Paulo, Brasil.

Dr. Giorgio Solimano, Associate Professor, Public Health-Nutrition, Columbia University, New York, New York.

Dr. J. Joseph Speidel, Chief, Research Division, Office of Population/AID, Department of State, Washington, D. C.

Dr. Zenas M. Sykes, Jr., Office of Population Research, Princeton University, Princeton, New Jersey.

Dr. Lance Taylor, Professor, Nutrition and Economics, Massachusetts Institute of Technology, Cambridge, Massachusetts.

Dr. Michael S. Teitelbaum, International Division, The Ford Foundation, New York, New York.

Dr. James Trussell, Princeton University, Office of Population Research, Princeton, New Jersey.

Dr. Henri L. Vis, Professor of Pediatrics, Free University of Brussels Hospital Universitaire St. Pierre, Bruxelles, Belgium.

Dr. Beverly Winikoff, Nutrition Specialist, Health Sciences Division, Rockefeller Foundation, New York, New York.

Dr. Howard Zacur, Postdoctoral Fellow, Department of Gynecology and Obstetrics, Johns Hopkins School of Medicine, Baltimore, Maryland.

PARTICIPANTS FROM THE NATIONAL INSTITUTES OF HEALTH

Dr. Wendy Baldwin, Sociologist, Behavioral Sciences Branch, CPR, NICHD.

Dr. Heinz Berendes, Chief, Contraceptive Evaluation Branch, CPR, NICHD.

Dr. Gabriel Bialy, Chief, Contraceptive Development Branch, CPR, NICHD.

Ms. Dolores Bryla, Statistician, Epidemiology and Biometry Research Program, NICHD.

Mr. Arthur Campbell, Deputy Director, CPR, NICHD.

Dr. Ronald Chez, Chief, Pregnancy Research Branch, CPR, NICHD.

Dr. Philip A. Corfman, Director, CPR, NICHD.

Dr. V. Jeffery Evans, Economist, CPR, NICHD.

Dr. Thorston Fjellstedt, Medical Officer, Center for Research for Mothers and Children, NICHD.

Mr. Benjamin Fulton, Administrative Officer, NICHD.

Dr. Henry Gabelnick, Chemical Engineer, Contraceptive Development Branch, CPR, NICHD.

Mr. George Gaines, Program Analyst, Office of Planning and Evaluation, NICHD.

Mr. James G. Hill, Chief, Office of Planning and Evaluation, NICHD.

Dr. Richard Horton, Medical Officer, Geographic Medicine Branch, NIAID.

Dr. Earl Huyck, Sociologist, Behavioral Sciences Branch, CPR, NICHD.

Dr. Marvin Karten, Chemist, Contraceptive Development Branch, CPR, NICHD.

Dr. H. K. Kim, Chemist, Contraceptive Development Branch, CPR, NICHD.

Dr. Norman Kretchmer, Director, NICHD.

Dr. Jonathan Lanman, Director, Center for Research for Mothers and Children, NICHD.

Ms. Julia Lobotsky, Biologist, Population and Reproduction Grants Branch, CPR, NICHD.

Dr. Helmut Muller, Medical Officer, Contraceptive Evaluation Branch, CPR, NICHD.

Ms. Janyce Notopoulos, Consultant, Office of Planning and Evaluation, NICHD.

Dr. Dolores Patanelli, Biologist, Contraceptive Development Branch, CPR, NICHD.

Dr. William Sadler, Chief, Population and Reproduction Grants
    Branch, CPR, NICHD.
Dr. James J. Schlesselman, Chief, Biometry Branch, NICHD.
Dr. Artemis Simopoulos, Chief, Developmental Biology and Nutrition,
    Center for Research for Mothers and Children, NICHD.
Mr. Rolf Versteeg, Program Liaison Officer, CPR, NICHD.
_____

CPR = Center for Population Research.
NICHD = National Institute of Child Health and Human Development.